INTERNATIONAL YEARBOOK OF NEPHROLOGY 1993

EDITORIAL BOARD

INTERNATIONAL YEARBOOK OF NEPHROLOGY 1993

Editors

Vittorio E. Andreucci
Department of Nephrology
University of Naples
Naples, Italy

and

Leon G. Fine
University College
Middlesex School of Medicine
The Rayne Institute
London, United Kingdom

Springer-Verlag
London Berlin Heidelberg New York
Paris Tokyo Hong Kong
Barcelona Budapest

ISBN-13: 978-1-4471-1950-0 e-ISBN-13: 978-1-4471-1948-7
DOI: 10.1007/ 978-1-4471-1948-7

Library of Congress Data available

Softcover reprint of the hardcover 1st edition 1992

Typesetting: Camera ready by author
28/3830-543210 Printed on acid-free paper

PREFACE

Nephrology, initially born as a small branch of medicine, has, in the last few decades, become an extraordinary large field of medicine. The recent development of renal medicine is mirrored by the numerous nephrological journals published, a natural consequence of the increasing number of basic and clinical research studies performed continuously all over the world.

Undoubtedly the progress which has occurred in the different, specific fields of renal medicine has given rise to subspecialities which range from renal physiology and pathology to hemo- and peritoneal dialysis and renal transplantation. Even the diagnostic methodology in nephrology, very useful in the clinical practice, has become a speciality within the speciality.

Thus, the problem for clinical nephrologists, as well as for internists, is to remain continuously up-dated in all fields of nephrology. Nephrology textbooks are published continuously and in great number. However, the time required for having authors appointed, chapters completed, manuscript edited, galley proofs corrected and the whole book printed makes many textbooks already out of date when they go on sale and their half lives are very short. On the other hand, nephrological journals are so many and the articles so numerous and detailed, that it is often impossible to rely on them for up-dating practicing clinicians.

The purpose of the International Yearbook of Nephrology is just to satisfy this requirement. The 1993 International Yearbook of Nephrology is the 5th in a successful series of yearly books aimed at keeping practising nephrologists and nephrologists-in-training abreast with rapidly changing areas of nephrology. As in the past 4 issues, the Yearbook is divided into sections; each section has a primary focus on what has been considered of greatest interest by the members of the Editorial Board. The principal aim of the Yearbook is, in fact, to provide reviews which are more current than those which appear in Nephrology textbooks and which can be in the hands of the readers a few months after the authors have completed the manuscripts. The appointed authors of the Yearbook are always experts in the field, who are asked to provide an objective review of the topic, up-dating the readers on the world-wide literature. A hallmark of prior issues has been the extensive and current bibliography of references to primary sources. This important feature has been maintained in the 1993 Yearbook with a complete, accurate and up-to-date list of important recent references.

Some readers have followed our request to suggest topics for upcoming issues of the Yearbook. This has been taken into consideration and has become an important element in selecting topics for the present issue. We continue to invite readers to provide such suggestions.

Credit for the success of the Yearbook rightfully belongs to the members of the Editorial Board. To all we express our deepest gratitude for their splendid cooperation. The Editorial Board of the International Yearbook will be reviewed periodically in order to renew the experts who provide the suggestions for relevant topics from year to year.

We express our sincere appreciation to the authors included in the present volume of the Yearbook, for their excellent reviews and for having met the deadline in forwarding their manuscripts for timely publication.

Vittorio E. Andreucci
Leon G. Fine

CONTENTS

CONTRIBUTING AUTHORS

John W. Adamson,
New York Blood Center,
New York, NY, USA

Stephen Batsford,
Institut für Medizinische
Mikrobiologie und Hygiene,
Abteilung Immunologie,
Hermann-Herder-Str.11,
D-7800 Freiburg i.Br., Germany

Ariela Benigni,
Mario Negri Institute for
Pharmacological Research,
Division of Nephrology,
Ospedali Riuniti,
Bergamo, Italy

Jonas Bergström,
Department of Renal Medicine,
Karolinska Institute,
Huddinge University Hospital,
Stockholm, S-141 86 Huddinge,
Sweden

Richard Chan,
Division of Nephrology,
Department of Medicine,
Lenox Hill Hospital,
New York, New York 10021, USA

Dominique Chauveau,
Département de Néphrologie,
Hôpital Necker,
149, rue de Sèvres,
75015 Paris, France

Norman Deane,
National Nephrology Foundation,
South Bronx Kidney Center,
1834 Webster Avenue,
New York, N.Y. 10457, USA

Peter M.J.M. de Vries,
Department of Internal Medicine,
Free University Hospital,
Amsterdam, The Netherlands.

Gerald F. DiBona,
Department of Internal Medicine,
University of Iowa College of Medicine
and Veterans Administration
Medical Center,
Iowa City, Iowa 52242, USA

Ab J.M. Donker,
Department of Internal Medicine,
Free University Hospital,
Amsterdam, The Netherlands.

Joseph W. Eschbach,
University of Washington
School of Medicine,
Seattle, WA, USA

Richard N. Fine,
Department of Pediatrics,
State University of New York
at Stony Brook,
Stony Brook, NY 11794-8111, USA

Eli A. Friedman,
Renal Disease Division,
Department of Medicine,
State University of New York,
Health Science Center at Brooklyn,
Brooklyn, New York 11203, USA

Dominique Ganeval,
Département de Néphrologie,
Hôpital Necker,
149, rue de Sèvres,
75015 Paris, France

Martin C. Gregory,
Divisions of Internal Medicine
and Nephrology,
Department of Medicine,
University of Utah
School of Medicine,
Salt Lake City, Utah, 84132, USA

Carmen Hinojosa-Laborde,
Department of Internal Medicine,
University of Iowa
College of Medicine and
Veterans Administration Medical Center,
Iowa City, Iowa 52242, USA

Bernard S. Kaplan,
Division of Nephrology,
Department of Pediatrics,
The Children's Hospital of Philadelphia,
University of Pennsylvania,
Philadelphia, Pennsylvania, 19104, USA

Ulla C. Kopp,
Department of Internal Medicine,
University of Iowa College of Medicine
and Veterans Administration Medical Center,
Iowa City, Iowa 52242, USA

Peter M. Kouw,
Department of Internal Medicine,
Free University Hospital,
Amsterdam, The Netherlands.

Brian Leaker,
Department of Medicine,
University College,
Middlesex School of Medicine,
The Rayne Institute,
London WC1 6JJ, England

Mary B. Leonard,
Division of Nephrology,
Department of Pediatrics,
The Children's Hospital of Philadelphia,
University of Pennsylvania,
Philadelphia, Pennsylvania, 19104, USA

Michael F. Michelis,
Division of Nephrology,
Department of Medicine,
Lenox Hill Hospital,
New York, New York 10021, USA

Anne Marie V. Miles,
Renal Disease Division,
Department of Medicine,
State University of New York,
Health Science Center at Brooklyn,
Brooklyn, New York 11203, USA

Tetsuo Morioka,
Institut für Medizinische Mikrobiologie
und Hygiene, Abteilung Immunologie,
Hermann-Herder-Str.11,
D-7800 Freiburg i.Br., Germany

Jørgen S. Petersen,
Department of Internal Medicine,
University of Iowa College of Medicine
and Veterans Administration
Medical Center,
Iowa City, Iowa 52242, USA

Thomas G. Pickering,
The New York Hospital
Cornell Medical Center,
Cardiovascular Center,
525 East 68th Street, Starr-4,
New York, NY 10021, USA

Kaety Plos,
Division of Clinical Immunology,
Department of Medical Microbiology,
Lund University, Lund, Sweden

Giuseppe Remuzzi,
Mario Negri Institute for
Pharmacological Research,
Division of Nephrology,
Ospedali Riuniti, Bergamo, Italy

Eduardo Ruchelli,
Department of Pathology,
The Children's Hospital of Philadelphia,
University of Pennsylvania,
Philadelphia, Pennsylvania, 19104, USA

Mark Siegler,
Department of Medicine,
Center for Clinical Medical Ethics,
University of Chicago,
Chicago IL 60637-1470, USA

Catharina Svanborg,
Division of Clinical Immunology,
Department of Medical Microbiology,
Lund University, Lund, Sweden

Zbylut J. Twardowski,
Division of Nephrology,
Department of Medicine,
University of Missouri,
Harry S. Truman Veterans
Administration Hospital,
Dalton Research Center,
Columbia, Missouri, U.S.A.

Peter A. Ubel,
Department of Medicine,
Center for Clinical Medical Ethics,
University of Chicago,
Chicago IL 60637-1470, USA

Robert J. Wineman,
National Nephrology Foundation,
South Bronx Kidney Center,
1834 Webster Avenue, New York,
N.Y. 10457, USA

Arnold Vogt,
Institut für Medizinische Mikrobiologie
und Hygiene, Abteilung Immunologie,
Hermann-Herder-Str.11,
D-7800 Freiburg i.Br., Germany

Rainer Woitas,
Institut für Medizinische Mikrobiologie
und Hygiene, Abteilung Immunologie,
Hermann-Herder-Str.11,
D-7800 Freiburg i.Br., Germany

Also available from Springer-Verlag

INTERNATIONAL YEARBOOK OF NEPHROLOGY 1992

CONTENTS

RENAL PHYSIOLOGY AND PATHOPHYSIOLOGY

Chapter 1

RENAL NERVES AND CATECHOLAMINE REGULATION OF RENAL FUNCTION

JØRGEN S. PETERSEN, CARMEN HINOJOSA-LABORDE, ULLA C. KOPP, AND GERALD F. DIBONA.

Department of Internal Medicine, University of Iowa College of Medicine and Veterans Administration Medical Center, Iowa City, Iowa 52242, USA

INTRODUCTION

There is considerable evidence that the renal nerves play an important role in the control of the renal circulation, tubular solute and water transport, and renin secretion. The purpose of this chapter is to review the physiology and pharmacology of the neural control of these aspects of renal function and to elaborate on how these mechanisms are altered during various pathophysiological states such as hypertension and edema forming disorders. This topic has been recently reviewed (1) and, due to space limitations, work published subsequent to that review (1) will be preferentially referenced.

CONTROL OF THE RENAL CIRCULATION

Alterations in renal nerve activity

Under normal resting physiological conditions, removal of renal nerve influences either by renal denervation or maneuvers which decrease renal nerve activity do not affect renal hemodynamics in humans, dogs and rats (1) indicating that basal efferent renal sympathetic nerve activity (ERSNA) is too low to influence renal hemodynamics. However, dramatic effects on renal hemodynamics can be observed when ERSNA is increased above resting levels. The threshold frequency of renal nerve stimulation required to cause a reduction in renal blood flow (RBF) and glomerular filtration rate (GFR) is greater than that required to affect renal tubular transport processes and renin secretion. This threshold frequency is about 1 Hz in rats, 1.5 Hz in dogs (2), and 1-2 Hz in primates. Increases in the intensity of electrical renal nerve stimulation cause progressive reductions in renal hemodynamics. In dogs, this relationship has been shown to be affected by the level of dietary sodium intake such that a low sodium diet suppressed the renal vasoconstrictor response to renal nerve stimulation while a normal or increased sodium diet potentiated the renal vascular responses to renal nerve stimulation. The role of the renal nerves in the autoregulation of RBF is controversial. Electrical renal nerve stimulation in dogs at frequencies from 0.5 to 2.0 Hz which caused modest reductions in RBF did not alter the RBF autoregulatory curves. However, reflex increases in renal nerve activity (produced by common carotid artery occlusion) which did not decrease resting levels of RBF and GFR resulted in impaired autoregulation of RBF and GFR (3).

Effector loci of renal nerves

The effector loci for neural control of the renal circulation are the afferent and efferent glomerular arterioles. Recent measurements of blood flow changes in glomerular arterioles in hydronephrotic rat kidneys indicate that renal nerve stimulation caused greater vasoconstriction in afferent arterioles compared to efferent arterioles (4). Renal nerve stimulation causes frequency dependent vasoconstriction of these arterioles which results in a decrease in the glomerular transcapillary hydrostatic pressure gradient and a decrease in the glomerular capillary ultrafiltration coefficient (5). The decrease in capillary ultrafiltration coefficient has been shown to be partially due to contraction of the glomerulus during renal nerve stimulation which causes a decrease in glomerular capillary surface area. The resultant renal hemodynamic effects of renal nerve stimulation are a decrease in single nephron plasma flow (SNPF) and a decrease in single nephron glomerular filtration rate (SNGFR). Similar to the observations in the whole kidney, basal ERSNA is too low to affect SNGFR or SNPF. However, when ERSNA is elevated as observed during sodium depletion there is a reduction in SNGFR (6) which can be restored to control levels by volume repletion or renal denervation.

Although the cellular mechanisms involved in the neural control of renal hemodynamics have not been elucidated, it has been shown that calcium plays an important role. Studies in isolated perfused kidneys indicate that the renal vasoconstrictor response to renal nerve stimulation can be abolished by calcium channel blockers. *In vitro* micropuncture studies have shown that calcium channel blocking agents attenuate the afferent and efferent glomerular arteriolar vasoconstrictor response to renal nerve stimulation; this prevented the fall in SNGFR.

Adrenergic receptors

The four principal subtypes of adrenergic receptors found in the kidney are α_1, α_2, β_1, and β_2. Neural modulation of renal vascular tone is mediated via α-adrenergic receptors. Studies indicate that α_1-adrenoceptors are the primary receptor subtype mediating renal vasoconstriction; however, the ratio between α_1 and α_2 mediated responses is species dependent (1, 7). There is evidence that presynaptic α_2-adrenoceptors inhibit norepinephrine release during renal nerve stimulation. This effect may be dependent on the length and/or intensity of renal nerve stimulation since a role for presynaptic α_2-adrenoceptors is not observed when the renal nerves are stimulated for a shorter duration of time. Presynaptic β-adrenoceptors have been shown to modulate neurally mediated renal vasoconstriction. Studies in isolated, perfused rat kidneys have shown that stimulation of presynaptic β-adrenoceptors with isoproterenol or physiological doses of epinephrine caused an enhancement of the renal vasoconstrictor response to renal nerve stimulation which was blocked by a specific β_2-adrenoceptor antagonist. These findings suggest that an increase in circulating levels of epinephrine as observed during stress may enhance neurogenic renal vasoconstriction.

The contribution of dopaminergic renal nerves to the control of the renal circulation is a controversial subject. There is considerable evidence for the existence of nerves in the kidney which contain dopamine (8) and for renal vasodilator effects of exogenous dopamine (9). However, the controversy arises from the lack of functional evidence that electrical stimulation of the renal nerves produces a renal response which can be antagonized by dopamine receptor antagonists (i.e. proof that dopamine is the neurotransmitter) (10). Central nervous system mechanisms may be necessary to activate dopaminergic renal nerves since it has been shown that electrical stimulation of the midbrain or intracerebroventricular administration of ouabain will elicit renal hemodynamic responses that appear to be mediated by the renal nerves and are antagonized by dopamine receptor antagonists. The receptor responsible for the vasodilator response to exogenous dopamine is the postsynaptic DA_1 receptor (9). The cellular mechanisms responsible for dopamine induced renal vasodilation involve an increase in CAMP production. In rats, SNGFR and glomerular ultrafiltration pressure were increased by dopamine and a specific DA_2 agonist suggesting a preferential DA_2 receptor mediated preglomerular vasodilation. In dogs, a specific DA_2 agonist, quinpirole, caused an increase in RBF but this effect was not abolished by pretreatment with selective DA_2 dopamine receptor antagonists suggesting that quinpirole-mediated vasodilation was not occurring via postsynaptic DA_2 receptors (11). The function of renal dopamine receptors has recently been reviewed (9).

Interactions between renal nerves and other circulating vasoactive substances

Renal nerve stimulation is known to increase renin secretion rate and angiotensin II generation. Angiotensin II can directly stimulate the release of norepinephrine from renal sympathetic nerve terminals, causing a magnification of the renal vasoconstrictor response to renal nerve stimulation. The interaction between renal sympathetic nerves and angiotensin II has recently been reviewed (12, 13). Studies in this area have led to the hypothesis that angiotensin II has a preferential efferent arteriolar vasoconstrictor effect while neurogenically released norepinephrine preferentially constricts the afferent glomerular arteriole. There is evidence that angiotensin II contributes to the renal vasoconstrictor responses to renal nerve stimulation. However, ERSNA can also influence renal hemodynamics independently of angiotensin II.

Vasodilator prostaglandins act as local modulators of the vasoconstrictor effects produced by renal nerve stimulation. Reflex increases in ERSNA produced by chronic sodium depletion or thoracic inferior vena cava constriction increased renal venous outflow of PGE_2 in dogs. Renal arterial administration of exogenous prostaglandins has been shown to attenuate the renal vasoconstrictor response to both renal nerve stimulation and norepinephrine. A micropuncture study in rats showed that renal nerve stimulation during prostaglandin inhibition with indomethacin resulted in an enhanced decrease in SNGFR caused by greater glomerular afferent arteriole vasoconstriction and a greater decline in the glomerular ultrafiltration coefficient as compared to responses observed without indomethacin.

Neuropeptide Y, a potent renal vasoconstrictor which is released during exercise and stress, may play a role in the sympathetic control of renal blood flow. There is evidence that neuropeptide Y is found in renal nerve fibers and may mediate slowly developing nonadrenergic reductions in renal blood flow produced by high intensity renal nerve stimulation during α-adrenoceptor blockade.

The evidence for the role of atrial peptides in renal function has been recently reviewed (14). It is hypothesized that neural influences may play an important role in modulating the renal actions of atrial peptides, since renal sympathetic nerves and atrial peptides have opposite effects on renal function. When the renal effects of atrial peptide were compared between innervated and denervated kidneys in cats, it was found that the renal effects of atrial peptide were blunted in innervated kidneys (15). Blunted renal excretory responses to atrial peptides have also been demonstrated in pathophysiological states characterized by elevated levels of ERSNA. Recent evidence indicates that renal sympathetic nerves alter the renal effects of atrial peptides by modulating glomerular atrial peptide receptor characteristics (16).

CONTROL OF RENAL TUBULAR SOLUTE AND WATER TRANSPORT

Renal denervation

To investigate the role of the renal nerves in renal tubular solute and water transport renal denervation has been used to decrease ERSNA and direct electrical stimulation of the renal nerves has been used to increase ERSNA. Following acute renal denervation, the proximal tubular reabsorption of sodium, chloride, bicarbonate, phosphate, and water is decreased. These changes occur in the absence of changes in whole kidney or single nephron RBF or GFR, renal interstitial hydrostatic pressure or peritubular capillary hydrostatic and oncotic pressures. The increased distal nephron delivery of fluid and solutes after acute renal denervation results in an increased sodium reabsorption in the loop of Henle and the distal tubule due to the high reabsorptive capacity of these nephron segments. However, in spite of increased distal nephron sodium reabsorption, acute renal denervation is associated with ipsilateral natriuresis and diuresis. *In vivo* perfusion of the loop of Henle and the distal tubule have shown that acute renal denervation decreases sodium reabsorption, suggesting that decreased neural stimulation of sodium reabsorption in the loop of Henle and the distal tubule contributes to denervation natriuresis and diuresis.

The occurrence of denervation natriuresis and diuresis in conscious rats with chronic renal denervation clearly indicates that the renal response to renal denervation is not due to the removal of an artificially increased ERSNA as is present in anesthetized surgically stressed animals. The effect of renal denervation has been observed for up to 35 weeks after renal denervation suggesting that it is not of transient nature.

In the hypertrophied kidney one week following uninephrectomy acute renal denervation does not elicit a diuretic and natriuretic response. This has been ascribed to decreased ERSNA and an attenuated sensitivity to low frequency renal nerve stimulation in the hypertrophied kidney of anesthetized rats.

In consideration of the effect of renal denervation on urinary excretion of sodium and water, the potentially confounding effect of supersensitivity of the vasculature and tubules to circulating catecholamines in the chronically denervated kidney is important. However, the plasma norepinephrine concentrations required to demonstrate this are high, producing vasoconstriction with resultant increases in mean arterial pressure and/or decreases in GFR and RBF which could mask the effect of renal denervation on urinary flow rate and sodium excretion. Although physiological increments in plasma norepinephrine concentration (less than 100% increase) can produce decreases in urinary sodium and water excretion without affecting mean arterial pressure, GFR or RBF in both dogs and humans, there is no evidence suggesting that supersensitivity can mask the effect of renal denervation at prevailing basal plasma norepinephrine concentrations.

Direct and reflex activation of the renal nerves

Studies using direct renal nerve stimulation have shown that there is a frequency dependent effect on renin release, tubular sodium reabsorption and RBF. The frequency response curve for renin release lies to the left of that for sodium reabsorption which in turn is to the left of that for RBF. Using a stimulation frequency below threshold for renal vasoconstriction the antinatriuretic response to renal nerve stimulation is abolished by renal α-adrenoceptor blockade with phenoxybenzamine, selective α_1-adrenoceptor blockade with prazosin or renal adrenergic blockade with guanethidine whereas there is no effect of renal α_2- or β-adrenoceptor blockade. The antinatriuretic response is unaffected by blockade of angiotensin II receptors or prostaglandin synthesis inhibition suggesting that the response is not mediated by either angiotensin II or prostaglandins which are known to be released in response to renal nerve stimulation. It has been shown that the antinatriuretic and decreased urinary bicarbonate excretion responses to low frequency renal nerve stimulation are decreased by inhibition of renal bicarbonate reabsorption with either acetazolamide or intrarenal bicarbonate infusion. These results suggest that neurogenic antinatriuresis is partly mediated by a mechanism that is dependent on intact renal tubular bicarbonate reabsorption.

Further studies using micropuncture methodology have demonstrated an increased absolute and fractional sodium and water reabsorption in the proximal tubules in the absence of changes in whole kidney GFR, SNGFR or RBF during low frequency renal nerve stimulation. In a study using direct renal nerve stimulation during *in vivo* microperfusion of the loop of Henle it was demonstrated that sodium chloride reabsorption in the loop of Henle is stimulated without significant changes in water reabsorption. This suggests that the thick ascending limb is the major site of action of the renal nerves in the loop of Henle.

Whereas neither stimulation of renin release nor the antinatriuretic or antidiuretic responses show tachyphylaxis during a 120 min nerve stimulation period RBF recovers to almost pre-stimulation values during a two hour stimulation period (17).

Reflex increases in ERSNA produce changes in renal sodium and water handling similar to those seen after direct electrical renal nerve stimulation. Activation of ERSNA by stimulation of the carotid baroreceptors decreases urinary sodium and water excretion without changes in GFR, RBF or intrarenal blood flow distribution. During these conditions the antidiuretic and antinatriuretic responses are prevented by intrarenal administration of phenoxybenzamine, phentolamine or guanethidine as well as by renal denervation or carotid sinus nerve section. These findings in anesthetized surgically stressed animals have been confirmed during head-up tilt in conscious chronically instrumented dogs indicating that reflex increases in ERSNA directly increase tubular sodium and water reabsorption causing antinatriureis and antidiuresis. In further support for a role of reflex ERSNA in increasing tubular sodium reabsorption in conscious animals, Petersen et al demonstrated that the compensatory response of increased proximal tubular sodium reabsorption during acute furosemide-induced volume depletion was impaired in conscious chronically instrumented rats with renal denervation (18) and in rats treated with the selective β_1-adrenoceptor antagonist doxazosin (19).

Conversely, reflex decreases in ERSNA by left atrial balloon inflation or stellate ganglion stimulation are associated with a natriuresis and diuresis in the absence of changes in renal perfusion pressure, RBF or GFR. During left atrial distention atrial receptors with myelinated vagal afferent fibers are stimulated which result in a reduction of plasma vasopressin concentration and suppression of ERSNA. The increased urine flow and decreased urine osmolality in response to left atrial distention are abolished in hypophysectomized dogs receiving constant intravenous infusion of vasopressin suggesting that the diuretic response during left atrial distention is due to suppression of vasopressin release. That reflex inhibition of ERSNA is involved in the natriuretic response to left atrial distention has been demonstrated by an attenuated natriuretic response after renal denervation. Similar diuretic and natriuretic responses have been demonstrated in response to right atrial balloon inflation and in agreement with a contributory role of reflex suppression of ERSNA, the natriuretic response was reversibly attenuated after cooling of the right cervical vagus. In a study of the renal responses to head-out water immersion in conscious chronically instrumented dogs Miki et al (20) provided evidence for a physiological role of decreased ERSNA as a mechanism of increasing sodium and water excretion in response to increased intrathoracic blood volume and atrial pressure. During head-out water immersion

ERSNA decreased abruptly by 45% which was sustained for 2 hours and associated with a reversible 2-3 fold increase in urinary flow rate and sodium excretion without changes in GFR. When these experiments were repeated following bilateral denervation, the diuretic and natriuretic responses were completely abolished, indicating that the diuretic and natriuretic responses were totally dependent on withdrawal of ERSNA. In further support for a physiologically important natriuretic and diuretic effect of withdrawal of ERSNA several studies in conscious rats, dogs, sheep and monkey have demonstrated that prior bilateral renal denervation attenuates the diuretic and natriuretic response to acute intravascular volume expansion. In a recent study Peterson et al (21) extended these observations by showing that the postprandial natriuresis after a high sodium meal in conscious monkeys was attenuated when the experiment was repeated following bilateral renal denervation.

Adrenergic receptors

Studies of renal tubular reabsorption of sodium, bicarbonate, calcium and water in response to renal nerve stimulation indicate that these responses are mediated by postsynaptic α_1-adrenoceptors located at neuroeffector junctions on the basolateral membrane of the renal tubules. Autoradiographic studies have demonstrated high concentrations of α_1-adrenoceptors in the proximal tubules whereas studies demonstrating α_1-adrenoceptors in the thick ascending limb of Henle's loop, the distal convoluted tubule and the collecting duct are lacking (22). However, functional studies suggest that α_1-adrenoceptors are distributed throughout the nephron; α_2-adrenoceptors are also predominantly located in the proximal tubules and outnumber α_1-adrenoceptors by 3:1. Whereas α_1-adrenoceptors are postsynaptic and mediate tubular responses to renal nerve stimulation, α_2-adrenoceptors are considered to be extrasynaptic and coupled via inhibitory G proteins to parathyroid hormone (proximal tubule) and vasopressin (collecting tubule) sensitive adenylate cyclase (22).

Renal tubular dopamine receptors of the subtype DA_1 have been demonstrated in the proximal tubule and in the collecting duct. Available evidence argues against a role for tubular DA_1-receptors in the antinatriuresis following low frequency renal nerve stimulation (10). However, several lines of evidence suggest that dopamine produced in the kidney acts as an autocrine or paracrine substance inhibiting tubular sodium reabsorption by inhibiting Na^+-K^+-ATPase and Na^+-H^+ antiporter activities (9). Studies in rats and dogs have shown an attenuating effect of dopamine receptor antagonists on the natriuretic response to intravenous volume expansion. This effect is pronounced at lower levels of hypervolemia (2% body weight), whereas it seems of less significance at high levels of volume expansion (10% body weight) (23). Compatible with a natriuretic effect of endogenous dopamine during intrathoracic volume expansion, dopamine antagonists attenuate the natriuretic response to lower body positive pressure and head-out water immersion in man.

Tubular interaction between the renal nerves and angiotensin II

Studies in the isolated perfused kidney indicate that angiotensin II facilitate norepinephrine release from sympathetic nerve terminals via a presynaptic effect. Suppression of the renin-angiotensin system by DOCA and NaCl administration or by pharmacological blockade attenuates the antinatriuretic effect of renal nerve stimulation in anesthetized rats (12). The attenuated antinatriuretic response to renal nerve stimulation during suppression of angiotensin II formation can be normalized by intravenous administration of angiotensin II suggesting that a minimum level of angiotensin II is required for a neurogenic antinatriuresis to occur (12). However, long term studies in chronically instrumented dogs suggest that this interaction may only be of significance during conditions with increased basal renal nerve activity.

ROLE OF RENAL NERVES IN SODIUM AND WATER HOMEOSTASIS

Studies in conscious chronically instrumented dogs have provided strong evidence for a significant role of ERSNA in the acute regulation of sodium and water homeostasis in conscious animals.

To test the role of the renal nerves in long term regulation of sodium homeostasis investigators have examined the ability of the denervated kidney to conserve sodium during dietary sodium restriction. Severe sodium restriction represents a sufficient challenge to maximally engage all mechanisms required for a normal renal adaptive response in order to avoid negative sodium balance. Under such conditions, the absence or malfunction of any one of these redundant mechanisms cannot be made up for by another and a negative sodium balance results. Thus, under these circumstances, renal denervation eliminates an essential mechanism which is revealed by the development of negative sodium balance. Studies in several species support the argument that the dependence of intact renal innervation is related to the magnitude of dietary sodium restriction, i.e. only during severe sodium restriction is intact renal innervation required to maintain sodium balance. Studies in humans with idiopathic or guanethidine-induced autonomic insufficiency have demonstrated that intact renal innervation is essential for the human kidney to maximally reabsorb sodium in response to a reduction in dietary sodium intake (24, 25). In a recent study, Greenberg et al (26) showed that sodium excretion following a change from low sodium intake to normal or high sodium intake is attenuated in rats with bilateral renal denervation. This effect is maintained for at least 72 hours also suggesting that withdrawal of ERSNA may be of significance in long term regulation of sodium balance.

RENORENAL REFLEX CONTROL OF RENAL FUNCTION

Renorenal reflexes are defined as responses occurring in one kidney as a result of interventions on the same (ipsilateral) or the opposite (contralateral) kidney that are mediated by neurohumoral mechanisms. Two classes of renal sensory receptors have been identified neurophysiologically: renal mechanoreceptors (MR) responding to increases in intrarenal pressure and renal chemoreceptors (CR) responding to renal ischemia (R1) and/or changes in the chemical environment in the renal interstitium (R2) (27).

In the rat, unilateral renal denervation results in an ipsilateral natriuresis and diuresis and a contralateral antinatriuresis and antidiuresis in the absence of systemic or renal hemodynamic changes. This response is associated with increased contralateral efferent renal nerve activity. Since the contralateral antinatriureis and antidiuresis are abolished by contralateral renal denervation, these findings indicate that the afferent renal nerves exert a tonic inhibition of contralateral sympathetic neural outflow promoting sodium and water excretion from the opposite kidney. The contralateral natriuresis and diuresis following acute unilateral nephrectomy is abolished by either ipsilateral or contralateral renal denervation suggesting involvement of a renorenal reflex. In a recent study Humphreys et al (28) demonstrated that the contralateral natriuresis and diuresis following uninephrectomy was associated with a rise in plasma concentration of γ-melanocyte stimulating hormone (γ-MSH) and were absent in rats treated with antibodies to γ-MSH. Conversely, plasma immunoreactive γ-MSH concentration was reduced in rats with acute renal denervation and did not increase after uninephrectomy in denervated rats, suggesting that afferent renal nerve activity may exert a permissive effect on both tonic and stimulated γ-MSH secretion.

Several studies designed to examine the functional significance of renorenal reflexes have used the approach of direct electrical stimulation of afferent renal nerves. However, the results of these studies have been variable. The non-uniform and conflicting responses have been ascribed to differences in species and anesthesia, and simultaneous stimulation of inhibitory and excitatory afferent renal nerve fibers. A more successful approach has been to study the effects of selective activation of renal sensory receptors. Renal MR have been localized in the cranial, central, caudal and pelvic areas of the kidney. These receptors respond to increases in intrarenal pressure produced by increased renal arterial, venous, and pelvic pressure. With regard to the renal CR, the R1 chemoreceptor is characterized by having no basal activity and responding to renal ischemia. The R2 chemoreceptors are spontaneously active with the resting discharge being higher in nondiuretic conditions. Besides being activated by ischemia, the R2 chemoreceptors are activated by renal pelvic administration of solutions of NaCl at concentrations 450-900 Mm, KCl at concentrations of 50-150 Mm, and to a lesser extent, urea and mannitol. The renorenal reflex responses to stimulation of renal MR or CR are highly species dependent. In dogs, renal MR stimulation results in a contralateral excitatory renorenal reflex response with a fall in contralateral renal blood flow and urinary sodium excretion at unchanged mean arterial pressure whereas there is no effect of ureteropelvic perfusion with hypertonic saline (R2 stimulation). In cats, renal MR or CR stimulation increases mean arterial pressure and produces variable effects on contralateral renal excretion with antidiuretic and antinatriuretic responses being associated with greater increases in mean arterial pressure. The variability in contralateral urine flow rate and sodium excretion suggests an interaction between local (renorenal reflex) and central (sinoaortic baroreceptor reflex) mechanisms involved in the ERSNA response to renal MR and CR stimulation. This hypothesis is supported by the fact that the responses of ERSNA and renal vasoconstriction to chemical activation of the mesenteric afferent renal nerves are enhanced following sinoaortic denervation plus vagotomy. In contrast to the dog and cat, in the rat, renal MR or CR stimulation produces a decrease in contralateral ERSNA associated with increased urinary flow rate and sodium excretion in the absence of changes in mean arterial pressure or renal hemodynamics. Findings in rats demonstrating a contralateral inhibitory renorenal reflex response produced by ipsilateral MR or CR stimulation, together with those showing a contralateral excitatory renorenal response following unilateral denervation, suggest that renorenal reflexes play a physiological role in the renal regulation of body fluid volume with each kidney exerting a tonic inhibition of sympathetic neural outflow to the opposite kidney. In addition, it has been demonstrated that ERSNA exerts a facilitory effect on renorenal reflexes elicited by renal MR or CR stimulation. It has been demonstrated that inhibitory renorenal reflexes are attenuated in rats treated with capsaicin to deplete sensory neurons of substance P and that the inhibitory renorenal reflex response could be reconstituted by renal pelvic administration of substance P (29). In addition, it has also been demonstrated that the inhibitory renorenal reflex response to pelvic MR or CR stimulation is also attenuated by renal pelvic perfusion of prostaglandin synthesis inhibitors and restored after renal pelvic administration of PGE_2 (30). These studies suggest that renal prostaglandins and substance P are involved in the inhibitory renorenal reflex responses to renal MR and CR stimulation in rats.

CONTROL OF RENIN SECRETION

Alterations in renal nerve activity

Three mechanisms primarily responsible for the release of renin by the kidneys are the renal vascular baroreceptor, the renal tubular *macula densa* receptor and the renal sympathetic nerves. Increases in ERSNA increase renin release. However increases in ERSNA are also capable of affecting the baroreceptor and *macula densa* mechanisms of renin release. Therefore multiple mechanisms are capable of contributing to the renin release response to efferent renal sympathetic nerve stimulation.

Low intensity renal nerve stimulation causes an increase in renin secretion without affecting renal hemodynamics or renal excretion of sodium (1). The secretion of renin in response to nerve stimulation is frequency dependent with a threshold stimulation frequency between 0.3-0.5 Hz in most species and somewhat higher (0.5-1.0 Hz) in monkeys. At these frequencies, renin release is due to direct neural stimulation of juxtaglomerular granular cells without alterations in the *macula densa* or baroreceptor mechanisms. At higher frequencies of renal nerve stimulation which affect sodium excretion and renal hemodynamics, the release of renin may be affected by input from the *macula densa* receptor and renal baroreceptor (31).

Other factors which indirectly alter renin release by affecting ERSNA are high (sinoaortic) and low (cardiopulmonary) pressure baroreceptors and dietary sodium intake. Renin secretion rate increases when there is a decrease in the inhibitory input from any one of the baroreceptor stations if such a withdrawal does not alter the activity of the other two (32). In addition, the increase in renin secretion rate that occurs with dietary sodium restriction in human subjects has been found to be associated with an increase in renal norepinephrine spillover which is an index of an elevated ERSNA.

Adrenergic receptors

There is considerable evidence that the adrenergic receptors responsible for low frequency renal nerve stimulation of renin release are β_1-adrenoceptors and not β_2-adrenoceptors (31-33). The increase in renin secretion produced by higher frequency stimulation of the renal nerves which decreases urinary sodium excretion and renal blood flow is partly mediated by activation of α_1-adrenoceptors in the renal vasculature and tubules and β_1-adrenoceptors located on the juxtaglomerular cells. Although the contribution of α-adrenoceptors to the release of renin during low intensity renal nerve stimulation is minimal, the role of these receptors in the overall control of renin release remains unclear. Dopamine mediates increases in renin release by activation of DA_1 receptors. Studies indicate that dopamine mediated renin release is related to direct stimulation of DA_1 receptors and is not associated with the conversion of dopamine to norepinephrine or the stimulation of renal nerves (9, 34).

Interaction between neural and non-neural mechanisms

There is considerable evidence for an interaction between the renal nerves and the baroreceptor and *macula densa* mechanisms in the control of renin secretion rate. Early studies revealed that increases in renin secretion mediated by non-neural mechanisms was greater in innervated kidneys than in denervated kidneys. Subsequent studies showed that this interaction is dependent on the level of renal arterial pressure and on the intensity of renal nerve stimulation. Similar findings have been demonstrated in humans in which reflex renal nerve stimulation produced by cold pressor stress enhanced the increase in renal venous plasma renin activity produced by renal arterial pressure reduction. Circulating epinephrine has also been shown to modulate the renin secretion rate response of non-neural stimuli by a presynaptic neural mechanism.

ROLE OF THE RENAL NERVES IN PATHOPHYSIOLOGICAL STATES

Hypertension

A major hypothesis for the development of hypertension is that abnormal renal function is critical for the initiation, development, or maintenance of primary hypertension (35). The maintenance of sodium and water balance by the kidneys is believed to be primary in long term control of arterial pressure. An increase in arterial pressure leads to an increased urinary sodium and water excretion with consequent reductions of blood volume until arterial pressure is returned to normal. In hypertension, it is hypothesized that factors disrupt the maintenance of sodium and water balance by the kidneys such that an elevated arterial pressure is required to reestablish and maintain normal sodium and water balance. Several types of renal dysfunction could contribute to the hypertensive state, including increased renal vascular resistance, increased renal retention of sodium and water, and increased release of renin, catecholamines, or other vasoactive substances. The extensive sympathetic innervation of the kidney is known to be important in the physiological regulation of these renal functions.

There is clear evidence that ERSNA is increased in essential hypertension. The increase in renal blood flow in response to the renal arterial administration of the α-adrenoceptor antagonist, phentolamine, has been shown to be significantly greater in hypertensive subjects than in normotensive subjects. In addition, the renal spillover of norepinephrine to plasma, which is used as an index of ERSNA, was shown to be increased in human essential hypertension.

All of the effects of an elevated ERSNA can contribute to the initiation, development, and maintenance of hypertension. Stimulation of renin secretion rate would lead to increases in both intrarenal and circulating angiotensin II, whose multiple and widespread effects are well known to participate in hypertension. Increased renal tubular sodium and water reabsorption as well as decreased renal blood flow (i.e., increased renal vascular resistance) and glomerular filtration rate would lead to renal sodium and water retention resulting in an increase in blood volume. Recently Takabatake et al (36) showed that the enhanced activity of the tubuloglomerular feedback (TGF) in spontaneously hypertensive rats is reduced following renal denervation whereas renal denervation does not affect TGF in normotensive Wistar Kyoto rats. Renal denervation affects the TGF curve in spontaneously hypertensive rats by increasing the turning point, decreasing the maximal slope and decreasing the maximal response. This suggests a role of increased ERSNA in the increased TGF response of spontaneously hypertensive rats; however, the intrarenal site of action of the renal nerves in the enhanced TGF response in spontaneously hypertensive rats is unknown. Thus, a primary defect consisting of increased ERSNA would produce sodium and water retention through the interaction of multiple renal mechanisms; the resultant increase in arterial pressure would promote pressure diuresis and natriuresis, allowing blood volume and arterial pressure to return to normal.

Strong evidence for the participation of the renal nerves in hypertension derives form the studies of complete renal denervation in several experimental forms of hypertension in animals.

The technique for complete renal denervation combines surgical and pharmacological disruption of the entire renal nerve population. It has been shown that complete renal denervation will delay the development and/or attenuate the magnitude of the hypertension in various experimental forms of hypertension (37-39). The uniform effect of complete renal denervation on the hypertension in such a diverse groups of animal models of hypertension implies a universally important role for the renal nerves in hypertension.

Three major interdependent causative elements in the physiology of primary hypertension have been identified as hereditary predisposition, environmental influences, and vascular structural adaptations to hypertension (40). Two components of environmental influences are excitatory environmental (psychoemotional) stress and dietary sodium intake. The development of hypertension in rats with a genetic predisposition to hypertension is accelerated by high dietary sodium intake alone or by environmental stress alone; however, the combination of genetic predisposition, high dietary sodium intake, and environmental stress resulted in a level of hypertension which was more severe than that associated with only one factor. Complete renal denervation prevents the development of stress hypertension, further emphasizing the important role of the renal nerves in the pathophysiology of hypertension.

The interaction between genetic predisposition to hypertension, environmental stress, and dietary sodium has been examined in various forms of experimental models of hypertension.

The acute environmental stress used in these studies is air jet stress which consists of a jet of air directed to the dorsum of the rat's head. Studies in spontaneously hypertensive rats, Dahl NaCl-sensitive rats, and more recently in borderline hypertensive rats (41), animal models known to be genetically predisposed to hypertension, indicate that air jet stress caused increases in ERSNA which decreased renal sodium excretion. Air jet stress had no or minor effects on the normotensive control animals. The effects on renal function in the hypertensive animals were abolished by prior renal denervation. These studies also demonstrated that high dietary sodium intake enhanced the effects of air jet stress on ERSNA and renal function in the hypertensive animals. A similar interaction between dietary sodium intake and stimuli which cause reflex activation of the sympathetic nervous system has also been demonstrated in humans.

Sodium retaining, edema forming states

Measurement of renal norepinephrine spillover, which correlates well with the frequency of direct sympathetic nerve stimulation, has been used to demonstrate increased ERSNA in patients with congestive heart failure and hepatic cirrhosis. Floras et al (42) recently demonstrated an inverse correlation between muscle sympathetic nerve activity and fractional sodium excretion in patients with hepatic cirrhosis. In a follow-up study the same investigators examined the natriuretic response to intravenous administration of atrial natriuretic peptide in cirrhotic patients with varying degree of ascites, and correlated the renal responses to muscle sympathetic nerve activity and the presence of ascites (43). The main finding of this study was a significant inverse correlation between the natriuretic response to atrial natriuretic peptide and muscle sympathetic nerve activity prior to administration of atrial natriuretic peptide. Furthermore, there was a strong inverse relationship between muscle sympathetic nerve activity and the fractional excretion of lithium, suggesting that cirrhotic patients with ascites who had the highest muscle sympathetic nerve activity and did not respond to atrial natriuretic peptide also had a higher fractional proximal tubular reabsorption of sodium than cirrhotic patients who responded to atrial natriuretic peptide administration. These results are in agreement with findings in cirrhotic rats in which the markedly attenuated natriuretic response to atrial natriuretic peptide was restored by prior bilateral renal denervation. Similar results have been obtained after administration of atrial natriuretic peptide in animal models of nephrotic syndrome and congestive heart failure. In patients with nephrotic syndrome, plasma norepinephrine concentration is increased indicating an increase in systemic sympathetic nerve activity.

The contribution of increased ERSNA to the renal sodium and water retention in edema forming states have been determined from the renal responses to interventions which selectively decrease ERSNA. The fractional sodium excretion is increased in patients with congestive heart failure following systemic α-adrenoceptor blockade without significant changes in RBF or GFR. In patients with hepatorenal syndrome bilateral lumbar sympathetic blockade to produce bilateral renal denervation causes a diuretic and natriuretic response associated with increased RPF and GFR.

In animal models of congestive heart failure, nephrotic syndrome and hepatic cirrhosis the ability to excrete an acute oral or intravenous load of saline is reduced and the impaired excretory response is significantly improved by bilateral renal denervation in each of these models. Furthermore, measurement of ERSNA during administration of an acute intravenous volume load has shown an attenuated reduction in ERSNA in each of these models of edema formation as compared with the reflex suppression of ERSNA observed in normal animals. These findings suggest that the impaired ability to excrete an acute isotonic saline load in these experimental models is partially dependent on an increase in basal ERSNA that fails to suppress normally in response to the isotonic saline load.

In recent studies, the role of ERSNA in the renal adjustment to chronic changes in sodium intake in these pathological models have been studied. In animal models of all of these edema forming disorders the cumulative sodium balance while consuming a low sodium diet is decreased by bilateral renal denervation (44). Thus, taken together these results indicate an important role for increased ERSNA in the chronic sodium and water retention and edema formation which characterizes congestive heart failure, nephrotic syndrome and hepatic cirrhosis.

REFERENCES

1. Kopp UC, DiBona GF: The neural control of renal function. In: "The kidney: physiology and pathophysiology" (Eds DW Seldin and G Giebisch), Raven Press, Ltd, New York, 1992, pp 1157-1204.
2. Poucher SM, Karim F: The renal response to electrical stimulation of renal efferent sympathetic nerves in the anesthetized greyhound. J Physiol, 434: 1-10, 1991.
3. Persson PB, Ehmke H, Nafz B, Kirchheim HR: Sympathetic modulation of renal autoregulation by carotid occlusion in conscious dogs. Am J Physiol, 258: F364-F370, 1990.
4. Fleming JT, Zhang C, Chen J, Porter JP: Selective preglomerular constriction to nerve stimulation in rat hydronephrotic kidneys. Am J Physiol, 262: F348-F353, 1992.
5. Kon V: Neural control of renal circulation. Miner Electrolyte Metab, 15: 33-44, 1989.
6. Steiner RW, Tucker BJ, Blantz RC: Glomerular hemodynamics in rats with chronic sodium depletion: Effect of saralasin. J Clin Invest, 64: 503-512, 1979.
7. DiBona GF: The functions of the renal nerves. Rev Physiol Biochem Pharmacol 94: 75-181, 1982.
8. Bell C: Dopamine release from sympathetic nerve terminals. Prog Neurobiol, 30: 193-208, 1988.
9. Lokhandwala MF, Amenta F: Anatomical distribution and function of dopamine receptors in the kidney. FASEB J, 5: 3023-3030, 1991.
10. DiBona GF: Renal dopamine containing nerves: what is their functional significance. Am J Hypertension, 3: 64S-67S, 1990.
11. Horn PT, Kohli JD: Absence of postsynaptic DA_2 dopamine receptors in the dog renal vasculature. Eur J Pharmacol, 197: 125-130, 1991.
12. Johns EJ: Role of angiotensin II and the sympathetic nervous system in the control of renal function. J Hypertension, 7: 695-701, 1989.
13. Blantz RC, Gabbai FB, Thomson SC, Tucker BJ: Adrenergic influences and interactions with angiotensin II. Kidney Int, 38: S84-S86, 1990.
14. Goetz KL: Physiology and pathophysiology of atrial peptides. Am J Physiol, 254: E1-E15, 1988.
15. Genovesi S, Protasoni G, Assi C, Golin R, Stella A, Zanchetti A: Interactions between the sympathetic nervous system and atrial natriuretic factor in the control of renal function. J Hypertension, 8: 703-710, 1990.
16. Awazu M, Kon V, Harris RC, Imada T, Inagami T, Ichikawa I: Renal sympathetic nerves modulate glomerular ANP receptors and filtration. Am J Physiol, 261: F29-F35, 1991.

17. Van Vliet BN, Smith MJ, Guyton AC: Time course of renal responses to greater splanchnic nerve stimulation. Am J Physiol, 260: R894-R905, 1991.
18. Petersen JS, Shalmi M, Lam HR, Christensen S: Renal response to furosemide: Effects of acute instrumentation and peripheral sympathectomy. J Pharmacol Exp Ther, 258: 1-7, 1991.
19. Petersen JS, Shalmi M, Abildgaard U, Christensen S: Alpha-$_1$ blockade inhibits compensatory sodium reabsorption in the proximal tubules during furosemide-induced volume contraction. J Pharmacol Exp Ther, 258: 42-48, 1991.
20. Miki K, Hayashida Y, Sagawa S, Shiraki K: Renal sympathetic nerve activity and natriuresis during water immersion in conscious dogs. Am J Physiol, 256: R299-R305, 1989.
21. Peterson TV, Benjamin BA, Hurst NL, Euler CG: Renal nerves and postprandial renal excretion in the conscious monkey. Am J Physiol, 261: R1197-R1203, 1991.
22. Jeffries WB, Pettinger WA: Adrenergic signal transduction in the kidney. Min Elect Metab, 15: 5-15, 1989.
23. Hansell P, Fasching A: The effect of dopamine blockade on natriuresis is dependent on the degree hypervolemia. Kidney Int, 39: 253-258, 1991.
24. Gill JR, Bartter FC: Adrenergic nervous system in sodium metabolism. II. Effects of guanethidine on the renal response to sodium deprivation in normal man. New Engl J Med, 275: 1466-1471, 1966.
25. Wilcox CS, Aminoff MJ, Slater JDH: Sodium homeostasis in patients with autonomic failure. Clin Sci, 53: 321-328, 1977.
26. Greenberg S, Terschner S, Osborn JL: Neurogenic regulation of rate of achieving sodium balance after increasing sodium intake. Am J Physiol, 261: F300-F307, 1991.
27. Stella A, Zanchetti A: Functional role of renal afferents. Physiol Rev, 71: 659-682, 1991.
28. Humphreys MH, Lin SY, Wiedemann E: Renal nerves and natriuresis following unilateral renal exclusion in the rat. Kidney Int, 39: 63-70, 1991.
29. Kopp U, Smith LA: Inhibitory renorenal reflexes: a role for substance P or other capsaicin-sensitive neurons. Am J Physiol, 260: R232-R239, 1991.
30. Kopp U, Smith LA: Inhibitory renorenal reflexes: a role for renal prostaglandins in activation of renal sensory receptors. Am J Physiol, 261: R1513-R1521, 1991.
31. Kopp UC: Interaction of sympathetic nerves with baroreceptor and *macula densa* receptor mechanisms for renin secretion. In: "The juxtaglomerular apparatus" (Eds AEG Persson and U Boberg), Elsevier, Amsterdam, 1988, pp 221-227.
32. Thames MD: Renin release: reflex control and adrenergic mechanisms. J Hypertension, 2 (suppl): 57-66, 1984.
33. Osborn JL, Johns EJ: Control of renin and prostaglandin release. Min Elect Metab, 15: 51-58, 1989.
34. Felder RA, Felder CC, Eisner GM, Jose PA: Renal dopamine receptors. In: "Peripheral action of dopamine" (Eds C Bell and B McGarth), MacMillan, New York, 1988, pp 124-140.
35. Cowley AC, Roman RR: Renal dysfunction in essential hypertension - implications of experimental studies. Am J Nephrol, 3: 59-72, 1983.
36. Takabatake T, Ushiogi Y, Ohta K, Hattori N: Attenuation of enhanced tubuloglomerular feedback activity in SHR by renal denervation. Am J Physiol, 258: F980-F985, 1990.
37. Baines AD: Renal nerves in the pathogenesis of hypertension: A review. Clin Exp Hypertension, A11 (suppl 1): 125-132, 1989.
38. Janssen BJA, Smits JFM: Renal nerves in hypertension. Miner Elect Metab, 15: 74-82, 1989.
39. Kline RL: Renal nerves and experimental hypertension: evidence and controversy. Can J Physiol Pharmacol, 65: 1540-1547, 1987.
40. Folkow B: Physiological aspects of primary hypertension. Physiol Rev, 62: 347-504, 1982.
41. DiBona GF, Jones SY: Renal manifestations of NaCl sensitivity in borderline hypertensive rats. Hypertension, 17: 44-53, 1991.
42. Floras JS, Legault, Morali GA, Hara K, Blendis M: Increased sympathetic outflow in cirrhosis and ascites: direct evidence from intrarenal recordings. Ann Int Med, 114: 373-380, 1991.

43. Morali GA, Floras JS, Legault L, Tobe S, Skorecki KL, Blendis LM: Muscle sympathetic nerve activity and renal responsiveness to atrial natriuretic factor during the development of hepatic ascites. Am J Med, 91: 383-392, 1991.
44. DiBona GF, Sawin LL: Role of renal nerves in sodium retention of cirrhosis and congestive heart failure. Am J Physiol, 260: R298-R305, 1991.

GLOMERULONEPHRITIS

Chapter 2

CHANGING CONCEPTS IN THE PATHOGENESIS OF LUPUS NEPHRITIS

ARNOLD VOGT, STEPHEN BATSFORD, TETSUO MORIOKA, RAINER WOITAS

Institut für Medizinische Mikrobiologie und Hygiene, Abteilung Immunologie, Hermann-Herder-Str.11, D-7800 Freiburg i.Br., Germany.

Lupus nephritis is a frequent and prognostically unfavourable organ manifestation of Systemic Lupus Erythematosus (SLE) (1-6). Granular deposits of immunoglobulin and complement along the glomerular capillary wall point to an immune complex disease (7-9). The aim of the present survey is to discuss a selection of relevant findings which may give us clues as to how these glomerular immune complexes arise. The volume of literature on this subject is now so large that attempts to encompass all aspects are futile. We have therefore restricted ourselves to ideas which appeal to us and devoted most detail to the areas in which our laboratory has been actively involved.

SLE research really began with the discovery of the LE cell phenomenon (10) and the description of particular serum autoantibodies (11-14). Since then a large volume of data has been gathered but the debate on the pathogenesis of lupus nephritis is still not settled. This is all the more surprising since several excellent animal models in mice exist which either spontaneously (15) or after grafting (16) develop a syndrome closely resembling the human disease.

Why it is so difficult to arrive at a convincing, unshakable concept of lupus nephritis and what can one learn from the rather frustrating efforts lying behind us? Why were we led to incorrect interpretations? Which findings can be judged to be hard facts that have to be incorporated into any concept of lupus nephritis?

At first one has to bear in mind the simple fact that SLE is a syndrome rather than one defined disease and that there is probably more than one antigen-antibody system that can lead to lupus nephritis.

This probably holds true also for the animal models. For example in renal and glomerular eluates of MLR/l mice and of GvH mice nephritogenic anti-laminin antibodies were recently detected (17-19); these may contribute significantly to the development of nephritis. It is not known (and even unlikely) that autoantibodies of this specificity play a role in human lupus nephritis. A distinct pathomechanism which is involved in one of the animal models may not necessarily be relevant to the human disease. It does make us aware that there may be nephritogenic autoantigens and autoantibodies involved in the pathogenesis of human lupus nephritis awaiting identification. Another lesson one should not forget is that one will only find the specifities which one searches for. On the other hand if there are antigens or antibodies consistently found in human lupus nephritis and in lupus mice, it seems to be justified to consider them as nephritogenic candidates. Such a candidate is obviously the autoantibody with specificity for DNA.

ROLE OF ANTI-DNA ANTIBODIES

Anti-DNA-antibodies have been shown to be present in renal and glomerular eluates obtained from SLE patients and lupus mice (20-25).

The central question is by what mechanism were they deposited within the glomeruli?

Circulating DNA-anti-DNA complexes are unlikely to accumulate within the glomerular basement membrane (GBM), as in *in vivo* experiments their clearance from the circulation is very rapid (26, 27). This dilemma seemed to be solved when an affinity of DNA for the GBM *in vitro* was reported (28), suggesting an *in situ* mechanism for the formation of glomerular DNA-anti-DNA complexes. However, *in vivo*, DNA fragments of various sizes do not possess a significant affinity for the GBM (29, 30).

Contrary statements (31, 32) do not stand up to closer examination. The amount of DNA fragments which can be found in the isolated glomeruli after renal perfusion is minimal. It is comparable to glomerular deposition of control antigens, like albumin, and amounted to about 0.2% (or 200 ng) of the injected dose when 100 μg of the probes were perfused (30). The amounts of DNA reported by other groups to be fixed to the glomeruli after renal perfusion are even lower and documentation of a glomerular capillary localization of the administered DNA, or the subsequently given antibody, is not convincing (31, 32).

This point has caused considerable confusion; it is necessary to define nephritogenic quantities; we believe that, under similar experimental conditions, these will lie in the microgram, not nanogram range. It should not be forgotten that DNA is rapidly cleared from the circulation by the liver (33, 34).

The lack of affinity of DNA for the GBM may be also assessed from the fact that about the same amount of DNA can be found in glomeruli isolated from both the perfused and non-perfused kidneys (32).

The *in vitro* demonstration of affinity of DNA for the GBM and collagen can be explained by contamination with fibronectin, which is present in normal serum and which can bind to DNA as well as to collagen type IV (35).

Throughout the years an association of lupus nephritis (particularly diffuse proliferative) with circulating anti-DNA antibodies has been established (36-39).

Though serological findings are often quoted, they obviously provide only circumstantial evidence, in that they are incapable of demonstrating whether or not circulating antibodies or complexes have the potential to bind to the target tissue (35). In fact, one could even argue that the titer of nephritogenic antibody to be expected in the serum should be rather low, if the epitopes of the target antigen are not saturated. In reality an abrupt fall in anti-dsDNA antibody titers together with decreased serum complement levels has been observed before exacerbation of nephritis, which supports the latter idea (40).

DO OTHER AUTOANTIBODIES PLAY A ROLE?

Whether, in addition to anti-dsDNA antibodies, which are assumed to be disease specific, other autoantibodies present in sera of SLE patients play a role in the pathogenesis of lupus nephritis has not been a major topic in recent considerations. Some of these antibodies, like anti-histone antibody, are found in up to 70% of sera of SLE patients, more frequently than the 40% of anti-dsDNA antibody (41-43).

Anti-histone antibody as well as antibodies directed against ribonucleoproteins (44, 45), which also can be found in sera of SLE patients, are theoretically of interest, because their target antigens are marked by high positive charge (see below). The pI of histones is in the range of 10.5 to 11.0. About 90% of the ribosomal proteins possess a pI above 10.0, not seldom even above 11.0 (46). The pI values calculated from the primary aminoacid structure (transcribed from the DNA-sequence) for the small ribosomal associated 25KD protein N (SM-D) and the 70KD U1 sm RNP amount to 11.78 and 10.97 respectively (47, 48).

From the physiological role of the proteins, their ability to interact with DNA and RNA and their extreme positive charge, one can predict that they will possess an affinity for highly negatively charged structures like the GBM. This notion has been substantiated in the case of histone, which can be planted to the glomerular capillaries by renal perfusion and intravenous injection (49).

NEPHRITOGENICITY OF CATIONIC ANTIGENS

The GBM is negatively charged due to proteoglycans in both *laminae rarae* (50). Cationized proteins can be readily deposited at these structures by charge-charge interactions. These planted antigens are accessible for circulating antibody and can serve as the starting point of *in situ* immune complex formation (51).

The critical parameters influencing the interaction of proteins with the GBM are the size and degree of net positive charge. In the case of cationized proteins the critical minimum size and pI are about 40KD and pH 9.5 respectively (52).

A unilateral immune complex glomerulonephritis with massive proteinuria could be provoked by perfusing small amounts of highly cationized human IgG (as a model antigen) directly into the left renal artery of rats, followed by antibody intravenously 15 min later (53). The complexes were initially formed mainly at the endothelial site and were transferred to the subepithelial region within a few hours (52), where they persisted for weeks.

Lattice formation is a prerequisite for protracted persistence (54). Using differentially charged bovine gamma-globulin (BGG) as antigen in a murine model of chronic active serum sickness, it was shown that the more cationic the immunogen the more nephritogenic and the greater the tendency to form subepithelial deposits (55). Slightly anionic and slightly cationic antigens induced mesangial deposits, and with highly anionic BGG no glomerular deposits were observed.

Complexes formed in the circulation will also bind to the glomerular capillary wall, provided their overall net charge is high enough (56, 57). With slightly anionic or neutral immune complexes or macromolecules with a size larger than that of serum albumin which are excluded from the filtration process, only transient subendothelial and more persistent mesangial deposits develop (58).

A capillary deposition of anionic proteins can, however, be mediated by polycations.

Injection of the polycation polyethyleneimine prior to native, anionic ferritin, soluble BSA-anti BSA complexes or anionized peroxydase led to capillary deposition of these molecules and complexes, the actual localization depending on size (59, 60).

MULTIPLICITY OF PATHOGENETIC MECHANISMS?

Any concept of the pathogenesis of lupus nephritis must take into consideration that there is probably more than one pathomechanism leading to lupus nephritis. This can be deduced from the variety of clinical symptoms in SLE and the great variation in glomerular histopathology seen in lupus nephritis. The immune deposits are mainly located subendothelially but can be found subepithelially, and within the mesangium (61). One can assume that the deposits consist of nephritogenic antibodies or nephritogenic antigens or both. The hardest facts available for any concept of the pathogenesis of lupus nephritis are antigen and antibody specificities identified in glomerular deposits or eluates of lupus kidneys. In analogy to Koch's postulates the accused nephritogenic antibodies, antigens and antigen-antibody complexes should possess affinity for the GBM and localize within the glomeruli after passive transfer into an experimental animal. In addition one should be able to demonstrate that the glomerular deposition of the nephritogenic antibodies, or antigens plus antibodies, or circulating immune complexes will lead to kidney damage in the experimental animal. Here intravenous application is preferable to the more unphysiological technique of renal perfusion. In the natural course of lupus nephritis both events, a deposition of circulating nephritogenic immune complexes and *in situ* immune complex formation, seem to be possible.

In the centre of any concept one has to bear in mind that the majority of the antibodies in the renal eluates consist of antibodies to dsDNA. This holds true for eluates obtained from kidneys of SLE patients and from lupus mice. One of the main questions therefore is how these antibodies are deposited in the glomeruli. The most interesting and most pertinent situation is the initial sequence of events. On the basis of recent data and speculation the following mechanisms are at the forefront of discussion:

[a] glomerular deposits are the result of nephritogenic antibodies, which either cross-react with intrinsic structures of the glomerulus or cause the formation of circulating immune complexes, followed by passive glomerular entrapment;

[b] glomerular deposition of cationic antigens to which circulating antibodies are bound, forming persistent, large lattice complexes *in situ*;

[c] glomerular deposition of cationic circulating immune complexes, containing cationic antigen or cationic antibody;

[d] mediation of glomerular deposition of anionic antigens or anionic circulating immune complexes by planted, cationic antigens.

CROSS-REACTING ANTI-DNA ANTIBODY

This concept imputes that the antibodies found in the glomerular deposits are a subpopulation of serum anti-DNA antibodies (62). The polyreactivity of the anti-DNA antibodies are thought to influence the mechanism of glomerular immune deposit formation, in that binding to multiple antigens is more likely to lead to soluble circulating immune complexes that can be trapped passively within glomeruli (24). There are various reports on cross-reactivity of anti-DNA antibodies, especially with polynucleotides (63-67), phospholipids (64, 66, 67), proteoglycans (68, 69), cell surface proteins (70-72) and other nuclear antigens (73). Most of the antigens mentioned are anionic and do not possess affinity for the GBM. If such immune complexes arise in the circulation they, in all likelyhood, will not localize within the GBM but will end up in the mesangium (74). The second pathogenetic mechanism assumed, the direct binding of cross-reacting anti-DNA antibodies to intrinsic structures of the glomerulus, has been studied mainly with monoclonal antibodies derived from spleen cells of lupus mice. Normal mice sacrificed two weeks after intraperitoneal injections of $2x10^6$ H241 hybridoma cells, producing cross-reacting anti-DNA antibody, showed marked glomerular IgG-deposits (75). The deposits were mainly located in the mesangium. No or only scanty glomerular deposits were observed with three other anti-DNA hybridomas and a further control hybridoma. Intravenous injection of 1 mg of monoclonal antibody caused a significant glomerular deposition only with H241. The binding site in native DNA of this antibody, which reacts with ds-DNA as well as with ss-DNA, has been well studied; it recognizes the phosphodiester backbone of DNA (76). The target antigen of this antibody in the glomerulus is thought to be laminin, because its reactivity was shown to be inhibited by laminin in addition to ds and ssDNA (77).

Let us consider quantitative aspects. The glomerular binding of H241 is low. Less than 0.1% (5-20 ng) of intravenously injected ^{125}I labelled antibody was bound to the glomeruli (from both kidneys) when isolated 1 hr after the injection. Staining for deposited IgG by indirect immunofluorescence was relatively weak even when 1 mg had been administered. This is surprising for an antibody that is thought to react directly with glomerular constituents and also as mice kidneys are prone to take up injected proteins unspecifically. In this connection the story of cross-reactivity of anti-DNA antibodies with heparansulfate (68, 69) may also be informative. Cross-reactivity with heparansulfate had been observed in human sera from SLE patients, in sera of MRL/l mice, with monoclonal antibodies derived from lupus mice and in glomerular eluates (68, 69, 78). When such a cross-reacting monoclonal antibody was more carefully analysed it turned out that the cross-reactivity was mediated via histone-DNA-complexes (79). Obviously dying cells release DNA-histone fragments, derived from nuclear antigens, into the culture supernatant which can bind to the monoclonal antibody synthesized. It is conceivable that similar complexes may occur in the circulation of SLE patients.

When the monoclonal anti-DNA antibodies are purified under dissociating conditions on protein A/Sepharose 4B columns, the binding to heparansulfate is completely abolished. The binding capacity to heparansulfate can be reconstituted by adding DNA together with histone (80). These observations raise the question whether the *in vivo* binding of the H241 monoclonal antibody to glomerular structures is also mediated by a DNA-histone complex. A fine granular binding to the GBM, both *in vitro* and *in vivo*, of anti-DNA mediated by histone-DNA has been mentioned in a recent paper (80). In this connection the finding that treatment of MLR/l mice with heparin delays and ameliorates the development of lupus nephritis may be relevant (81). This was interpreted by the authors in terms of cross-reactivity of nephritogenic anti-DNA antibodies, but may be explained equally well by assuming that the polyanion heparin prevents glomerular binding of histone-mediated DNA-anti DNA complexes.

Reports on direct renal binding of cross-reacting anti-DNA antibodies, including that observed after perfusion of isolated kidneys (82) should be interpreted with caution when studies are performed with anti-DNA antibodies not purified under dissociating conditions.

Another problem (in our feeling not solved) may well be fictitious cross-reactivity caused by contamination of anti-DNA antibodies with other antibody populations. Given the present state of the art, the most convincing way for demonstrating the existence of nephritogenic antibody is to test renal eluted globulin for antibody activity, study their *in vivo* binding to normal glomeruli followed by analysis of the specificity of the latter after a second renal elution under dissociating conditions. Studying the specificity of the antibodies bound in the glomeruli has the advantage of selection for potentially nephritogenic antibodies. It circumvents the problems of interpreting the various specifities identified in the serum.

Approaches using this idea have been reported recently. Separation of antibody from serum of GvH mice by affinity purification on a Sepharose 4B-RTE (renal tubular epithelial antigen) column into anti-RTE antibodies and antinuclear antibodies showed that only the first one, not cross-reacting with DNA, reacted with the glomerular capillary when transferred *in vivo* to a normal mouse, and induced immune complex nephritis and proteinuria (18). In addition *in vivo* transfer of glomerular eluates from GvH mice which contained autoantibodies with specificity for laminin and dipeptidyl peptidiase IV, both components of the GBM, bound in a granular pattern along the GBM. Intensive staining was still observed at day 19, when only 90 µg of protein from the glomerular eluates was injected. In another recent study renal perfusion via the aorta with 40 µg and 100 µg of glomerular eluates from diseased MRL/l mice and GvH mice respectively caused strong IgG deposition along the glomerular capillaries, the former remained linear in pattern while the latter became granular after 5 days (83). The eluates contained, beside anti-DNA and anti-histone, anti-laminin antibodies. The antibody specificities had been identified after purification of the IgG under dissociating conditions. Whether anti-laminin antibody or other non-nuclear autoantibodies are involved in the pathogenesis of lupus nephritis in humans should be studied in binding experiments as outlined above.

CATIONIC ANTIGENS PROMOTE IMMUNE COMPLEX FORMATION IN THE GBM

The basis of this concept is that the autoantibodies present in the glomerular eluates did not bind directly to intrinsic structures of the glomeruli but were introduced via the corresponding antigen. Several mechanisms are plausible:

[a] the autoantibody reacts with an antigen previously planted by charge-charge interactions to the GBM;

[b] glomerular deposition of a circulating cationic antigen-antibody complex;

[c] glomerular deposition of a circulating anionic antigen-antibody complex is mediated by a planted cationic antigen;

[d] stepwise *in situ* reaction by charge-charge interaction of a cationic nuclear antigen followed by anionic antigens and the corresponding autoantibodies.

AUTOANTIBODIES TO NUCLEAR ANTIGENS

The most prominent feature of SLE is the occurrence of autoantibodies to nuclear antigens of extreme opposite charge. Nuclear antigens like DNA and RNA are strongly anionic molecules while those like histones and most of the ribonucleoproteins are highly cationic.

Autoantibodies against histones are present in the serum of SLE patients in about 70% of cases (41), autoantibodies against ribonucleoproteins are found in the sera of 15 to 60% (84). For several reasons these autoantibodies have hardly been considered as pathogenetic. In contrast to anti-dsDNA antibodies they are not disease specific. Anti-histone antibodies are, for example, observed in more than 95% of the sera of cases of drug induced SLE, where lupus nephritis is absent or very rare (85). If histones and histone antibodies participate in the pathogenesis of lupus nephritis obviously co-factors or other additional pathomechanisms are involved. Nevertheless the idea that cationic antigens are nephritogenic and that cationic nuclear proteins play a decisive role in lupus nephritis is attractive. This concept can easily explain how DNA and anti-DNA, both without any affinity for the GBM, can be found in glomerular deposits and glomerular eluates.

Patients with lupus nephritis have glomerular deposits in the mesangial, subendothelial and subepithelial areas (61). The latter localization is thought to be an indication that cationic antigens are involved (86).

Anti-histone antibodies have recently been identified in glomerular eluates from diseased MRL/l- and GvH-mice (83). In addition histones have been detected by indirect immunofluorescence in glomerular deposits of renal biopsies from patients with lupus nephritis (87) and in kidneys from diseased lupus mice (88).

There are also data pointing to ribonuclear proteins and the corresponding autoantibodies as nephritogenic factors, as antibodies to sm and to Ro have been detected in renal eluates (89, 90). In a recent paper the ratio of serum antibodies to U1RNP and sm has been shown to have predictive value for the development of lupus nephritis (91). The 70KD U1RNP exhibiting a pI of 10.97 (48) is, as far as size and charge are concerned, an ideal candidate for a nephritogenic antigen, as can be inferred from the findings with cationized proteins (52).

Finally recent studies suggest that the 7kD heat shock protein ubiquitin has to be added to the list of potentially pathogenic auto-antigens in SLE.

In one series antibody to ubiquitin was found in over 70% of sera from SLE patients (92). Moreover deposition of ubiquitin, in particular ubiquitinated histone H2A (U-H2A), was seen in about 50% of biopsies from patients with lupus nephritis (87). Thus a further antigen-antibody system can be introduced to the renal glomerulus by histone, in this case not by direct charge-charge interaction (see below), but "riding piggyback".

CATIONIC NUCLEAR AUTOANTIGENS

Considering the fact that highly cationic nuclear antigens are characteristic autoantigens in SLE and that subepithelial immune deposits in lupus nephritis are common, it seemed promising to regard cationic nuclear proteins as candidates for nephritogenic antigens. As a model antigen we chose histones. The content of histones in the nuclei is relatively high and the frequency of anti-histone antibody in the serum of SLE patients can be 70% (41); even higher than that of anti-DNA antibodies. The structure which is most likely to be released into the circulation from dying cells is the nucleosome (93). There is indirect evidence that both core histone-DNA complexes and histone complexes free of DNA can circulate in sera of SLE patients. Circulating DNA could be precipitated by IgG with anti-histone activity, suggesting that extracellular DNA might circulate in blood as nucleosomes (93). Also autoantibodies with reactivity for histone epitopes not exposed in intact nucleosomes nor in histone dimer-DNA or histone tetramer-DNA have been observed in sera of SLE patients (94).

HISTONES HAVE AFFINITY FOR THE GBM

We started our experimental studies for identifying antigens of nuclear origin with affinity for the GBM, with histone aggregates. Histone aggregates bind to the negatively charged structures of the GBM by charge-charge interactions. When 200 g of various ^{125}I labelled histone subfractions were injected into the left renal artery of rats via the aorta, 13 to 32 μg of the administered material was found in the isolated glomeruli after 15 min (49) compared to 0.4 μg of lysozyme, which was used as cationic control antigen. The affinity for the GBM correlated with the ability of the histone subfractions to form aggregates (mol wt>100,000) (49, 95) and possession of regions of clustered basic residues. The highest glomerular deposition, about 16% of the injected dose, was observed with the arginine rich histone H3, the lowest (6.5%) with H1. Kinetic studies revealed that histones planted in the GBM persist long enough to serve as targets for circulating antibody.

That histones may be involved in the pathogenesis of lupus nephritis is supported by recent findings. In the majority of kidneys of proteinuric lupus mice (NZB/NZW F1 and GvH) we were able to demonstrate the presence of histones in the glomerular deposits (88). In renal biopsies from cases of human lupus nephritis granular deposits of histones were found along the glomerular capillaries and/or in the mesangium in more than 60 percent of the cases (87). What is the likelihood that *in situ* complex formation, as outlined above, is also occurring in the natural course of lupus nephritis? The prerequisite of *in situ* formation of glomerular immune complexes is alternating release of antigen and antibody into the circulation. This is conceivable and the observation of a marked fall of anti-dsDNA antibody titers in serum before disease exacerbation could point in this direction (40). At this stage of our knowledge we feel that the best approach is to test all the substructures of chromatin which may occur in the circulation for their affinity for the GBM.

During recent months we have also tested the glomerular affinity of histone octamers and tetramers by renal perfusion experiments (these oligomeric structures are physiological). Both structures could be deposited along the glomerular capillaries, showing that they possess the expected affinity for the GBM. We are still awaiting the answer to the question of whether circulating histone octamer-DNA and histone tetramer-DNA, both subnucleosome particles, will bind to the GBM. If the answer is yes, this could easily explain the frequently confirmed presence of anti-DNA antibodies in glomerular eluates.

HISTONE-MEDIATED POLYANION DEPOSITION

Another mechanism worthy of consideration is polycation mediation of polyanion deposition. A simple way of looking at this is to assume that planted polycations may neutralize the anionic charge of, or even render a transitory positive charge to the GBM. In agreement with this notion, it could be shown that planted histone mediates the glomerular deposition of subsequently injected DNA (49). In quantitative studies, when 200 µg histone H3 were injected into the left kidneys via the aorta followed by 100 µg of ^{125}I labeled ss- or dsDNA fragments of 500 to 7000 basepairs, 39 µg and 35 µg of the injected DNA respectively were bound to the glomeruli at 15 min (30). As with the planted histones, the deposited DNA was accessible for circulating antibody.

A ROLE FOR PRE-FORMED IMMUNE COMPLEXES?

The anti-DNA antibody could also be introduced into the glomerulus as part of a preformed complex, the binding of the complex (DNA-anti-DNA) being mediated by histone. DNA breakdown in the circulation is very rapid, only DNA fragments of size not exceeding 15 bases remain longer in the circulation (34). Immune complexes containing exposed DNA are also removed rapidly from the circulation. *In vivo* processing does appear to yield immune complexes containing small DNA fragments. They may therefore persist long enough in the circulation to have a chance to interact with cationic antigens present as target molecules in the GBM. From *in vitro* studies it could be inferred that such immune complexes are likely to be composed of up to 3 to 4 anti-DNA antibodies fixed to 1 DNA fragment (96). We recently found that such small complexes (obtained from soluble DNA anti-DNA complexes prepared with a monoclonal antibody in DNA excess and treated with nuclease) bound to glomerular planted histone H3 when injected intrarenally. Significant quantities of mouse globulin accumulated along the glomerular capillaries. However, the amount of DNA in the immune complexes however was too small to be detectable by available methods (intercalating dyes or by indirect immunofluorescence). If the above mechanism is also valid in lupus nephritis in man and in mice this would explain the rare reports of the successful detection of DNA in glomerular deposits. Over 20 years ago one group reported detection of ssDNA in glomerular deposits in most biopsies of lupus nephritis (97) as well as in glomerular lesions of lupus mice (98) by indirect immunofluorescence, using antisera to nucleosides. In another report, DNA could be identified in 2 of 15 cases of lupus nephritis and then only following prior treatment of the kidney sections with 2M NaCl (7). No confirmatory data were reported thereafter and we, too, failed to detect DNA in glomerular deposits in lupus and lupus-like nephritis, using intercalating dyes and/or indirect immunofluorescence.

WHAT ADDITIONAL DATA ARE REQUIRED?

One observation which at first sight seems to speak against the idea that histones (or other cationic nuclear antigens) play a decisive role in the pathogenesis of lupus nephritis, is the high frequency of anti-histone antibodies observed in drug induced SLE, where kidney involvement is rare. In our opinion this does not seriously weaken the case. It tells us that additional antigen-antibody systems like DNA- anti-DNA are a prerequisite for development of immune complex nephritis in SLE. It may be of relevance that in drug induced SLE, serum antibodies with reactivity to dsDNA and sm nuclear antigens are very rare or even absent (85, 99, 100). Further evidence will have to be gathered before the concept of the pathogenicity of cationic nuclear antigens can be considered to be established, this includes:

[a] demonstration of the presence of cationic nuclear antigens in glomerular deposits. This can be achieved only with the limitations of immune histological methods, since when

working with glomerular eluates one has great difficulty in discriminating between antigens present in glomerular deposits and contaminating antigens extracted from glomerular cells.

[b] identification of antibody in glomerular eluates that retain specificity for nuclear antigens under dissociating conditions.

[c] identification of chromosomal substructures and soluble immune complexes containing nuclear antigens possessing affinity for the GBM.

[d] establishment of an animal model, according to the above concept, leading to immune complex nephritis and causing proteinuria.

IDIOTYPIC AND CATIONIC ANTI-DNA ANTIBODIES

This concept assumes that not all anti-DNA antibodies are nephritogenic and that certain idiotypes can serve as markers for pathogenicity (23, 101-103). This opinion is based on the observation that particularly anti-DNA antibody idiotypes are associated with nephritis in murine and human SLE and can be detected in glomerular deposits (104-107). In addition in NZB/W F1 mice the onset of lupus nephritis can be down regulated and suppressed by administering anti-idiotypic antibody to anti-DNA (108, 109). On the other hand, administration of two out of several monoclonal anti-dsDNA antibodies with the IdGN2 idiotype derived from NZB/W F1 mice has been shown to accelerate the onset of nephritis in young NZB/W mice (110). It is even possible to induce a lupus-like disease in normal C3H.SW mice following immunization with human monoclonal anti-DNA antibody bearing the public idiotype 16/6, which is found in 50% of SLE patients (111). These observations are most readily explained by abnormal immunoregulation, the idiotype immunization causing disturbances of idiotype-anti-idiotype networks resulting in the occurrence of pathogenic anti-DNA antibodies, without providing insight into the mechanism of glomerular deposition of these antibodies.

CATIONIC ANTI-DNA ANTIBODY

In addition to the concept of histone-mediated immune deposit formation, it is conceivable that cationic antibody may bind by charge-charge interaction to the *laminae rarae internae* and *externae* and may capture circulating antigen (112) or may mediate glomerular deposition of circulating immune complexes. The suspicion that cationic antibodies might indeed play a pathogenic role in lupus nephritis arose when 2 laboratories independently showed that anti-DNA antibodies found in glomerular eluates from NZB/W F1 lupus mice were more cationic than antibodies to DNA in the circulation of these mice (22, 113). Intravenously injected, highly cationized immunoglobulin readily binds to the glomerular capillaries but does not persist unless lattice formation with specific antigens occurs (58).

Several reports point strongly in the direction that in lupus nephritis cationic anti-DNA antibodies could be involved in the formation of glomerular deposits. Compared to serum antibody the IgG antibodies with reactivity for DNA in the renal and glomerular eluates of lupus kidney have been found to be more cationic (22, 114). There is one exception to this (115). From the studies with cationized antibody, one can infer that the degree of positive charge and the proportion of cationic IgG in the circulating immune complexes are critical parameters. A proportion of 20% of cationized anti-HSA antibodies having a pI of 9.3 or higher in the preformed immune complex was sufficient to render deposition along the glomerular capillaries (116). Reviewing the relevant publications it is not clear whether highly cationic anti-DNA antibodies were present in the glomerular eluates in such quantities. Concrete values can be derived from detailed studies in SNF1 lupus mice derived by crossing autoimmune NZB with normal SWR mice (114, 117). The progeny develop uniformly lethal glomerulonephritis; in the glomerular eluates restricted idiotypic diversities are found and thought to be nephritogenic.

Among 65 monoclonal antibodies established from SNF1 and NZB mice, cross-reactive idiotype families could be identified, of which 5 were highly cationic. The majority of the monoclonal antibodies that were highly cationic in charge had the allotype of the normal SWR parents and were of isotype Ig2b. The highest pI observed among the antibodies was a pH 8.8 (114).

This is also mirrored in the immunoblotting of isoelectrofocused kidney eluate-Ig. A small, but relevant fraction of the renally eluted IgG, stained with anti-mouse Ig antibody or with anti-idiotype antibodies, migrated in IEF up to a pI of 9.0 or 8.8 respectively (117).

The critical point is whether the degree of positive charge and the proportion of these cationic anti-DNA antibodies is high enough to mediate glomerular deposition when present in circulating DNA-anti-DNA immune complexes. This question could be tested by *in vivo* transfer of soluble DNA-anti-DNA complexes prepared from renal eluates from lupus mice and small DNA fragments in excess. If the cationic anti-DNA antibodies present in the renal eluates are nephritogenic by virtue of their high positive charge, the preformed immune complexes should possess affinity for the GBM and deposit within the glomerular capillaries.

OUTLOOK

Critical appraisal of studies on the pathogenesis of lupus nephritis does not support the notion that DNA alone is the crucial element. Attention is drawn rather to anti-dsDNA antibodies, which account for about 50% of known autoantibody specificity. Several ideas have emerged, substantiated by relevant data, which may give us an understanding of the mechanism by which anti-DNA antibodies can be deposited in the glomeruli of lupus kidneys and how the formation of glomerular deposits are initiated. All three concepts, cross-reacting anti-DNA antibody, mediation by cationic nuclear antigens like histones and ribonucleoproteins and cationic anti-DNA antibodies are feasible. It should be shown that the putative nephritogenic antigens, antibodies, or antigen-antibody complexes possess affinity for the GBM and that a lupus-like disease can be established. The necessary methodology and techniques are now available for this task to be accomplished.

REFERENCES

1. Pollak VE, Kant KS: Systemic lupus erythematosus and the kidney. In: "Systemic Lupus Erythematosus" (Ed RG Lahita), John Wiley & Sons, New York, 1987, pp 643-671.
2. Wallace D, Podell J, Weiner J, Klineberg JR, Forouzesh S, Dubois EL: Systemic Lupus Erythematosus - survival patterns. Experience with 609 patients. JAMA, 245: 934-938, 1981.
3. Lee P, Urowitz MB, Bookman AAM, Koehler BE, Smythe HA, Gordon DA, Ogryzlo MA: Systemic Lupus Erythematosus: a review of 110 cases with reference to nephritis, the nervous system, infections, aseptic necrosis and prognosis. Q J Med, 46: 1-32, 1977.
4. Cameron JS, Turner DR, Ogg CS, Williams DG, Lessof MH, Chantler C, Leibowitz S: Systemic lupus with nephritis: a long term study. Q J Med, 48: 1-24, 1979.
5. Estes DE, Christian CL: The natural history of SLE by prospective analysis. Medicine (Baltimore), 50: 85-95, 1971.
6. Rosner S, Ginzler EM, Diamond HS, Weiner M, Schlesinger M, Fries JF, Wasner C, Medsger TA Jr, Ziegler G, Klippel JH, Hadler NM. Albert DA, Hess EV, Spencer-Green G, Grayzel A, Worth D, Hahn BH, Barnett EV: A multi-center study of outcome in systemic lupus erythematosus. II. Cause of death. Arthritis Rheum, 25: 612-617, 1982.
7. Koffler D, Schur PH, Kunkel HG: Immunological studies concerning the nephritis of systemic lupus erythematosus. J Exp Med, 126: 607-624, 1967.
8. Mellors RC, Ortega LG, Holman HR: Role of gamma globulins in pathogenesis in renal lesions in systemic lupus erythematosus and chronic membranous glomerulonephritis, with an observation on the lupus erythematosus cell reaction. J Exp Med, 106: 191-202, 1957.
9. Vasquez JJ, Dixon FJ: Immunohistochemical study of lesions in rheumatic fever, systemic lupus erythematosus and rheumatoid arthritis. Lab Invest, 6: 205-217, 1957.
10. Hargraves MM: Discovery of the LE cell and its morphology. Mayo Clin Proc, 44: 579-599, 1969.
11. Cepellini R, Polli E, Celada FA: DNA-reacting factor in serum of a patient with lupus erythematosus diffusus. Proc Soc Exp Biol Med, 96: 572-574, 1957.
12. Holman HR, Kunkel HG: Affinity between the lupus erythematosus serum factor and cell nuclei and nucleo protein. Science (Washington, D.C.), 126: 162-163, 1957.
13. Miescher P, Straessle R: New serological methods for the detection of the LE factor. Vox Sang, 2: 283-287, 1957.
14. Robbins WC, Holman HR, Deicher HR, Kunkel HG: Complement fixation with cell nuclei and DNA in lupus erythematosus. Proc Soc Exp Biol Med, 96:575-579, 1957.

15. Dixon FJ: Murine lupus: A model for human autoimmunity. Arthritis Rheum, 28:1081-1088, 1985.
16. Lewis RM, Armstrong MYK, André-Schwartz J, Muftouglu A, Beldotti L, Schwartz RS: Chronic allogeneic disease. I.Development of glomerulonephritis. J Exp Med, 128: 653-667, 1968.
17. Bruijn JA, Hogendoorn PCW. Corver WE, van den Broek LJCM, Hoedemaeker PJ, Fleuren GJ: Pathogenesis of experimental lupus nephritis: a role for anti-basement membrane and anti-tubular brush border antibodies in murine chronic graft-versus host disease. Clin Exp Immunol, 79: 115-122, 1990.
18. Bruijn JA, van Leer EHG, Baelde HJJ, Corver WE, Hogendoorn PCW, Fleuren GJ: Characterization and *in vivo* transfer of nephritogenic autoantibodies directed against Dipeptidyl Peptidase IV and laminin in experimental lupus nephritis. Lab Invest, 63: 350-359, 1990.
19. Termaat RM, Assmann KJM, van Son JPHF, Dijkman HBPM. Koene RAP, Berden JHM. Antigen specificity of antibodies bound to glomeruli of mice with SLE-like syndromes. JASN, 1: 542, 1990.
20. Lambert PH, Dixon FJ: Pathogenesis of the glomerulonephritis of NZB/W mice. J Exp Med, 127: 507-522, 1968.
21. Winfield JB, Faiferman I, Koffler D: Avidity of anti-DNA antibodies in serum and IgG glomerular eluates from patients with systemic lupus erythematosus. J Clin Invest, 59: 90-96, 1977.
22. Ebling FM, Hahn BH: Restricted subpopulations of DNA antibodies in kidneys of mice with systemic lupus. Arthritis Rheum, 23: 392-403, 1980.
23. Kalunian KC, Panosian-Sakakian N, Ebling FM, Cohen AH, Louie JS, Kaine J, Hahn BH: Idiotypic caracteristics of immunoglobulins associated with systemic lupus erythematosus. Studies of antibodies deposited in glomeruli of humans. Arthritis Rheum, 32: 513-522, 1989.
24. Pankewycz OG, Migliorini P, Madaio MP: Polyreative autoantibodies are nephritogenic in murine lupus nephritis. J Immunol, 139: 3287-3294, 1987.
25. Sabbaga J, Pankewycz OG, Lufft V, Schwartz RS, Madaio MP: Cross-reactivity distinguishes serum and nephritogenic anti-DNA antibodies in human lupus from their natural counterparts in normal serum. J Autoimmunity, 3: 215-235, 1990.
26. Emlen W, Mannik M: Clearance of circulating DNA/anti-DNA immune complexes in mice. J Exp Med, 155: 1210-1217, 1982.
27. Taylor RP, Kujala G, Edberg JC, Foreman P, Davis IV JS, Wright E: The kinetics of clearance of human antibody/dsDNA immune complexes from rabbit circulation. Effects of dsDNA size, rheumatoid factor, and reduction and alkylation of the antibodies, J Immunol, 136: 3785-3792, 1986.
28. Izui S., Lambert PH, Miescher PA: *In vitro* demonstration of a particular affinity of glomerular basement membrane and collagen for DNA. A possible basis for a local formation of DNA-anti-DNA complexes in systemic lupus erythematosus. J Exp Med, 144: 428-443, 1976.
29. Cukier R, Osborne-Pellegrin M, Tron F: Absence de fixation *in vivo* de l'acide désoxy-ribonucléique sur la membrane basale glomérulaire chez la souris C57BL/6. C R Acad Sci (III) 303: 109-112, 1986.
30. Stöckl FW, Schmiedeke T, Sugisaki Y, Mertz A, Batsford S, Vogt A: DNA has no affinity for the GBM *in vivo*; binding is mediated by histone. Kidney Int, 37: 434, 1990.
31. Carlson JA, Hodder SR, Ucci AA, Madaio MP: Glomerular localization of circulating single-stranded DNA in mice. Dependence on the molecular weight of DNA. J Autoimmunity, 1: 231-241, 1988.
32. Horgan C, Johnson RJ, Gauthier VJ, Mannik M, Emlen W: Binding of double-stranded DNA to glomeruli of rats *in vivo*. Arthritis Rheum, 32: 298-305, 1989.
33. Chused TM, Steinberg AD, Talal N: The clearance and localization of nucleic acids by New Zealand and normal mice. Clin exp Immunol, 12: 465-476, 1972.
34. Emlen W, Mannik: Effect of DNA size and strandedness on the *in vivo* clearance and organ localization of DNA. Clin Exp Med Immunol, 56: 185-192, 1984.
35. Lake RA, Morgan A, Henderson B, Staines NA: A key role for fibronectin in the sequential binding of native dsDNA and monoclonal anti-DNA antibodies to components of the extracellular matrix: its possible significance in glomerulonephritis. Immunology, 54: 389-395, 1985.
36. Tan EM, Schur PH, Carr RI, Kunkel HG: Deoxyribonucleic acid (DNA) and antibodies to DNA in the serum of patients with lupus erythematosus. J Clin Invest, 45: 1372-1740, 1966.

37. Winfield JB, Koffler D, Kunkel HG: Role of DNA/anti-DNA complexes in the immunopathogenesis of tissue injury in systemic lupus erythematosus. Scand J Rheum, 11: 59-62, 1975.
38. Tron F, Bach JF: Relationship between antibodies to native DNA and glomerulonephritis in systemic lupus erythematosus. Clin Exp Immunol, 28: 426-432, 1977.
39. Asero R, Banfi G, Radelli L, Origgi L, Bertetti E, Vanoli M, Riboldi P: Relationship between antibodies to dsDNA and to soluble cellular antigens and histologically defined glomerulonephritis in patients with SLE. Autoimmunity, 7: 13-21, 1990.
40. Swaak AJG, Aarden LA, Statius van Eps LW, Feltkamp TEW: Anti-dsDNA and complement profiles as prognostic guides in systemic lupus erythematosus. Arthritis Rheum, 22: 226-235, 1979.
41. Tan EM: Autoantibodies to nuclear antigens (ANA): Their immunobiology and medicine. Adv Immunol, 33: 167-240, 1982.
42. Gioud M, Kaci MA, Monier JC: Histone antibodies in systemic lupus erythematosus. A possible diagnostic tool. Arthritis Rheum, 25: 407-413, 1982.
43. Muller S, Bonnier D, Thiry M, Van Regenmortel MHV: Reactivity of autoantibodies in systemic lupus erythematosus with synthetic core histone peptides. Int Arch Allergy Appl Immunol, 89: 288-296, 1989.
44. Hardin JA: The lupus autoantigens and the pathogenesis of systemic lupus erythematosus. Arthritis and Rheum, 29: 457-460, 1986.
45. St.Clair EW, Query CC, Bentley R, Keene JD, Polisson RP, Allen NB, Caldwell DS, Rice JR, Cox C, Pisetsky DS: Expression of autoantibodies to recombinant (U1) RNP-associated 70K antigen in systemic lupus erythematosus. Clin Immunol Immunopathol, 54: 266-280, 1990.
46. Garrett RA, Wittmann HG: Structure of bacterial ribosomes. In: "Advances in Protein Chemistry" (Eds CB Anfinsen, JT Edsall, FM Richards), Harcourt Brace Jovanovich Publishing, New York and London, 1973, pp 277-347.
47. Schmauss C, McAllister G, Ohosone Y, Hardin JA, Lerner MR: A comparison of snRNP-associated Sm-autoantigens: human N, rat N and human B/B'. Nucleic Acids Res, 17: 1733-1743, 1989.
48. Theissen H, Etzerodt M, Reuter R, Schneider C, Lottspeich F, Argos P, Lührmann R, Philipson L: Cloning of the human cDNA for the U1 RNA-associated 70K protein. The EMBO Journal, 5: 3209-3217, 1986.
49. Schmidedeke TJM, Stöckl FW, Weber R, Sugisaki Y, Batsford SR, Vogt A: Histones have high affinity for the glomerular basement membrane. J Exp Med, 169: 1879-1894, 1989.
50. Kanwar JS, Farquhar MG: Anionic sites in the glomerular basement membrane. *In vivo* and *in vitro* localisation to the *laminae rarae* by cationic probes. J Cell Biol, 81: 137-153, 1979.
51. Batsford SR, Takamiya H, Vogt A: A model of *in situ* immune complex glomerulonephritis in the rat employing cationized ferritin. Clin Nephrol, 14: 211-216, 1980.
52. Vogt A, Rohrbach R, Shimizu F, Takamiya H, Batsford S: Interaction of cationized antigen with rat glomerular basement membrane: *in situ* immune complex formation. Kidney Int, 22: 27-35, 1982.
53. Oite T, Batsford SR, Mihatsch MJ, Takamiya H, Vogt A: Quantitative studies of *in situ* immune complex glomerulonephritis in the rat induced by planted cationized antigen. J Exp Med, 155: 470-474, 1982.
54. Mannik M, Agoda LYC, David KA: Rearrangement of immune complexes in glomeruli leads to persistence and development of electron dense deposits. J Exp Med, 157: 1516-1528, 1983.
55. Gallo GR, Caulin-Glaser T, Emancipator SN, Lamm ME: Nephritogenicity and differential distribution of glomerular immune complexes related to immunogen charge. Lab Invest, 48: 353-462, 1983.
56. Caulin-Glaser T, Gallo GR, Lamm ME: Non-dissociating cationic immune complexes can deposit in glomerular basement membrane. J Exp Med, 158: 1561-1572, 1982.
57. Gallo GR, Caulin-Glaser T, Lamm ME: Charge of circulating immune complexes as a factor in glomerular basement membrane localization in mice. J Clin Invest 67: 1305-1313, 1981.
58. Mannik M: Mechanisms of tissue deposition of immune complexes. J Rheumat Dis, 14: 35-42, 1987.
59. Barnes JL, Radnik RA, Gilchrist EP, Vankatachalam MA: Size and charge selective permeability defects induced in glomerular basement membrane by a polycation. Kidney Int, 25: 11-19, 1984.

60. Barnes JL, Venkatachalam MA: Enhancement of glomerular imune complex deposition by a circulating polycation. J Exp Med, 160: 286-293, 1984.
61. Zollinger HU, Mihatsch MJ: Renal Pathology in Biopsy. Springer Verlag, Berlin, Heidelberg, New York, 1978.
62. Eilat D: Cross-reactions of anti-DNA antibodies and the central dogma of lupus nephritis. Immunology Today, 6: 123-127, 1985.
63. Andrzejewski Jr C, Rauch J, Lafer E, Stollar BD, Schwartz RS: Antigen binding diversity and idiotypic cross-reactions among hybridoma autoantibodies to DNA. J Immunol, 126: 226-231, 1981.
64. Lafer EM, Rauch J, Andrzejewski Jr C, Mudd D, Furie B, Schwartz RS, Stollar DB: Polyspecific monoclonal lupus autoantibodies reactive with both polynucleotides and phospholipids. J Exp Med, 153: 897-909, 1981.
65. Pisetsky DS, Caster SA: Binding specificities of monoclonal anti-DNA antibody. Mol Immunol, 19: 645-650, 1982.
66. Shoenfeld Y, Rauch J, Massicotte M, Stollar BD, Schwartz, RS: Polyspecificity of monoclonal lupus autoantibodies produced by human-human hybridomas. N Engl J Med, 308: 414-420, 1983.
67. Gavalchin J, Nicklas JA, Eastcott JW, Madaio MP, Stollar BD, Schwartz RS, Datta SK: Lupus prone (SWRxNZB)F1 mice produce potentially nephritogenic autoantibodies inherited from the normal SWR parent. J Immunol, 134: 885-894, 1985.
68. Faaber P, Rijke GPM, Van de Putte LBA, Capel PJA, Berden JHM: Crossreactivity of human and murine anti-DNA antibodies with heparan sulphate: the major glycosaminoglycan in glomerular basement membranes. J Clin Invest, 77: 1824-1830, 1986.
69. Faaber P, Capel PJA, Rijke GPM, Vierwinden G., Van de Putte LBA, Koene RAP: Crossreactivity of anti-DNA antibodies with proteoglycans. Clin Exp Immunol, 55: 502-510, 1984.
70. Jacob L, Tron F, Bach JF, Louvard D: A monoclonal anti-DNA antibody also binds to cell-surface protein(s). Proc Natl Acad Sci USA, 81: 3843-3845, 1984.
71. Tron F, Jacob L, Bach JF: Binding of murine monoclonal anti-DNA antibody to Raji cells. Implications for the interpretation of the Raji cell assay for immune complexes. Eur J Immunol, 14: 283-386, 1984.
72. Faaber P, v.d.Broek MF, Rijke GPM, Capel PJA, Berden JHM: Direct binding of monomeric anti-DNA antibodies to Raji-cells. Scand J Immunol, 22: 539-548, 1985.
73. Migliorini P, Ardman B, Kaburaki J, Schwartz RS: Parallel sets of autoantibodies in MRL-lpr/lpr mice. An anti-DNA, anti-SmRPM, anti-GP70 network. J Exp Med, 165: 483-499, 1987.
74. Mannik M: Pathophysiology of circulating immune complexes. Athritis Rheum, 25: 783-787, 1982.
75. Madaio MP, Carlson J, Cataldo J, Ucci A, Migliorini P, Pankewycz O: Murine monoclonal anti-DNA antibodies bind directly to glomerular antigens and form immune deposits. J Immunol, 138: 2883-2889, 1987.
76. Stollar BD, Zon G, Pastor RW: A recognition site on synthetic helical oligonucleotides for monoclonal anti-native DNA autoantibody. Proc Natl Acad Sci USA, 83: 4469-4473, 1986.
77. Sabbaga J, Peres Line SR, Potocnjak P, Madaio MP: A murine nephritogenic monoclonal anti-DNA autoantibody binds directly to mouse laminin, the major non-collageneous protein component of the glomerular basement membrane. Eur J Immunol, 19: 137-143, 1989.
78. Smeenk RJT, Brinkman K, Van den Brink HG,, Westgeest AAA: Reaction patterns of monoclonal antibodies to DNA. J Immunol, 140: 3786-3792, 1988.
79. Termaat RM, Brinkman K, van Gompel F, van den Heuvel LPW, Veerkamp JH, Smeenk RJT, Berden JHM: Cross-reactivity of monoclonal anti-DNA antibodies with heparan sulphate is mediated via bound DNA/histone complexes. J Autoimmunity, 3: 531-545, 1990.
80. Termaat RM, Brinkmann K, Nossent JC, Swaak AJG, Smeenk RJT, Berden JHM: Anti-heparan sulphate reactivity in sera from patients with systemic lupus erythematosus with renal or non-renal manifestations. Clin Exp Immunol, 82: 268-274, 1990.
81. Naparstek Y, Ben-Yehuda A, Madaio MP, Bar-Tana R, Schuger L, Pizov G, Neeman Z, Cohen IR: Binding of anti-DNA antibodies and inhibition of glomerulonephritis in MRL-lpr/lpr mice by heparin. Arthritis Rheum, 33: 1554-1559, 1990.
82. Raz E, Brezis M, Rosenmann E, Eilat D: Anti-DNA antibodies bind directly to renal antigens and induce kidney dysfunction in the isolated perfused rat kidney. J Immunol, 142: 3076-3082, 1989.

83. Termaat RM: Nephritogenicity of anti-DNA antibodies. Thesis of the Katholieke Universiteit van Nijmegen, 1991.
84. Koffler D: Laboratory evaluation of systemic lupus erythematosus. In "Systemic Lupus Erythematosus" (Ed RG Lahita) John Wiley & Sons, New York, 1987, pp 497-521.
85. Lahita R, Kluger J, Drayer DE, Koffler D, Reidenberg MM: Antibodies to nuclear antigens in patients treated with procainamide or acetylprocainamide. N Engl J Med, 301: 1382-1385, 1979.
86. Vogt A: New aspects of the pathogenesis of immune complex glomerulonephritis: formation of subepithelial deposits. Clinical Nephrology, 21: 15-20, 1984.
87. Stöckl F, Schmiedeke T, Muller S, Atanassov C, Waldherr R, Rodriguez-Iturbe B, Sugisaki Y, Nakabayashi F, Nagasawa T, Batsford S, Andrassy K, Vogt A: Glomerular Histone and Ubiquitin deposits in biopsies of SLE patients. J Am Soc Nephrol, 1: 541, 1990.
88. Schmiedeke T, Stöckl F, Muller S, Mertz A, Vogt A: Detection of Histone H3 and H2A in glomerular deposits of lupus-mice. Kidney Int, 37: 430, 1990.
89. Maddison PJ, Reichlin M: Deposition of antibodies to a soluble cytoplasmic antigen in the kidneys of patients with systemic lupus erythematosus. Arthritis and Rheum, 22: 858-863, 1979.
90. Paller MS, Moore SW, Tan E, Schrier RW: Anti-cytoplasmic antibodies in antinuclear antibody-negative lupus erythematosus. Am J Med, 75: 529-533, 1983.
91. Reichlin M, Van Venrooij WJ: Autoantibodies 3 to the URNP particles: relationship to clinical diagnosis and nephritis. Clin Exp Med, 83: 286-290, 1990.
92. Muller S, Briand JP, Van Regenmortel MHV: Presence of antibodies to ubiquitin during the autoimmune response associated with systemic lupus erythematosus. Proc Natl Acad Sci USA, 75: 8176-8180, 1988.
93. Fournié GJ: Circulating DNA and lupus nephritis. Kidney Int, 33: 487-497, 1988.
94. Burlingame RW, Rubin RL: Subnucleosome structures as substrates in enzyme-linked immunoadsorbent assays. J Immunol Methods, 134: 187-199, 1990.
95. Thomas JO, Kornberg RD: An octamer of histones in chromatin and free in solution. Proc Natl Acad Sci USA, 72: 2626-2630, 1975.
96. Emlen W, Burdick G: Clearance and organ localization of small DNA anti-DNA immune complexes in mice. J Immunol, 140: 1816-1822, 1988.
97. Andres GA, Accini L, Beiser SM, Christian CL, Ginotti GA, Erlanger BF, Hsu KC, Seegal BC: Localization of fluorescein-labeled antinucleoside antibodies in glomeruli of patients with active systemic lupus erythematosus nephritis. J Clin Invest, 49: 2106-2118, 1970.
98. Seegal BC, Accini L, Andres GA, Beiser SM, Christian CL, Erlanger BF, Hsu KC: Immunologic studies of autoimmune disease in NZB/NZW F1 mice. I. Binding of fluorescein-labeled antinucleoside antibodies in lesions of lupus-like nephritis. J Exp Med, 130: 203-216, 1969.
99. Blomgren SE, Condemi JJ, Vaughan JH: Procainamide-induced lupus erythematosus. Clinical and laboratory observations. Am J Med, 52: 338-348, 1972.
100. Northway JD, Tan EM: Differentiation of antinuclear antibodies giving speckled staining patterns in immunofluorescence. Clin Immunol Immunopathol, 1: 140-152, 1972.
101. Hahn BH, Ebling FM: Idiotypic restriction in murine lupus; high frequency of three public idiotypes on serum IgG in nephritic NZB/NZW F1 mice. J Immunol 138: 2110-2118, 1987.
102. Shoenfeld Y, Isenberg D: DNA antibody idiotypes: a review of their genetic, clinical and immunopathological features. Sem Arthritis Rheum, 16: 245-252, 1987.
103. Solomon G, Schiffenbauer J, Keiser HD, Diamond B: Use of monoclonal antibodies to identify shared idiotypes on human antibodies to DNA from patients with systemic lupus erythematosus. Proc Natl Acad Sci USA, 80: 850-854, 1983.
104. Isenberg DA, Collins C: Detection of cross-reactive anti-DNA antibody idiotypes on renal tissue-bound immunoglobulins from lupus patients. J Clin Invest, 76: 287-294, 1985.
105. Muryoi T, Sasaki T, Hatakeyama A, Shibata S, Suzuki M, Seino J, Yoshinaga K: Clonotypes of anti-DNA antibodies expressing specific idiotypes in immune complexes of patients with active lupus nephritis. J Immunol, 144: 3856-3861, 1990.
106. Rauch J, Hazeltine M, Tannenbaum H, Danoff D, Isenberg DA, Wild J, Samples J, Esdaile JM: Association of anti-DNA idiotype markers with clinical and serological manifestations in patients with systemic lupus erythematosus. J Rheumatol, 17: 178-185, 1990.
107. Diamond B, Schwartz MM: The glomerular immune deposits in patients with systemic lupus erythematosus glomerulonephritis contain a common IgG idiotype. Kidney Int, 31: 336, 1987.

108. Weisbart R, Noritake DT, Wong AL, Chan G, Kacena A, Colburn KK: A conserved anti-DNA antibody idiotype associated with nephritis in murine and human systemic lupus erythematosus. J Immunol, 144: 2653-2658, 1990.
109. Hahn BH, Ebling FM: Suppression of murine lupus nephritis by administration of anti-idiotypic antibody to anti-DNA. J Immunol, 132: 187-190, 1984.
110. Tsao BT, Ebling FM, Roman C, Panosian-Sahakian N, Calame K, Hahn BH: Structural characteristics of the variable regions of immunoglobulin genes encoding a pathogenic autoantibody in murine lupus. J Clin Invest, 85: 530-540, 1990.
111. Mendlovic, S, Brocke S, Shoenfeld Y, Ben-Bassat M, Meshorer A, Bakimer R, Mozes E: Induction of a systemic lupus erythematosus-like disease in mice by a common human anti-DNA idiotype. Proc Natl Acad Sci, 85: 2260-2264, 1988.
112. Batsford S, Oite T, Takamiya H, Vogt A: Anionic binding sites in the glomerular basement membrane: possible role in the pathogenesis of immune complex glomerulonephritis. Renal Physiol, 3: 336-340, 1980.
113. Dang H, Harbeck R: The *in vivo* and *in vitro* glomerular deposition of isolated anti double-stranded-DNA antibodies in NZB/W mice. Clin Immunol Immunopathol, 30: 265-278, 1984.
114. Galvalchin J, Seder RA, Datta SK: The NZB x SWR model of lupus nephritis. I. Cross-reactive idiotypes of monoclonal anti-DNA antibodies in relation to antigenic specificity, charge, and allotype. Identifiction of interconnected idiotype families inherited from the normal SWR and the autoimmune NZB parents. J Immunol, 138: 128-137, 1987.
115. Yoshida H, Yoshida M, Izui S, Lambert S, Lambert PH: Distinct clonotypes of anti-DNA antibodies in mice with lupus nephritis. J Clin Invest 76: 685-694, 1985.
116. Gauthier VJ, Mannik M: A small proportion of cationic antibodies in immune complexes is sufficient to mediate their deposition in glomeruli. J Immunol, 145: 3348-3352, 1990.
117. Gavalchin S, Datta SK: The NZB x SWR model of lupus nephritis. II. Autoantiboies deposited in renal lesionss show a distinctive and restricted idiotype diversity. J Immunol, 138: 138-148, 1987.

Chapter 3

LIGHT-CHAIN DEPOSITION DISEASE: DIAGNOSIS, PROGNOSIS AND THERAPY

DOMINIQUE CHAUVEAU, DOMINIQUE GANEVAL

Département de Néphrologie, Hôpital Necker, 149, rue de Sèvres, 75015 Paris, France

Light-chain deposition disease (LCDD) is a systemic disease characterized by monotypic light-chain (LC) deposits. Although various organs may be affected, it is usually heralded by renal involvement. Diagnosis is made on immunohistologic findings: deposits are reactive with one anti-light-chain antiserum (kappa or lambda) and lack amyloid characteristics. LCDD is always associated with B-cell dyscrasias, but in one third of reported cases the lymphoplasmacytic proliferation does not fit the usual criteria for malignancy. In this article we review the prominent pathological and clinical features that are currently important to consider in the clinical care of patients with LCDD.

Under normal circumstances, the small amount of LC physiologically detected in the serum which passes the glomerular barrier is reabsorbed by proximal tubular cells and catabolized there. It must be clearly stated that toxicity of monoclonal light chains, the - so-called Bence-Jones proteins- is not uniform. LC can eventually lead to four pathologic lesions within the kidney. The commonest is cast nephropathy or myeloma kidney, the hallmark of which is intratubular deposition of casts. Its incidence was 32% in a necropsy study (1) in myeloma patients. The casts contain various plasma proteins, Tamm-Horsfall protein and LC. In rare patients Bence-Jones proteins, almost exclusively kappa LC, form crystalline deposits within tubular cells that are associated with varying degrees of proximal tubular dysfunction (the Fanconi syndrome). Finally two types of tissue deposits can be recognized: AL amyloid and light chains. In the autopsy study cited above, LCDD was found in 5% and amyloidosis in 11% of the patients (1). Most patients with the former disorder have Bence-Jones protein of the lambda type, as the latter is most common with kappa light chains. Usually, the various types of histopathological lesions tend to occur independently, although association of several different lesions can also be seen. Generally speaking, the term light-chain disease refers to the systemic toxic potential of Bence-Jones proteins, including the four renal lesions described above. For convenience, we will consider here only light-chain deposition disease. Other aspects of LC-associated features have been covered extensively elsewhere (2-5).

PATHOLOGICAL CHANGES

The most characteristic and constant renal histopathological feature is the linear fixation of antisera directed against a single class of LC along tubular basement membranes (TBM). Prior to immunofluorescence study, the diagnosis can be suspected in the presence of bright, refractile, ribbon-like, PAS-positive thickening of TBM by light microscopy (6). Distal and collecting tubules are predominantly involved. Tubular atrophy is frequent. On occasion, TBM deposits are surrounded by macrophagic cells similar to those encountered around myeloma casts (5). In some cases, a positive immunofluorescence can be seen along the *vasa recta* or lying free in the interstitium. By electron microscopy tubular deposits appear as finely granular electron-dense material within the basement membrane or along its external aspect (6). In rare instances electron-dense deposits are not detected despite positive immunofluorescence (7).

Vessel walls are commonly involved by similar electron-dense material of monoclonal LC that lies along endothelial basement membranes or surrounds smooth-muscle cells. Glomerular involvement is heterogeneous (6, 8) and quite uncommon in the absence of TBM deposits. In most cases, the fluorescence is nodular in the mesangium and linear along the glomerular basement membrane (GBM). However, in milder forms no glomerular fixation of LC antisera can be found on immunofluorescence. By light microscopy, thickening of the GBM and Bowman's capsule are common features. Usually, PAS-positive mesangial deposits are associated with a moderate increase in mesangial matrix. In one third of the cases, this substantial mesangial increase leads to a nodular glomerulosclerosis (9) with a pattern similar to that observed in Kimmelstiel-Wilson diabetic nephropathy, including PAS-positivity. The mesangial nodules and deposits are nonCongophilic. Unusual lesions have been reported including capillary microaneurysms (10), endocapillary proliferation and crescentic glomerulonephritis (8). Electron microscopy shows punctate electron-dense deposits located in the *lamina rara interna* of the GBM or mesangial aggregates of variable size. The intensity and distribution of dense deposits do not always correlate with the pattern on immunofluorescence (9, 11).

Diagnosis of LCDD is made on immunohistologic findings. The most distinguishing feature is linear staining along basement membranes for kappa or more rarely lambda LC. In diabetes, although histologic appearance may be similar, the linear staining is for albumin and IgG. Morphologically the amyloid deposits that are associated with B-cell dyscrasias (AL amyloidosis) have the same topography as LC deposits. Both may even be associated in 5-10% of the cases. However, amyloid deposits bind Congo red and have a beta-pleated fibrillar ultrastructure. Another fibrillary glomerulopathy has recently attracted attention: it is characterized by extracellular deposits mimicking amyloidosis on ultrastructural examination. However deposits fail to react with Congo red. This entity has been labeled fibrillary glomerulonephritis or immunotactoid glomerulopathy (12). Of interest, monoclonal LC mesangial deposits are found in 10% of the patients, as IgG and C3 positive staining are constant findings. Apart from the typical aspect of light chain without heavy chain deposit disease, light- and heavy-chain deposition disease is recognized upon demonstration of linear staining of both light and heavy chains of a single immunoglobulin class. It could account for 10% of monoclonal immunoglobulin deposition disease (8, 13). One case of nodular glomerulosclerosis has also been observed with linear staining of heavy gamma chain, without detectable light chain (G. Touchard, personal communication).

Extrarenal involvement in LCDD was demonstrated in the initial report by Randall et al (14). Its precise incidence in various tissues remains unknown, as evidence of tissue deposits is far more common than are clinical manifestations. Virtually all organs may be involved. Deposits are preferentially found in vessel walls of the liver, heart and spleen (9, 14, 15) as well as in endocrine glands, the gastrointestinal tract and the pancreas. Peliosis hepatis, characterized by the presence of multiple small blood-filled cavities in the liver substance can be found in association with liver deposits (1, 16, 17). Central nervous system involvement is a common finding at autopsy. LC deposits have been noted along peripheral nerves (18). Pulmonary nodules have also been reported as a primary presentation (19). The usefulness of skin biopsy to diagnose LCDD in patients with heavy proteinuria and a monoclonal component in serum or urine has been suggested (15) but never adequately evaluated.

CLINICAL MANIFESTATIONS

LCDD involves predominantly males, with a sex ratio ranging from 2:1 to 4:1 in different series. Age at diagnosis varies from 35 to 75. The usual renal manifestations consist of proteinuria and renal failure. Proteinuria exceeds 2 g/day in 90% of patients. The nephrotic syndrome is noted in one quarter of these cases. Proteinuria is composed of monoclonal immunoglobulins including Bence-Jones protein, or albumin, or both in various proportions. Some 85 to 100% of patients present with renal failure (9, 15, 20, 21). Renal impairment progresses rapidly to end-stage renal failure in untreated patients. Microscopic haematuria and moderate hypertension are not uncommon. Prominent tubular dysfunction is quite unusual (22).

The spectrum of systemic *sequelae* of LCDD include congestive heart failure, arrhythmias, conduction defects and infrequently myocardial infarction (23). Liver involvement is only rarely a major feature of the initial presentation, but hepatomegaly, liver function abnormalities and portal hypertension eventually progressing to liver failure are common in the clinical course (16, 24, 25). Peripheral neuropathy (18) and subcutaneous nodules (26) have been reported.

HEMATOLOGICAL FINDINGS

LCDD always reflects a clonal lymphoplasmacytic disorder. In two thirds of cases, conventional examination of bone marrow aspirates or biopsies discloses a malignant dyscrasia, multiple myeloma as a rule, or in rare cases another malignancy (Waldenström disease, non-Hodgkin lymphoma or plasma cell leukemia) (27). In most series, manifestations of LCDD lead to discovery of the malignancy. In rare cases, however, tissue deposition emerged in myeloma patients coincident with an aggressive phase of myelomatosis despite on-going chemotherapy (9). Such a rare presentation suggests the emergence of a specific clone prone to secrete particular light chains. In one third of LCDD cases which have no detectable malignancy at presentation and little or no apparent increase in plasma cells, an excess of monoclonal LC production is detectable in two ways: first, an abnormal kappa:lambda ratio is usually evidenced by immunofluorescence study of bone marrow-cells which enhances diagnosis accuracy by showing restricted monoclonal LC production. Of course the LC isotype is the same within tissue deposits and clonal plasma cells. Second, *in vitro* immunoglobulin biosynthesis and secretion experiments have indicated abnormalities in most patients [see below] (28).

The reported proportions of patients with monoclonal proteins in the serum and urine are close to 60 and 75%, respectively (9, 15). Conversely in 15 to 20% of proven LCDD no monoclonal component can be detected in serum or urine despite the use of sensitive methods such as immunoelectrophoresis of concentrated urines or immunofixation. This figure includes cases of pseudo-nonsecretory myeloma characterized by rapid disappearance of LC due to their rapid deposition in various organs (29).

PROGNOSIS AND TREATMENT

The deposition of monoclonal immunoglobulins in various tissues is one of the most serious complications of the B-cell dyscrasias. Its natural history remains unclear and its course depends upon systemic deposition and the degree of malignancy. In our experience, in the absence of chemotherapy, renal insufficiency always progressed to end-stage renal failure. Progressive renal impairment within 2 years, even in patients without overt malignancy, has also been noted in this setting in 15 patients (21). With chemotherapy, we and others (30, 31) have documented stabilization or even improvement of renal function in up to 80% of patients on a 3 year follow-up. In the absence of overt dyscrasia, we have even documented the reversal of renal deposits paralleling the regression of renal impairment. On renal replacement therapy, 5/18 patients who were followed in our hospital died of other organ failure related to protein deposition (two and three cases of hepatic and cardiac involvement, respectively). However, one patient had a 10-year survival without chemotherapy. From available data, it is not clear whether chemotherapy prevents extrarenal deposition.

We feel, however, that it is logical to try to reduce immunoglobulin synthesis and subsequent deposition by using chemotherapy in anuric patients, whether or not the underlying hematological disease is malignant. We would also extend these recommendations to all cases of symptomatic deposition disease.

Symptomatic management of renal failure in LCDD patients may have a favourable effect on renal function. This includes suppression of nephrotoxic drugs, including non-steroidal antiinflammatory drugs, treatment of renal infection or hypercalcemia, prevention of cast-induced tubular obstruction by abundant alkaline diuresis, and control of hypertension. Chronic renal replacement therapy must be offered as often as indicated. In patients with overt malignancy and end-stage renal failure it is worthwhile to use regular dialysis until one can assess the response to chemotherapy.

As mentioned previously, cyclical therapy with melphalan and prednisone is of value in some patients, even in the absence of overt malignancy. To avoid the myelotoxicity of melphalan in patients with renal failure, lowering of doses is warranted. Whether cyclophosphamide plus prednisone or polychemotherapy may improve the prognosis of renal disease and overall survival in LCDD remains to be elucidated. Clearly an aggressive approach must be regarded cautiously because of potential toxicity of drugs eliminated through the kidney. Moreover, use of adriamycin or its derivatives should be avoided in patients with possible cardiac deposits. To our knowledge, bone-marrow transplantation has been successfully performed in 2 patients with myeloma-related LCDD and moderate renal failure; on short term follow-up both have experienced complete remission of the hematological disorder despite persistent renal impairment.

Finally, kidney transplantation should be offered to those patients with no evidence of malignancy who require chronic replacement therapy. LCDD may recur in some cases, several years after kidney transplantation and can result in graft failure (32, 33).

MECHANISMS OF LC DEPOSITION

The mechanisms of LC deposition remain unknown. A striking finding is that only 5-10% of patients with multiple myeloma develop such a disease, although a monoclonal urinary protein is initially detected in 50% of patients. The propensity to form linear precipitates might depend upon local tissue factors or structural abnormalities of monoclonal components. Local tissue factors probably come into play since, for unclear reasons, deposits have both a predilection for kidney tissue and an affinity for basement membranes.

Structural abnormalities of the monoclonal immunoglobulin are suggested by the following: [1] recurrence of LCDD on kidney grafts has been reported after renal transplantation in several cases (see review in 32). In one case, myeloma-related LCDD developed with *de novo* multiple myeloma 3 years after transplantation; [2] Solomon et al (7) have developed an *in vivo* experimental model by injecting Bence-Jones protein from 40 patients with dysglobulinemia into mice. They demonstrated that the kidney lesions produced in mice tend to mimic those in the kidneys of the patients from whom the proteins were obtained; of the 18 patients with renal tissue available for the study, the findings in 14 were comparable to those in the mice. This implicates the protein as being responsible for the pathological changes. However the findings reported by Solomon et al included cast nephropathy and AL amyloidosis as well as LCDD. In the group with LCDD, dissociations were frequently recognized. The injection of the Bence-Jones protein from 6/18 patients with LCDD led to basement membrane nephropathy in only three mice, and conversely three animals developed LCDD changes that were not detectable in the corresponding patients. These discrepancies may, in turn, depend upon the characteristics of the protocol used; [3] The role of the isoelectric point and isotype (kappa or lambda) of the light chain to determine kidney lesions has been disputed (7); [4] Direct studies of the monoclonal Ig deposited in tissues and within bone marrow-cells demonstrated that in a substantial number of cases, gross abnormalities of light chains, being either too short or, more commonly, glycosylated and thus too large, may predispose to tissue deposition. In the remaining patients, molecular weight of the LCs lies within normal range and their overall structure is normal (28).

Data on the primary structure of LC are available in only 3 patients. In the first case, it was related to V_KI subgroup (34) and in the other two, the kappa chain belonged to V_KIV subgroup (35, 36). In these latter patients, sequencing of the variable (V) segment demonstrated several mutations that resulted in abnormal glycosylation and increased molecular weight in one case, but neither of these changes in the other. Thus, the molecular approach ultimately demonstrated that structural abnormalities may be involved in tissue deposition.

REFERENCES

1. Ivanyi B: Frequency of light chain deposition nephropathy relative to renal amyloidosis and Bence-Jones cast nephropathy in a necropsy study of patients with myeloma. Arch Pathol Lab Med, 114: 986-987, 1990.
2. Fang LST: Light-chain nephropathy. Kidney Int, 27: 582-592, 1985.
3. Kyle RA: Monoclonal gammopathies and the kidney. Ann Rev Med, 40: 53-60, 1989.
4. Sturgill BC, Tucker FL, Bolton WK: Immunoglobulin light chain nephropathies. Pathol Annu, 22: 133-150, 1987.
5. Hill GS: Dysproteinemias, amyloidosis and immunotactoid glomerulopathy. In: "Pathology of the kidney" (Ed RH Hepstinstall), Vol. 2, Little Brown, Boston, 1991, pp 1631-1713.
6. Noël LH, Droz D, Ganeval D, Grünfeld JP: Renal granular monoclonal light chain deposits: morphological aspects in 11 cases. Clin Nephrol, 21: 263-269, 1984.
7. Solomon A, Weiss DT, Kattine AA: Nephrotoxic potential of Bence-Jones proteins. N Engl J Med, 324: 1845-1851, 1991.
8. Sanders PW, Herrera GA, Kirk KA, Old CW, Galla JH: Spectrum of glomerular and tubulointerstitial renal lesions associated with monoclonal immunoglobulin light chain deposition. Lab Invest, 64: 527-537, 1991.
9. Ganeval D, Noel LH, Preud'homme JL, Droz D, Grünfeld JP: Light-chain deposition disease: its relation with Al-type amyloidosis. Kidney Int, 26: 1-9, 1984.
10. Sinniah R, Cohen AM: Glomerular capillary aneurysms in light-chain nephropathy. Am J Pathol, 118: 298-305, 1985.
11. Bangertner AR, Murphy WM: Kappa light chain nephropathy. Virchows Arch A, 410: 531-539, 1987.
12. Alpers CE: Immunotactoid glomerulopathy: an entity distinct from fibrillary glomerulonephritis. Am J Kidney Dis, 19: 185-191, 1992.
13. Gallo G, Picken M, Buxbaum J, Frangione B: The spectrum of monoclonal immunoglobulin deposition disease associated with immunocytic dyscrasias. Semin Hematol, 26: 234-245, 1989.
14. Randall RE, Williamson WC, Mullinax F, Tung MY, Still WJS: Manifestations of systemic light chain deposition. Am J Med, 60: 293-299, 1980.
15. Buxbaum JN, Chuba JV, Hellman GC, Solomon AL, Gallo GR: Monoclonal immunoglobulin deposition disease: light chain and light and heavy chain deposition diseases and their relation to light chain amyloidosis. Ann Int Med, 112: 455-464, 1990.

16. Droz D, Noel LH, Carnot F, Degos F, Ganeval D, Grünfeld JP: Liver involvement in nonamyloid light chain deposits disease. Lab Invest, 50: 683-689, 1984.
17. Voinchet O, Degott C, Scoazec JY, Feldmann G, Benhamou JP: Peliosis hepatis, nodular regenerative hyperplasia of the liver and light-chain deposition in a patient with Waldenström's macroglobulinemia. Gastroenterology, 95: 482-486, 1988.
18. Dalakas MC, Engel WK: Polyneuropathy with monoclonal gammopathies: studies of 11 patients. Ann Neurol, 10: 45-52, 1981.
19. Kijner CM, Yousem SA: Systemic light chain deposition disease presenting as multiple pulmonary nodules. Am J Surg Pathol, 12: 405-413, 1988.
20. Tubbs RR, Gephardt GN, McNahon JT, Hall PM, Valenzuela R, Vidt DG: Light chain nephropathy. Am J Med, 71: 263-269, 1981.
21. Confalioneri R, Barbiano di Belgiojoso G, Banfi G, Ferrario F, Bertani T, Pozzi C, Casanova S, Lupo A, de Ferrari G, Minetti L: Light chain nephropathy: histological and clinical aspects in 15 cases. Nephrol Dial Transplant, 2: 150-156, 1988.
22. Nakamato Y, Imai H, Hamanaka S, Yoshida K, Akihama T, Miura AB: IgM monoclonal gammopathy accompanied by nodular glomerulosclerosis, urine-concentrating defect and hyporeninemic hypoaldosteronism. Am J Nephrol, 5: 53-58, 1985.
23. Peng SK, French WJ, Cohen AH, Fausel RE: Light chain cardiomyopathy associated with small-vessel disease. Arch Pathol Lab Med, 112: 844-846, 1988.
24. Bedossa P, Fabre M, Paraf F, Martin E, Lemaigre G: Light chain deposition disease with liver dysfunction. Human Pathol, 19: 1008-1014, 1988.
25. Faa G, Van Eyken P, De Vos R, Fevery J, Van Damme B, De Groote J, Desmet VJ: Light chain deposition disease of the liver associated with AL-type amyloidosis and severe cholestasis. J Hepatol, 12: 75-82, 1991.
26. Maury CPJ, Teppo AM: Massive cutaneous hyalinosis. Am J Clin Pathol, 82: 543-551, 1984.
27. Rahman A, Mossey RT, Susin M, Budman D, Mailloux LU: Kappa-chain nephropathy associated with plasma cell leukemia. Arch Int Med, 144: 1689-1690, 1984.
28. Preud'homme JL: Immunoglobulin synthesis in plasma cell dyscrasias with renal lesions. In: "The kidney in plasma cell dyscrasias" (Eds L Minetti, G D'Amico, C Ponticelli), Kluwer Academic Publishers, Dordrecht, The Netherlands, 1988, pp 31-43.
29. Matsuzaki H, Yoshida M, Akahoshi Y, Kuwahara K, Satout T, Takatsuki K: Pseudo-nonsecretory multiple myeloma with light chain deposition disease. Acta Haematol, 85: 164-168, 1991.
30. Heilman RL, Holley K, Offord K, Velosa J, Kyle R: Apparent renal response to melphalan and prednisone (MP) in light chain deposition disease. Kidney Int, 35: 209A, 1988 (Abstract).
31. Gipstein RM, Cohen AH, Adams DA, Adams T, Grabie MT: Kappa light chain nephropathy without evidence of myeloma cells. Response to chemotherapy with cessation of maintenance hemodialysis. Am J Nephrol, 2: 276-281, 1982.
32. Alpers CE, Marchioro TL, Johnson RJ: Monoclonal immunoglobulin deposition disease in a renal allograft: probable recurrent disease in a patient without myeloma. Am J Kidney Dis, 13: 418-423, 1989.
33. Gerlag PGG, Koene RAP, Berden JHM: Renal transplantation in light chain nephropathy: case report and review of the literature. Clin Nephrol, 25: 101-104, 1986.
34. Picken MM, Frangione B, Barlogie B, Luna M, Gallo G: Light chain deposition disease derived from the K_1 light chain subgroup. Am J Pathol, 134: 749-754, 1989.
35. Cogne M, Preud'homme JL, Bauwens M, Touchard G, Aucouturier P: Structure of a monoclonal kappa chain of the V_KIV subgroup in the kidney and plasma cells in light chain deposition disease. J Clin Invest, 87: 2188-2190, 1991.
36. Khamlichi AA, Aucouturier P, Silvain C, Bauwens M, Touchard G, Preud'homme JL, Nau F, Cogne M: Primary structure of a monoclonal k chain in myeloma with light chain deposition disease. Clin Exp Immunol, 87: 122-126, 1992.

HYPERTENSION

Chapter 4

AMBULATORY BLOOD PRESSURE MONITORING IN CLINICAL PRACTICE: USES AND ABUSES

THOMAS G. PICKERING

The New York Hospital-Cornell Medical Center, Cardiovascular Center, 525 East 68th Street, Starr-4, New York, NY 10021, USA

Ambulatory blood pressure monitoring is a technique that was first developed 25 years ago, but is only now beginning to gain acceptance as a clinically useful procedure. The inherent variability of blood pressure and its susceptibility to transient emotional influences means that the conventional clinical measurements may not accurately reflect an individual's "true" level of blood pressure. These sources of error provide the rationale for ambulatory monitoring, which can be overcome by increasing the number of readings and taking them outside the clinic setting.

The development of reasonably accurate and reliable noninvasive recorders has provided the opportunity to use this technology for both clinical and research purposes. While the accuracy of any noninvasive automatic technique is less than optimal (particularly during physical activity), the technical errors are relatively small in comparison to the greater error of the estimate of true pressure based on a small number of clinic readings.

TECHNIQUES OF AMBULATORY MONITORING

The currently available monitors all take blood pressure either by the Korotkoff sound or the oscillometric techniques, from a sphygmomanometer cuff over the brachial artery (1). They are fully automatic, weigh less than 1 kg, and pump up and deflate the cuff at preset intervals (usually every 15 or 30 minutes) for a 24 to 48 hour period. The readings of blood pressure and heart rate are stored in the memory of the recorder, which can be played out at the end of the recording period into a personal computer. During the recording period the patients can go about their normal daily activities, although vigorous exercise should be avoided. To prevent artifact interfering with the blood pressure measurements, the patients are instructed to keep the monitored arm immobile while the cuff is inflated. It is also customary to ask them to keep a diary of their activities and position, because these have an important influence on blood pressure.

This procedure provides 50-100 readings over 24 hours. The data are usually expressed as the average values of systolic and diastolic pressure during the day, during the night, and for the whole 24 hours.

ACCURACY OF THE RECORDERS

A major concern when the noninvasive recorders were first introduced was whether they were sufficiently accurate and reliable to give clinically usable readings. All of the currently available models have undergone extensive validation testing, mostly in comparison with mercury sphygmomanometer readings, but also in many cases with intra-arterial recordings (2-4). In almost all cases the average discrepancy between the devices' and observers' readings are less than 5 mm Hg, with somewhat better accuracy for systolic than diastolic pressure. Not surprisingly, they are less accurate at the two extremes of blood pressure. The accuracy falls off markedly during physical exercise or in situations where there is vigorous movement of the arm (2).

Table 1. Clinical conditions associated with an abnormal diurnal rhythm of blood pressure.

Essential Hypertension (rarely)	
Black race	
Chronic Renal Failure	
Congestive Heart Failure	
Cushings Syndrome	
Steroid Treatment	
Pheochromocytoma	
Autonomic Neuropathy	- Idiopathic
	- Diabetes Mellitus
Toxemia of Pregnancy	

WHAT INFORMATION IS PROVIDED?

In principle, ambulatory monitoring can provide a better estimate of both the true or average level of blood pressure and its variability than clinic measurements. In many cases there is a substantial discrepancy between the clinic and ambulatory blood pressures. In hypertensive patients (but not in normotensives) the former is typically higher, and if the ambulatory pressure is normal, the patients may be classified as having white coat hypertension. In a minority of hypertensive patients (often smokers), the ambulatory pressure may be higher than the clinic pressure (5). The correlation coefficient between physician-measured pressures and the average daytime ambulatory pressure is around 0.7 (6), which means that clinic pressures account for only about 50% of overall blood pressure variance.

There is typically a marked diurnal profile of blood pressure, with the highest readings occurring during the morning hours (especially if the patient goes to work during the monitoring, which we encourage), and lower readings while at home in the evening (6, 7). The lowest pressures are seen at night during sleep. These changes can of course only be appreciated with a full 24 hour recording.

In hypertensive patients the entire diurnal profile of blood pressure is reset at a higher level, with a minor increase of variability (7). The profile may vary both as a result of psychosocial factors, and for other less well understood reasons. Thus, subjects who stay at home during the day of the monitoring will tend to have lower daytime pressures than if they go to work (8). And the pressure at home in the evening is likely to be higher in women who have children than in single women, even if they go to work during the day (9).

There are also variations in what happens at night. In most hypertensives there is a normal fall of blood pressure at night, but in some patients with both essential and various types of secondary hypertension (Table 1) the blood pressure remains elevated throughout the night (10-12). Although the pathological significance of this is unclear, there is evidence that when it occurs in patients with essential hypertension there is an increased prevalence of left ventricular hypertrophy (13), which we know carries a bad prognosis independently of blood pressure (14).

WHICH MEASURE OF BLOOD PRESSURE GIVES THE BEST PREDICTION OF RISK?

The main reason for measuring blood pressure in hypertensive patients is the evaluation of the risk of cardiovascular disease. Therefore, the ultimate determinant of the clinical value of ambulatory monitoring is the degree to which it improves this prediction. There are two ways of deciding whether ambulatory measurement gives a better prediction than clinic measurement. One is to compare the correlations of the two measures of blood pressure with target organ damage in cross-sectional studies, and the other is to compare the prediction of risk of cardiovascular morbidity in longitudinal studies. The latter process is clearly preferable on theoretical grounds, but is more difficult to achieve in practice, because it involves following a large number of patients for many years. We have reviewed elsewhere a considerable number of studies showing that ambulatory pressure does indeed correlate more closely with target organ damage, the most widely used index of which has been left ventricular hypertrophy (LVH) measured echocardiographically (1). Other comparisons have used ECG-LVH (15), arterial stiffness (16), and early markers of renal damage (17), and almost all have shown ambulatory pressure to be superior.

So far there is only one prospective study, conducted by Perloff and Sokolow in San Francisco, which has shown that in patients with mild hypertension the prediction of risk can be improved by ambulatory monitoring (18, 19).

Table 2. Clinical indications for ambulatory blood pressure monitoring.

- Hypertensives without target organ damage
- Disparity between clinic and home blood pressure
- Resistant hypertension
- Orthostatic hypotension (autonomic neuropathy)
- Intermittent symptoms possibly related to blood pressure changes
- Episodic hypertension
- Evaluation of treatment

CLINICAL APPLICATIONS OF AMBULATORY MONITORING

In Table 2 some common clinical situations where ambulatory monitoring might be beneficial are listed. When there are signs of target organ damage in a hypertensive patient, there is enough justification to recommend antihypertensive treatment without further testing (18). When high blood pressure is the only detectable abnormality, however, ambulatory monitoring may, at any rate in theory, provide an improved estimate of the "true" blood pressure.

White coat hypertension

For the clinician, perhaps the single most important application of ambulatory recording techniques is the detection of patients with "white coat hypertension", which we have defined as a persistently elevated clinic pressure together with a normal daytime ambulatory pressure (20).

The definitions of "elevated" and "normal" in this context are clearly quite arbitrary, and the prevalence of the condition will depend on the cutoff points used, as well as the population being studied, but in our own population is approximately 20%. Others have reported a prevalence of 38% (21) and 39% (22). This may be sought for in patients without signs of target organ damage, and when there is a large discrepancy between clinic and home readings. The pressor effect of a physician in a clinic setting has been recognized for many years (23-25), and may provoke a transient rise of pressure of as much as 30 or 40 mm Hg.

In the office, the pressure recorded by the physician is typically consistently higher than the pressure recorded by a nurse or technician in the same physical setting (20), which in turn is likely to be higher than the pressure recorded by an automatic recorder with no observer present. In a study of 702 patients evaluated by ambulatory monitoring (7) whom we divided into three groups (58 normotensive, 578 with borderline hypertension, and 66 with established hypertension) on the basis of their clinic pressures, we found that in the normotensives approximately 60% of readings obtained during ambulatory monitoring were higher than the clinic level, while in the borderline and established hypertensives the corresponding figures were 40 and 20%, as shown in Figure 1.

White coat hypertension is observed in both young and old patients, of either sex, though with perhaps a slight preponderance in women (20, 22). It may be an important contributor to systolic hypertension of the elderly (26). Contrary to what might be expected, patients with white coat hypertension do not appear to be generally more anxious than others with sustained hypertension (22, 27, 28). Our working hypothesis to explain the phenomenon is that it begins as a manifestation of the defense response, which can produce a rise of pressure in anyone when the blood pressure is first taken. Normally, this habituates with repeated exposure, which accounts for the well-known tendency of clinic pressures to decline after multiple visits (29). In some patients, however, we hypothesize that this habituation does not take place, and the response may become permanent as a result of classical and cognitive conditioning.

This view implies that the white coat effect should be specific to the clinic setting, and not simply a manifestation of generally increased blood pressure lability or reactivity. Our own data, though limited, are in accord with this view, since our patients with white coat hypertension did not show an increased lability of pressure during ambulatory monitoring, and Floras has obtained similar results (30).

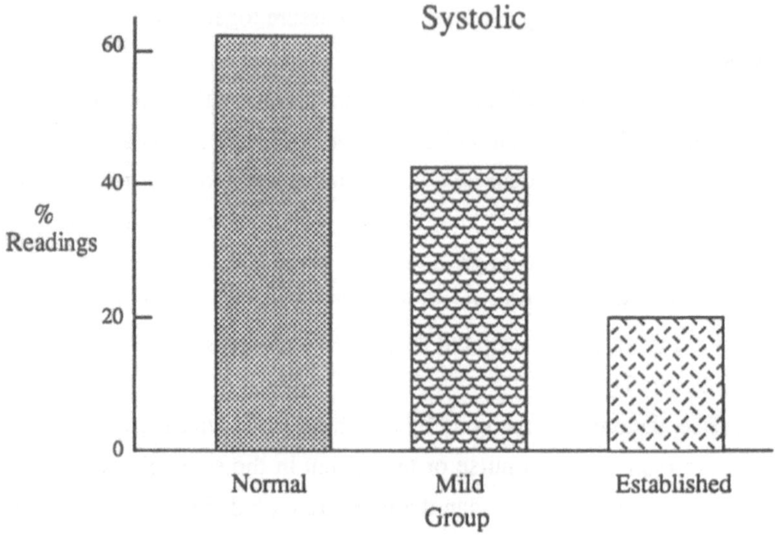

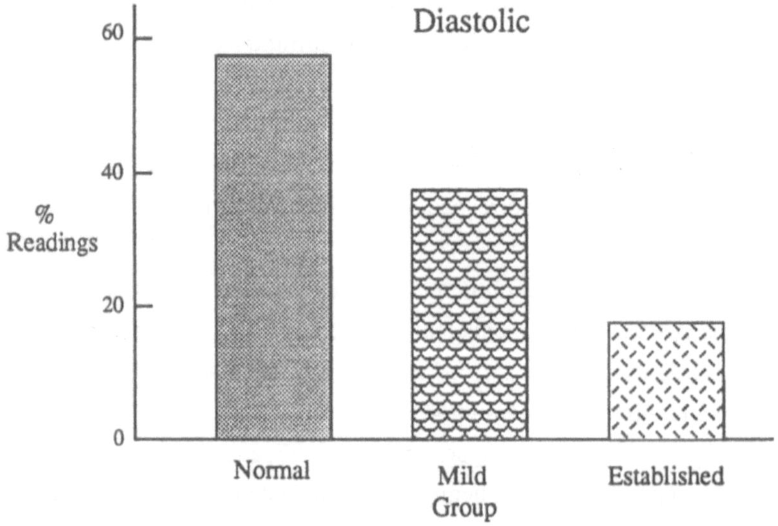

Figure 1. Average percentage of readings of systolic (upper panel) and diastolic (lower panel) blood pressure obtained during ambulatory monitoring which were higher than the individuals' clinic pressures, in three groups of subjects [Reproduced with permission from Harshfield GA, Pickering TG, James GD, Blank SG: Blood pressure variability and reactivity in the natural environment. In: "Blood pressure measurements" (Eds W Meyer-Sabellek, M Anlauf, R Gotzen, L Steinfeld), Steinkopff-Darmstadt, 1990, pp 241-251].

The important practical question is whether such patients are at less risk of developing cardiovascular morbidity than others whose pressure is elevated both during clinic visits and at other times. As yet no conclusive answer can be given, but what evidence there is does indicate a lower risk. At least three studies have found that there is less target organ damage in patients with white coat hypertension in comparison to those with essential hypertension (24, 30, 31). In one of these, White et al (31) showed that for the same level of clinic pressure, patients with white coat hypertension had less left ventricular hypertrophy and better left ventricular function than those with sustained hypertension. The only published prognostic study, performed by Perloff et al (18, 19), did not deal specifically with white coat hypertension, but did show that patients without target organ damage whose ambulatory pressure was lower than their clinic pressures were at less risk than those in whom it was the same or higher.

Resistant hypertension

At the opposite end of the spectrum, ambulatory monitoring may be of diagnostic value in patients with apparently resistant hypertension. A study by Littler et al (32) investigated a group of patients whose blood pressures remained persistently elevated despite aggressive antihypertensive treatment, but who did not show an equivalent degree of target organ damage. These patients had much lower ambulatory pressures than would have been expected from their clinic pressures. In our experience, occasional patients with clinic pressures as high as 180/120 mm Hg may have ambulatory and home pressures that are unequivocally normal.

Autonomic neuropathy

A major management problem is the patient with autonomic neuropathy, which may be idiopathic, or associated with other conditions such as diabetes. In these patients the blood pressure may be too high at times, and too low at others. The normal diurnal pattern of blood pressure may be grossly deranged, with the highest pressures occurring during the night, and the lowest when the patient is upright during the day (33). Ambulatory monitoring may be of great value in adjusting the appropriate mix of hypertensive and antihypertensive medications in such patients.

Other clinical applications of ambulatory monitoring

Some patients may experience symptoms that could be related to transient changes of blood pressure. An extreme example of this is the patient with a pheochromocytoma, who may or may not show paroxysmal elevations of blood pressure (34), but much more common is the patient whose intermittent symptoms are found to be unrelated to blood pressure, and in whom the demonstration of a normal blood pressure profile may be reassuring. In our experience blood pressure monitoring has not proved to be of much value in diagnosing patients with syncope.

Interpretation of results

Although the large number of blood pressure readings provided by ambulatory monitoring is one of its principal strengths, the question arises as to how the recordings should be analyzed and interpreted. The traditional process of evaluating a hypertensive patient involves the decision whether the blood pressure is above or below a certain threshold level, which determines whether treatment is recommended or withheld. Since hypertension is a continuum, however, any threshold is arbitrary. For clinic pressure this threshold has been set at levels varying from 140/90 mm Hg to 160/100 mm Hg. There is abundant evidence that ambulatory pressures tend to be lower than clinic pressures in hypertensive subjects (35), so there is no *a priori* reason to choose the same threshold level for ambulatory pressures. This raises the question of how such a level should be defined. The most widely advocated procedure is to measure ambulatory pressures in a population of normotensive individuals and define an upper limit of normal using some statistically acceptable definition of the normal range, such as two standard deviations above the mean, or the 90th percentile. While the data from such studies have been used to define an upper range of "normal" (36), they have been criticized on the grounds that the prognostic significance of such dividing lines is unknown (37).

There is as yet no consensus on what the upper limit of normal for ambulatory recordings should be, but an average daytime value above 140/90 mm Hg may be considered probably abnormal, while one below 135/85 mm Hg probably normal.

CONCLUSIONS

Although originally introduced purely as an investigational procedure, ambulatory blood pressure monitoring has demonstrated that the conventional clinic measurement often gives a very imprecise estimate of the true level of blood pressure, particularly in hypertensive patients. This discrepancy is largely due to the phenomenon of white coat hypertension. While it is not yet proven that such patients are at low risk of cardiovascular morbidity, currently available evidence suggests that they may be. The main clinical application of ambulatory monitoring may thus be in the diagnosis of patients with white coat hypertension, but better criteria are needed for defining the normal range of ambulatory pressures. It is likely that in the near future there will be less reliance on the use of clinic pressures for diagnosing hypertension, and much greater use of ambulatory monitoring, which has the potential of becoming a routine diagnostic procedure.

SUMMARY

Noninvasive ambulatory blood pressure monitoring is a technique that can overcome many of the limitations of clinic blood pressure measurement in the evaluation of hypertensive patients, and give a more reliable estimate of the true level of blood pressure and its variability. Currently available recorders are unobtrusive and reasonably accurate, and can describe the normal diurnal profile of blood pressure. There is evidence that ambulatory blood pressures correlate more closely with target organ damage than clinic pressure, and also that they give a better prediction of the risk of cardiovascular morbidity. The main clinical application is in patients with mild hypertension, many of whom will be found to have normal pressures outside the clinic (white coat hypertension).

REFERENCES

1. Pickering TG: Ambulatory monitoring and blood pressure variability. Science Press, London, 1991.
2. White WB, Lund-Johansen P, Omvik P: Assessment of four ambulatory blood pressure monitors and measurements by clinicians versus intraarterial blood pressure at rest and during exercise. Amer J Cardiol, 65: 60-66, 1989.
3. Santucci S, Cates EM, James GD, Schlussel YR, Steiner D, Pickering TG: A comparison of two ambulatory blood pressure monitors, the Del Mar Avionics Pressurometer IV and the Spacelabs 90202. Am J Hypertens, 2: 797-799, 1989.
4. Graettinger WR, Lipson HL, Cheung DG, Weber MA: Validation of portable noninvasive blood pressure monitoring devices. Comparisons with intra-arterial and sphygmomanometer measurements. Am Heart J, 116: 1155-1160, 1988.
5. Mann SJ, James GD, Wang RS, Pickering TG: Elevation of ambulatory systolic blood pressure in hypertensive smokers. JAMA, 265: 2226-2228, 1991.
6. Harshfield GA, Pickering TG, Kleinert HD, Blank S, Laragh JH: Situational variations of blood pressure in ambulatory hypertensive patients. Psychosom Med, 44: 237-245, 1982.
7. Harshfield GA, Pickering TG, James GD, Blank SG: Blood pressure variability and reactivity in the natural environment. In: "Blood pressure measurements" (Eds W Meyer-Sabellek, M Anlauf, R Gotzen, L Steinfeld), Steinkopff-Darmstadt, 1990, pp 241-251.
8. Pieper C, Schnall P, Warren K, Pickering TG: Comparison of ambulatory blood pressure and heart rate on a work day and a non-work day: evidence of a "carry-over effect" (Submitted for publication).
9. James GD, Cates EM, Pickering TG, Laragh JH: Parity and perceived job stress elevate blood pressure in young normotensive working women. Am J Hypertens, 2: 637-639, 1989.

10. Verdecchia P, Schillaca G, Guerreri M, Galteschi C, Benemio G, Boldrini F, Porcellati C: Circadian blood pressure changes and left ventricular hypertrophy in essential hypertension. Circulation, 81: 528-536, 1990.
11. Pickering TG: The clinical significance of diurnal blood pressure variations: Dippers and nondippers. Circulation, 81: 700-702, 1990.
12. Hany S, Baumgart P, Frielingsdorf J, Vetter H, Vetter W: Circadian blood pressure variability in secondary and essential hypertension. J Hypertens, 5 (Suppl 5): S487, 1987.
13. Koren MJ, Devereux RB, Casale PN, Savage DD, Laragh JH: Relation of left ventricular mass and geometry to morbidity and mortality in uncomplicated essential hypertension. Ann Int Med, 114: 345-352, 1991.
14. Pickering TG, Deveeux RB: Ambulatory monitoring of blood pressure as a predictor of cardiovascular risk. Am Heart J, 114: 925-928, 1987.
15. Vermeersch P, Duprez D, Packet L, Clement DL: Left ventricular hypertrophy in mild hypertension: Value of ambulatory recordings. J Hypertens, 5 (Suppl 5): S495-S495, 1987.
16. Asmar RG, Brunel PC, Pannier BM, Lacolley PJ, Safar ME: Arterial distensibility and ambulatory blood pressure monitoring in essential hypertension. Am J Cardiol, 61: 1066-1070, 1988.
17. Opsahl JA, Abraham PA, Halstenson CE, Keane WF: Correlation of office and ambulatory blood pressure measurements with urinary albumin and N-acetyl-beta-D-glucosaminidase excretion in essential hypertension. Am J Hypertens, 1: 1175-1205, 1988.
18. Perloff D, Sokolow M, Cowan R: The prognostic value of ambulatory blood pressure. JAMA, 249: 2792-2798, 1983.
19. Perloff D, Sokolow M, Cowan RM, Juster RP: Prognostic value of ambulatory blood pressure measurements: further analysis. J Hypertens, 7 (Suppl 3): S3-S10, 1989.
20. Pickering TG, James GD, Boddie C, Harshfield GA, Blank S, Laragh JH: How common is white coat hypertension? JAMA, 259: 225-228, 1988.
21. Krakoff LR, Eison H, Phillips RH, Leiman SH, Lev S: Effect of ambulatory pressure monitoring on the diagnosis and cost of treatment for mild hypertension. Am Heart J, 116: 1152-1154, 1988.
22. Lerman CE, Brody DS, Hui T, Lazaro C, Smith DG, Blum MJ: The white coat hypertension response: prevalence and predictors. J Gen Int Med, 4: 225-231, 1989.
23. Ayman D, Goldshine AD: Blood pressure determinations by patients with essential hypertension: the difference between clinic and home readings before treatment. Am J Med Sci, 200: 465-474, 1940.
24. Sokolow M, Perloff D, Cowan R: Contribution of ambulatory blood pressure to the assessment of patients with mild to moderate elevations of office blood pressure. Cardiovasc Rev Reports, 1: 295-303, 1980.
25. Mancia G, Bertinieri G, Grassi G et al: Effects of blood pressure measurement by the doctor on patient's blood pressure and heart rate. Lancet, II: 695-697, 1983.
26. Ruddy MC, Bialy GB, Malka ES, Lacy CR, Kostis JB: The relationship of plasma renin activity to clinic and ambulatory blood pressure in elderly people with isolated systolic hypertension. J Hypertens, 6 (Suppl 4): S412-S415, 1988.
27. Schneider RH, Egan RM, Johnson EH et al: Anger and anxiety in borderline hypertension. Psychosom Med, 48: 242-248, 1986.
28. Gerardi RJ, Blanchard EB, Andrasik F: Psychological dimensions of "office hypertension". Behav Res Ther, 23: 609-612, 1985.
29. Watson RDS, Lumb R, Young MA, Stallard TJ, Davies P, Littler WA: Variation in cuff blood pressure in untreated out patients with mild hypertension - implications for initiating antihypertensive treatment. J Hypertens, 5: 207-211, 1987.
30. Floras JS, Jones JV, Hassan MO, Osikowska B, Sever PS, Sleight P: Cuff and ambulatory blood pressure in subjects with essential hypertension. Lancet, II: 107-109, 1981.
31. White WB, Schulman P, McCabe EJ, Dey HM: Average daily blood pressure, not office blood pressure, determines cardiac function in patients with hypertension. JAMA, 261: 873-877, 1989.
32. Littler WA, Honour AJ, Pugsley DJ, Sleight P: Continuous recording of direct arterial pressure in unrestricted patients. Its role in the diagnosis and management of high blood pressure. Circulation, 51: 1101-1106, 1975.
33. Mann S, Altman DG, Raftery EB, Bannister R: Circadian variation of blood pressure in autonomic failure. Circulation, 68: 477-483, 1983.

34. Littler WA, Honour AJ: Direct arterial pressure, heart rate, and electrocardiogram in unrestricted patients before and after removal of a pheochromocytoma. Quart J Med, 43: 441-449, 1979.
35. Pickering TG, Harshfield GA, Kleinert HD, Blank S, Laragh JH: Comparisons of blood pressure during normal daily activities, sleep, and exercise in normal and hypertensive subjects. JAMA, 247: 992-996, 1982.
36. Staessen J, Bulpitt CJ, Fagard R et al: Reference values for the ambulatory blood pressure and the blood pressure measured at home: a population study. J Human Hyperten, 5: 355-367, 1991.
37. Pickering TG: Ambulatory monitoring and the definition of hypertension. J Hypertens (in press).

URINARY TRACT INFECTIONS

Chapter 5

DETERMINANTS OF THE DEVELOPMENT OF ACUTE PYELONEPHRITIS AND PYELONEPHRITIC RENAL SCARRING

CATHARINA SVANBORG AND KAETY PLOS

Division of Clinical Immunology, Department of Medical Microbiology, Lund University, Lund, Sweden

Infections of the urinary tract vary in severity. The most frequent form is asymptomatic bacteriuria (ABU) which occurs in about 1% of young girls, 2% of pregnant women and 15-20% of elderly individuals. The frequency estimates for acute pyelonephritis and acute cystitis are less consistent. Both are common conditions in all age groups. Acute pyelonephritis is distinguished from acute cystitis by the involvement of the kidneys and systemic sites. Acute pyelonephritis is commonly diagnosed as significant bacteriuria accompanied by fever, loin pain, elevated acute-phase reactants and reduced renal concentrating capacity (1).

Acute pyelonephritis may be defined as a bacterial infection involving the kidneys. Despite this apparently simple definition, acute pyelonephritis is a heterogeneous disease entity, varying in severity as well as consequences. Prior to the advent of antibiotics, the mortality rate was 15-20%, and recurrent episodes of acute pyelonephritis and progressive renal scarring were a major cause of end stage renal diseases. Today, acute pyelonephritis remains a serious condition, and, despite adequate treatment, renal scarring still occurs in a subgroup of the patients with acute pyelonephritis (1).

The aims of this review are: [1] to summarize the information on bacterial virulence and kidney tropism; [2] to comment on host response mechanisms which are involved in the pathogenesis of acute pyelonephritis; [3] to discuss host and bacterial determinants of renal scarring

BACTERIAL VIRULENCE

Escherichia coli is the most frequent cause of acute pyelonephritis and renal scarring (1). This review of bacterial virulence will therefore be limited to Escherichia coli. This

Gram-negative bacterium is an inhabitant of the large intestine both in man and animals (2). Most Escherichia coli strains are members of the normal fecal flora in healthy individuals. A subset of Escherichia coli cause infection both in the intestine and at extraintestinal sites e.g. diarrhoea, urinary tract infection (UTI), neonatal meningitis and septicemia.

This difference in virulence between Escherichia coli strains was recognized as early as the turn of the century (3, 4). Several investigators subsequently tried to classify Escherichia coli hoping to find markers which would discriminate between the more or less virulent strains. Systematic studies of Escherichia coli virulence were made possible by the development of serotyping (5-7). Isolates which had particular pathogenicity in man were found to belong to certain O antigen types and to be hemolytic more often than other strains (8, 9).

The clonal structure of Escherichia coli populations

The extended use of serotyping techniques revealed that certain O antigens occurred in combination with a limited set of capsular (K) antigens and flagellar (H) antigens (7). Furthermore, strains of a given O:K:H antigen combination (serotype) resembled each other in the biochemical reactions used for biotyping.

These findings led to the concept that natural populations of Escherichia coli occur as lineages or clones (10). Orskov (10) used the work clone to denote "bacterial cultures isolated independently from different sources in different locations and at different times but sharing so many identical phenotypic and genotypic traits that the most likely explanation for this identity is a common origin". More recent work has shown that Escherichia coli strains of a specific O:K:H antigen combination share a number of independent phenotypic characteristics including outer membrane protein patterns (OMP), electrophoretic types of cytoplasmic enzymes (ET) and adherence properties (11-15). The identification of Escherichia coli isolates as members of the same clone should idealy be based on DNA sequence homology. For practical purposes the identification of clones among clinical isolates is mainly based on phenotypic characteristics such as O:K:H serotype, biotype and ET.

The multilocus enzyme electrophoresis technique deserves some special comments. Intracellular enzymes are separated according to their mobility in an electric field. Enzymatically active proteins are detected by their ability to convert a substrate to a coulored end product. Isoenzymes of the same substrate specificity but with different mobilities are identified and designated as electromorphs. Since the difference in mobility is due to allelic variation at the respective chromosomal loci encoding each enzyme, isolates with the same repertoir of electromorphs are considered to be more closely related than those with different electromorphs. It has been proposed that the electromorph difference can be taken as a measure of genetic relatedness between Escherichia coli clones. This is in contrast to serotyping, which provides the information that O1:K1:H7 isolates are different from O4:K12:H1 isolates, but does not permit estimates of relatedness.

The clonal model of the population structure of Escherichia coli holds that each clone gives rise to identical progeny and that all parts of the chromosome of a strain are descended from a single ancestor. Recombination affecting large regions of the chromosome must be too rare to break up these clones (16). Recombination affecting small chromosomal or plasmid DNA segments may still occur, with little effect on the overall clonal identity. The acquisition of new DNA will be favoured when the encoded phenotype provides a selective advantage. Electrophoretic studies of Escherichia coli have shown that 94% of the loci are polymorphic with a mean diversity of 0.34-0.54 (13, 17). Based on this diversity an immense number of possible combinations would be generated. In contrast, a limited number of clonotypes are recovered from urinary isolates (13, 18, 19).

The same ETs are found in different geographic areas and at different times. The existing clones have probably been selected throughout evolution because of special fitness, for various ecological nisches including the large intestine and the urinary tract (20, 21).

Escherichia coli virulence factors

The properties which distinguish pyelonephritogenic Escherichia coli clones have been identified by careful comparisons with isolates from patients with ABU or the fecal flora of healthy individuals (22-24).

Multiple properties are relatively more frequent in the pyelonephritis strains, than in other Escherichia coli. These include adherence factors, iron-binding proteins, toxins, capsules etc. During the last decade, studies on the molecular mechanisms of virulence have provided detailed information on the pathogenesis of acute pyelonephritis.

This information was recently reviewed in the monograph by Kunin (1) and in the review by Svanborg and de Man (25).

Some of the information is summarized below with the focus on P-fimbriae.

ADHERENCE

Uropathogenic Escherichia coli attach to epithelial cells from the human urinary tract. Adherence enhances the tropism of bacteria for the urinary tract, as well as the virulence (see below). Adherence is mediated by bacterial surface components, adhesins, which bind to specific receptors on host cells. The adhesins of Gram-negative bacteria are often associated with fimbriae (26). Fimbriae are functionally distinct from flagella which are thicker, longer and more flexible and responsible for mobility (26, 27) and sex pili which are thicker and function in conjugation but do not attach bacteria to other surfaces (28). The fimbriae can be classified according to the antigenic properties of the major fimbrial subunit (29), or according to their binding properties (30). Regardless of the variation in these functions, however, they share the basic structure. The fimbriae are hair-like filamentous polymers 0.5-2 μm long with a diameter of 5-7 nm and a central axial hole with a diameter of 0.2-0.25 μm (27, 31). It consists of 500-1,000 identical major protein subunits polymerized into a helix. The minor proteins include the adhesin protein, responsible for the binding specificity (32). They are bound to the fimbrial subunit either at the tip or along the fimbriae (33-37).

Uropathogenic Escherichia coli express several fimbriae associated adhesins, which have been isolated and characterized both phenotypically and genotypically (38-40). The attachment of Escherichia coli to uroepithelial cells is mainly caused by P-fimbriae. The symbol P was chosen because of the association with Pyelonephritis and the P blood group system. The P-fimbriae recognize as receptors oligosaccharide sequence in the globo-series of glycolipids (41). These structures are antigens in the P blood group system and are expressed on erythrocytes and uroepithelial cells depending on the P blood group phenotype of the individual. P-fimbriated Escherichia coli agglutinate erythrocytes from P1 and P2 individuals, but do not bind to erythrocytes or epithelial cells from individuals of the P blood group who lack these receptors (41, 42).

S fimbriae and type 1 fimbriae may contribute to adherence in the urinary tract if the appropriate receptors are expressed (43-45). Type 1 or mannose-sensitive (MS) fimbrial adhesins recognize mannose containing receptors. Their binding is blocked by solutions of D-mannose or α-methyl-D-mannoside (46, 47). Receptors for type 1 fimbriae are present on erythrocytes and uroepithelial cells from many species (48) and type 1 fimbriae are widely distributed among virulent and non-virulent Escherichia coli strains (49). In the human urinary tract, type 1 fimbriae bind mannose epitopes on secreted glycoproteins like the Tamm-Horsfall protein and secretory IgA (50-52). When these substances coat uroepithelial cells, they may provide receptor epitopes for bacterial surface colonization;

when secreted they may eliminate type 1 fimbriated Escherichia coli strains and prevent colonization or infection. Furthermore, type 1 fimbriae play a complex role in the interaction with human polymorphonuclear leucocytes (PMNLs). The adhesion of type 1 fimbriated Escherichia coli strains to PMNLs may promote bacterial killing. It has been suggested that type 1 fimbriae play an important role in the pathogenesis of renal scars (53) and also contribute to infection of the bladder (54-56).

GENETICS AND STRUCTURE

P-fimbriae are encoded by the chromosomal gene cluster termed pap (pyelonephritis associated pili) (57-59). The designation sfso, fst, fei, fel are sometimes used for pap gene clusters isolated from Escherichia coli isolates of different F serotypes (60-62). The gene organization of the pap gene cluster cloned from Escherichia coli strains of different F serotype has been shown to be quite similar except for the regions which encode the major pilin subunits and the minor pilin proteins including the adhesin protein (62, 63).

The pap gene cluster from Escherichia coli J96 (F13) (57), consists of 11 genes pap A-papK. The papA gene encodes the major subunit, which forms the filamentous structure (64, 65). The minor adhesin related subunits encoded by papE, papF and papG form the adhesin complex located at the tip of the fimbriae (36, 66). PapG is the actual adhesin molecule responsible for the receptor binding. Five other proteins are important in P-fimbrial biogenesis. PapD is present in the periplasmic space and plays a role in the transport of the subunits papE and papG from the inner membrane to the outer membrane and seems to stabilize them during the translocation (67, 68). The exact role of papC is not known but it has been proposed to form a pore through which the pilus is assembled (68, 69). PapH terminates fimbrial assembly and helps in anchoring the fimbriae (70). The role of papJ and papK is less clear. The papJ gene product has been suggested to facilitate the assembly of papA subunits into the pilus structure (71) and the papK gene product has been suggested to be a pilin like protein located at the pilus tip (71). PapB and papI encode regulatory proteins involved in positive transregulation of papA transcription (72, 73).

The pap gene clusters form a family with a high degree of similarity except for the adhesin specific G adhesin and the pap A sequences (37, 74-76). Marklund and co-workers (75) compared nucleotide sequences of papG and prsG genes from 11 different human and dog Escherichia coli urinary isolates. They found that three classes of adhesins with approximately 70% sequence homology could be distinguished. Adhesin gene sequences within each class were highly conserved (>97%) (75). Probes specific for the G adhesin sequences have recently been developed.

The type 1 fimbriae are encoded by the pil gene cluster which was first cloned from Escherichia coli J96 (57, 77). The fim gene cluster, which was characterized by Klemm (78), was derived from Escherichia coli PC-31. The pil and fim genes show a high degree of homology (78). The organization of the fim gene resembles that of pap (79). fimH encodes the specific adhesin proteins (33, 34), which are located at the tip as well as along the fimbriae (80). The fimA encodes the fimbrial subunit protein and can be expressed independently from the fimH encoded adhesin protein (81). However, it is interesting that the fimA gene product has to be present on the cells to confer the adhesive phenotype. This is in contrast to what has been found for the P-fimbriae. The fimB and fimE encode the proteins involved in regulation of the transcription of the fim gene cluster (78).

The expression of fimbriae is subject to phase variation (27, 32, 82-85). Changes in temperature, glucose concentration and other experimental conditional may switch on or off the fimbriae.

Little is known about *in vivo* growth conditions and the extent of fimbrial expression. Pere et al (86) studied fimbriae on bacteria in urine without subculture, using immunofluorescence techniques. The P-fimbriae were found to be expressed, while type 1 occurred less frequently. Genotypic studies are therefore required to determine the potential of a given strain to express fimbriae under favorable *in vivo* conditions.

PATHOGENESIS OF ACUTE PYELONEPHRITIS

The large intestine as a reservoir for Escherichia coli infecting the urinary tract

The Escherichia coli clones which infect the urinary tract usually originate from the patients own fecal flora (87). At the onset of symptomatic UTI the same clone may be recovered from the urinary tract and the fecal flora (88-92).

Two theories have been used to describe the spread of Escherichia coli strains from the fecal reservoir to the urinary tract (88). The prevalence theory suggested that the dominating strain will cause UTI as a consequence of its statistically increased chance of spreading to the urinary tract. The special pathogenicity theory proposed that the uropathogenic bacteria possess virulence factors which make them able to cause UTI. These theories can now be reconciled since it has been shown that attachment promotes bacterial persistence in the large intestine and virulence in the urinary tract (93).

P-FIMBRIAE AND THE COLONIZATION OF THE LARGE INTESTINE

It has recently become apparent that P-fimbriae influence the colonization of the large intestine. Receptors for P-fimbriae are expressed on human colonic epithelial cells (94). P-fimbriated Escherichia coli were found to establish a resident population in the large intestine and persist longer than other Escherichia coli strains (93). These findings suggested that P-fimbriae have evolved to enhance the fitness of Escherichia coli for their natural site of colonization in the large intestine. The occurrence of similar receptors in the urinary tract may coincidentally enhance the virulence of the same strains for the urinary tract.

P-fimbriae also enhance the ability of Escherichia coli to spread from the large intestine to the urinary tract. This was recently demonstrated in infants and children with their first episodes of acute pyelonephritis and ABU (95). Intestinal, urethral and urine cultures were taken at the onset of infection. The frequency of P-fimbriated strains was analyzed using oligonucleotide probes specific for the $papG_{IA2}$ and $prsG_{J96}$ regions as well as for the entire pap gene cluster. A pap positive strain was recovered from the urinary tract of every child who carried such a strain in the large intestine. This was independent of their simultaneous carriage of pap negative strains. Pap negative strains occurred in the urinary tract only of children who were not colonized with pap negative strains; all had ABU.

The role of P-fimbriae for bacterial persistence in the urinary tract is less clear. The high frequency of pap positive Escherichia coli strains not only in acute pyelonephritis but also in ABU suggested that the pap encoded phenotype enhances the persistence. This was supported by animal studies (96, 44, 55, 56). On the other hand, P-fimbriae were rarely expressed by ABU strains once isolated from the urinary tract. The role of P-fimbriae for bacterial persistence in the urinary tract was recently tested *in vivo*. Patients were deliberately colonized with Escherichia coli lacking or possessing the pap_{J96} DNA sequences. Interestingly, the wild-type strain lacking P-fimbriae was found to persist, while the pap positive transformant was eliminated. This emphasizes how little we know about the bacterial determinants of growth and persistence in the urinary tract.

P-FIMBRIAE AND THE INDUCTION OF ACUTE PYELONEPHRITIS

P-fimbriae enhance the virulence of Escherichia coli for the urinary tract. This has been shown both indirectly and directly. First, attaching P-fimbriated and pap DNA positive Escherichia coli have been found to occur more frequently in patients with acute pyelonephritis than in other patient groups (97). This association has been demonstrated in children (98-103) as well as in adults (25). Second, patients infected with P-fimbriated Escherichia coli were found to have higher levels of fever, C-reactive protein (CRP), erythrocyte sedimentation rate (ESR), pyuria and lower renal concentrating capacity than those infected with other Escherichia coli strains, regardless of clinical diagnosis (25). Third, isolated P-fimbriae have been shown to trigger an inflammatory response in the host. Interleukin-6 and leucocytes were found in the urine of mice after intravesical inoculation of adhesin positive but not adhesin negative P-fimbriae. Similarly, epithelial cells were triggered by P-fimbriae to secrete cytokines (104, 105).

Although P-fimbriae are virulence factors in their own right, the virulence of an Escherichia coli clone for the urinary tract depends on the P-fimbriae and on the clonally associated traits. The relationship between P-fimbriae and the bacterial clonotype has been analyzed using probes specific for the pap gene cluster. As expected pap positive strains dominated in acute pyelonephritis, but in addition about 60 per cent of strains from asymptomatic carriers were pap positive (106). This apparent contradiction was partly resolved using the $papG_{IA2}$ and $prsG_{J96}$ probes which differentiated between two types of G adhesins. The pap positive strains in the pyelonephritis group carried the $papG_{IA2}$ sequences. These sequences occurred less frequently in the pap positive cystitis and ABU strains (101). Furthermore, the majority of $papG_{IA2}$ positive ABU strains belonged to clonotypes other than the $papG_{IA2}$ positive pyelonephritis strains.

The accumulation of Escherichia coli clones with the $papG_{IA2}$ adhesins in patients with acute pyelonephritis may reflect the ability of these P-fimbriae to trigger an inflammatory response in the urinary tract. In contrast, the inflamatogenicity of the $prsG_{J96}$ adhesin has not been investigated. The $prsG_{J96}$ positive strains occur mainly in patients with acute cystitis or ABU. This suggested that strains expressing the $prsG_{J96}$ encoded adhesins are less likely than the $papG_{IA2}$ positive strains to cause inflammation in the host.

These observations suggest the following roles for P-fimbriae in the pathogenesis of acute pyelonephritis.

Pap positive isolates colonize the large intestine and establish a dominating and resident population. The likelihood of this occurring is increased in individuals who are prone to UTI. The pap positive strains then spread to the urinary tract with greater success than pap negative isolates. Once established the bacteriuria may cause a variety of host responses depending on the type of papG adhesin and the clonally associated traits. The $papG_{IA2}$ adhesin will trigger an inflammatory response, which explains the association of this genotype with disease. The papG$_{IA2}$ sequences will only be maintained in clones which resist the host response and consequently survive the acquisition of these sequences. The prsG adhesin will be less inflammatogenic which explains the lack of association with disease. The prs sequences can therefore be carried by a wide array of clones, also those which are not resistant to host defenses. Both the intestinal carriage and the urinary tract colonization will depend on adequate receptor expression by the host.

HOST FACTORS IN ACUTE PYELONEPHRITIS

The inflammatory response to infection

The host response during UTI has two different consequences. First, it determines the symptoms and signs of infection. The intensity of the host response is a direct measure of the severity of infection. Second, the host response influences the resistance to UTI. Recurrent episodes of acute pyelonephritis and ABU occur in a subset of the population, who are defective in the antibacterial defenses which determine the resistance to UTI; maybe in their inflammatory response to infection.

INDUCTION OF THE ACUTE INFLAMMATORY RESPONSE

Acute pyelonephritis is characterized by an inflammatory response to the infecting Escherichia coli strain. The local inflammation is apparent from the pyuria and excretion into the urine of kidney proteins, from the loin pain which is thought to be due to the renal edema, and from the reduction in distal tubular function as shown by reduced renal concentrating capacity. The systemic inflammatory response is characterized by fever, elevated CRP and ESR levels and is followed by the induction of specific immunity. Recently some mechanisms of this response have been identified (107). Acute pyelonephritis is accompanied by cytokine production; both locally and systemically (108, 109).

The term cytokine describes a diverse group of hormone-like proteins which are involved in the communication between cells. It includes interleukins, interferons, colony stimulating factors and tumor necrosis factor (TNF). The name interleukin (IL) was chosen since it was thought that these molecules were produced by leucocytes and mainly functioned in the generation of the immune response. It has, however, also become well established that the cytokines are major effector molecules in the inflammatory response.

IL-1, IL-6 and TNF participate in the generation of fever and acute phase responses. IL-8 is mainly a chemotactic peptide and a granulocyte activating factor.

Bacterial products stimulate cytokine production. Molecules like endotoxin can activate many different cell types to produce cytokines. Indeed, many of the clinical signs of Gram-negative septicemia may be prevented by compounds which inhibit the activity of TNF and IL-1. Septicemia is, however, a rare event even in acute pyelonephritis. In most patients, the bacteria remain localized to the urinary tract. Many of the cell types which can respond to endotoxin *in vitro* are rarely exposed to microbial products. We have therefore examined the local cytokine production in the urinary tract, and the ability of epithelial cells to produce cytokines in response to bacterial stimulation.

CYTOKINE PRODUCTION IN VIVO

The cytokine response to urinary tract infection *in vivo* has been studied in experimentally infected mice, deliberately colonized humans and patients with urinary tract infection. In mice, an IL-6 response occurred within minutes of intravesical instillation of Escherichia coli bacteria and isolated P-fimbriae (104, 108, 109). The mucosal and systemic responses appeared to be segregated. For example, the elevation in circulating IL-6 levels which resulted after intraperitoneal infection was not accompanied by the excretion of IL-6 into the urine. The instillation of bacteria into urinary tract gave rise to a urinary IL-6 response which preceded the subsequent rise in systemic IL-6 levels.

Evidence for a mucosal IL-6 response was obtained after deliberate colonization of the human urinary tract with Escherichia coli (108). The urinary IL-6 levels increased within the first hour after bacterial colonization. None of the patients had elevated circulating IL-6 levels, and none of them developed symptoms or elevated levels of circulating acute phase reactants like CRP.

Patients with natural episodes of Escherichia coli bacteriuria were also found to secrete IL-6 into the urine (109). Indeed, elevated IL-6 levels were found in most individuals with bacteriuria, regardless of the type of bacteria which caused the infection. Elevated circulating IL-6 levels were mainly seen in patients with acute pyelonephritis. In a subsequent study of children with urinary tract infection, the IL-6 levels were shown to be higher in children who were infected with P-fimbriated Escherichia coli than in those infected with P-fimbriae negative Escherichia coli (Benson et al, in preparation). These results demonstrated that IL-6 secretion is activated during mucosal infections. Possibly, the P-fimbriae enhance the spread of IL-6 from local to systemic sites. This could explain why patients infected with P-fimbriae positive Escherichia coli had higher levels of the IL-6 related responses such as fever and CRP than patients infected with other Escherichia coli strains.

EPITHELIAL CELLS PRODUCE CYTOKINES

The naive mucosal surfaces are dominated by epithelial cells and their products. The influx of inflammatory cells such as granulocytes during acute infection occurs after the cytokine response (110). We tested the hypothesis that epithelial cells might be a primary source of cytokine production (105). Human epithelial cell lines were used; A498 from human kidney, J82 from human urinary bladder, Caco2 and HT29 from the large intestine. Cytokine production was investigated by three methods: [1] the secreted cytokines were detected by bioassays or immunoassays; [2] the cellular content of individual cytokines was studied by immuno-fluorescence using monoclonal antibodies to the respective cytokines; [3] the RNA specific for the different cytokines was detected by PCR. The epithelial cells were cultured to confluency, and exposed to bacteria, bacterial components, or cytokines. The results may be summarized as follows.

The kidney and bladder epithelial cell lines constitutively produced cytokines. They were stimulated by Escherichia coli to increase their cytokine production above constitutive levels. Bacteria which attached to the kidney celline stimulated cells to produce more IL-6 than bacteria which did not adhere to the cells. This difference was not seen for the bladder epithelial celline which responded to all bacteria tested (105).

We subsequently tested ability of isolated fimbriae to trigger the cytokine response. Kidney epithelial cells were incubated with P-fimbriae prepared so as to either retain or have lost the receptor binding site. The adherence positive P-fimbriae triggered an IL-6 response; the adhesin negative fimbriae did not. To examine if the activation was due to endotoxin associated with the fimbrial proteins the endotoxin activity of the adhesin positive fimbriae was titrated using the limulus lysate assay. Purified lipid A with the corresponding activity was added to the cells. The IL-6 response to the fimbriae lps complex was significantly higher than the response lipid-A alone. This demonstrated that the epithelial cells produced cytokines, that they responded to bacterial stimulation, and that adherence influenced the response.

We further investigated the spectrum of cytokines produced in response to the bacterial stimulation (Agace et al, submitted for publication). Monoclonal antibodies to IL-1α, IL-1β, TNFα, TNFβ, IL-6, IL-8 and GMCSF were used for immunofluorescence staining. The epithelial cells were found to produce IL-1α, IL-6 and IL-8 but no TNF or

IL-1β. For comparison, human peripheral blood monocytes were exposed to Escherichia coli bacteria, and the spectrum of cytokine production was investigated by the same techniques. The monocytes responded with IL-1α, IL-6 and IL-8 production but also with IL-1β, and TNF production. These results suggested that the repertoir of cytokines produced by epithelial cells in response to bacterial stimulation is limited compared to that of monocytes. This may be of importance to maintain the integrity of the mucosal surfaces and protect other tissues.

Most cells with the ability to produce cytokines have also been shown to respond to stimulation by cytokines. We tested the ability of IL-1 and TNF to elicit a cytokine response in the epithelial cells. PCR was used to examine the induction of cytokine mRNA. The cells demonstrated the ability to produce a wide range of cytokines after IL-1α or TNFα stimulation (Hedges et al, in preparation). This may be essential for the chronic inflammatory processes which may follow after the acute pyelonephritis episodes.

Inflammation as a mechanism of bacterial clearance from the urinary tract

The resistance of the urinary tract to infection has been ascribed specific immunity, especially secretory IgA (111). More recently, however, the role of inflammation has come into focus. This followed when natural resistance to UTI was shown not to be impaired by immunodeficiency. In humans, acute pyelonephritis is not mainly a problem in patients with defects in the humoral immuneresponse (hypogamma-globulinemia). Mice with defects in cellular immuneresponses (nude or xid) or with severe combined immunodeficiencies were shown to clear infection as efficiently as their immunocompetent littermates (112).

The natural resistance to UTI was, however, impaired in lps non responder mice of the C3H and C57Bl backgrounds. The lps gene cluster is located on chromosome four in the mouse. The gene products are, however, not known. The C3H/HeJ and C57Bl/10/ScCr mice are designated as lps^d, lps^d based on their inability to respond to the lipid A moiety of endotoxin. The increased susceptibility to infection of the lps^d mice is accompanied by a defective inflammatory response; both the cytokine secretion and the granulocyte recruitment are impaired. The importance of the inflammatory response for resistance to UTI is further shown by the impairment of clearance which occurs in lps^n mice following treatment with anti-inflammatory agents (104, 110, 112). These findings emphasize the importance of inflammation for the resistance to UTI. They do, however, not negate a role for specific immunity as an induced host factor. This discussion is beyond the scope of this review.

Receptors for bacterial adhesins

The ability of a P-fimbriated strain to attach and colonize depends on the receptors offered by the host. Receptors for the P-fimbriae are expressed on epithelial cells both in the large intestine and in the urinary tract. Receptor epitopes for the papG_{IA2} adhesin class are provided by most of the members of the globo-series of glycolipids, including those with an internal rather than a terminal Galα1-4Galβ (41). They occur on uroepithelial cells and erythrocytes of most individuals, except those of blood group p. The globo-series of glycolipids are expressed on uroepithelial cells of all individuals except those of blood group P. This P blood group dependence might have been used to determine the role of receptor expression for the susceptibility to infection with P-fimbriated Escherichia coli. The frequency of p individuals is, however, too low for such an approach.

The receptor expression in the large intestine can therefore influence the tendency to carry uropathogenic Escherichia coli strains. The carrier frequency was recently compared between healthy children, and children from the same population who developed acute pyelonephritis or ABU (113). The fecal carriage of pap/prs positive Escherichia coli was significantly higher both in children with acute pyelonephritis and ABU than in the controls (95). This suggested that the proneness to develop UTI may be due to the tendency to become colonized by pap/prs positive Escherichia coli in the large intestine. Furthermore, the frequency of P1 individuals was significantly higher among infants carrying pap/prs positive Escherichia coli in the large intestine, than among those carrying pap/prs negative Escherichia coli isolates. It is tempting to assume that the difference in intestinal carriage relates to the adherence of P-fimbriae to the colonic epithelial cells and the receptor expression of the host. This remains to be demonstrated. The information on P blood group and intestinal glycolipid expression is limited. Receptors for P-fimbriae are known to occur on human colonic epithelial cells both when cultured *in vitro* and when derived from surgical specimens (94). The derivatization of the globo-series of glycolipids with ABH determinants at other mucosal sites is known to be influenced by ABH blood group and secretor state, but the variation of intestinal receptors with host blood group is not known. The findings of the present study may clarify a previous observation related to P blood group and UTI. P1 individuals have an increased tendency to attract recurrent pyelonephritis when infected with P-fimbriated Escherichia coli strains compared to P2 individuals (114). This difference may reflect the receptor expression in the large intestine and the tendency to become colonized with P-fimbriated strains.

The expression by epithelial cells of the globo-series of glycolipids is, however, also dependent on ABH blood group and secretor state (115). Secretor individuals elongate the oligosaccharides on the globo-series of glycolipids with the A or B blood group determinants depending on blood group. P1A1 secretor individuals therefore express the globo-A glycolipid, whereas non-secretors, B or O individuals do not. Globo-A is the receptor for the prsG encoded adhesins. Consequently, it was possible to analyze the blood group dependency in patients with UTI. The blood group A frequency was 100% among individuals infected with prs only strains, compared to 43% in the population at large (116). These observations indicated that bacteria infect hosts with appropriate receptor expression, and suggested that adherence is required also for bacterial persistence in the urinary tract. The most abundant type of P-fimbriae, encoded by the $papG_{IA2}$ sequences, bind to receptors present on most uroepithelial cells, which would not be expected to vary between hosts.

MECHANISM OF RENAL SCARRING

Renal scarring is seen in 13% of boys and 4.5% of girls with urinary tract infection (117, 118). There are several theories about the etiology of renal scarring as seen in association with urinary tract infection:

[a] the inflammatory response, especially the polymorphonuclear leucocytes, destroys the tissue by the release of oxygen radicals (119);

[b] changes in renal tissue antigenicity, induced by endotoxin or Escherichia coli antigens, triggers autoimmune processes leading to renal scarring (120, 121);

[c] high pressure sterile reflux has been proposed to cause renal scarring in experimental studies (122);

[d] the combination of reflux and infection induces renal scarring in the majority of cases (123). Children who develop renal scars frequently have infection in combination with reflux (124). Indeed new scar formation in children with reflux occurred only in the presence of infection (125).

Bacterial adherence and renal scarring

Acute pyelonephritis is thought to be a prerequisite for the development of renal scarring.

It was therefore expected that the most virulent bacteria, which caused the most severe acute pyelonephritis episodes, would cause the scars. Since bacterial adherence is a characteristic of the pyelonephritogenic clones, it was expected that bacterial attachment would be an important factor in the pathogenesis of renal scarring (126, 127) and that the patients with acute pyelonephritis due to adhering bacteria were at risk.

The studies of Lomberg et al (118, 128), in girls with recurrent pyelonephritis, showed the opposite. Bacteria isolated from the patients, who later were shown to developed renal scarring frequently, lacked the capacity to attach to the globo-series of glycolipids (128). Those strains also lacked the other characteristics of the pyelonephritogenic Escherichia coli clones (118).

The association between P-fimbriae and renal scarring was analyzed in 197 boys with first time urinary tract infection (129). The results revealed that boys who developed pyelonephritis with P-fimbriae negative bacteria often had renal abnormalities (41% renal scarring, 11% other renal abnormalities). Boys with pyelonephritis caused by P-fimbriated Escherichia coli ran only a 5% risk of renal scarring. The relative risk for renal abnormalities was 8.3 times higher for the boys with pyelonephritis and P-fimbriae negative bacteria, as compared to boys with pyelonephritis and P-fimbriated Escherichia coli .

Influence of vesicoureteric reflux

Vesicoureteric reflux is a major risk factor in renal scarring.

Lomberg et al (130) proposed that the low frequency of adhering strains in patients with renal scars was due to the reflux, which permitted non-attaching bacteria to be transported to the kidneys.

Boys with P-fimbriae negative pyelonephritis had reflux ≥ grade II in 55% while patients with pyelonephritis and P-fimbriated Escherichia coli had reflux > grade I in only 25% ($p < 0.001$).

Reflux did not solely explain the association between P-fimbriae negative Escherichia coli infections and renal abnormalities.

The frequency of renal abnormalities was 2% in patients without reflux who were infected with P-fimbriated Escherichia coli, 9% in patients without reflux who were infected with P-fimbriae negative bacteria, 21% in patients with reflux and P-fimbriated Escherichia coli, and 79% in patients with reflux and P-fimbriae negative bacteria. The risk for this last group was thus 39 times higher than that for non reflux patients infected with P-fimbriated Escherichia coli.

Strength of acute inflammation and renal abnormalities

Since the acute inflammatory response during acute pyelonephritis was thought to determine the renal scarring, we compared the strength of the acute inflammatory response between acute pyelonephritis episodes in patients with and without scarring. Below 2 months of age, patients with renal abnormalities had significantly lower body temperature and CRP levels. There were no significant differences in these responses in the older patients with or without renal scars.

It therefore appeared that the high acute inflammatory response induced by P-fimbriated Escherichia coli did not lead to renal scarring. These observations in the boys and the previously noted higher incidence of P-fimbriated Escherichia coli in girls with recurrent pyelonephritis without renal scarring, as compared to girls with renal scarring suggested that acute pyelonephritis and renal scarring are determined by different processes (118, 130).

SUMMARY

Renal scarring occurs in a subset of children with acute pyelonephritis. By definition these children have increased susceptibility to infection. With the exception of vesicoureteric reflux, the determinants of this susceptibility are poorly understood. What can be said about the bacterial determinants of renal scarring?

[1] The increased host susceptibility may be such that any organism entering the urinary tract can cause pyelonephritis. The rare occurrence of virulent bacteria could then be a statistical effect, secondary to how often they occur in the introital area of these patients. In patients resistant to infection, selection against the non-virulent bacteria would result in a higher frequency of attaching and virulent strains.

[2] The strains inducing renal scarring may carry as yet undefined determinants which increase their ability to cause tissue damage. The MS adhesins have been suggested as one such mechanism (127). At present, we have no markers which suggest that the clonotype or pap genotype are special among the scarring compared to the non-scarring strains (130).

[3] Common to the more or less virulent clones of Escherichia coli is the content of endotoxin and outer membrane proteins with an inflammatogenic/immunogenic potential (131). In the absence of bacterial adhesins, and in the presence of reflux, bacteria may be flushed into the kidney and deliver toxins to the tissues.

[4] The natural history of pyelonephritis is changed by treatment. In the absence of treatment scars might have developed also after infection with P-fimbriae positive bacteria. Now, the development of scars probably is a function of the time between onset of infection and treatment. This may, in turn, be determined by the intensity of the symptoms. Infections with bacteria of low virulence in a susceptible host may give rise to atypical clinical states, and delayed onset of treatment. The importance of early antibiotic treatment to reduce development of renal scarring is well documented both from experimental studies (123) and from the clinic (125, 126). Asymptomatic infections of the upper urinary tract have been suggested to occur with a high frequency (131).

REFERENCES

1. Kunin CM: Detection prevention and management of urinary tract infections. Philadelphia, Lea and Febiger, 1987.
2. Cooke EM: Escherichia coli: distribution in nature, epidemiology. In "Escherichia coli and man" (Ed EM Cooke), Churchill Livingstone, Edinburgh, UK, 1974, pp 13-30.
3. Smith T: Studies on pathogenic B. coli from bovine sources. J Exp Med, 46: 141-153, 1927.
4. Uhlenhuth P: Pathogenität des Bacterium coli. Zentralblatt Hyg und Microbiol, 26: 476-484, 1897.
5. Kauffman F: The serology of the the coli group. J Immun, 57: 71-100, 1947.
6. Kauffmann F: Zur serologie der coli-gruppe. Acta Path Microbiol Scand, 21: 20-45, 1944.
7. Orskov I, Orskov F, Jann B, Jann K: Serology, chemistry and genetics of O and K antigens of Escherichia coli. Bacteriol Rev, 41: 667-710, 1977.
8. Sjöstedt S: Pathogenicity of certain serological types of E. coli. Their mouse toxicity, hemolytic power, capacity for skin necrosis and resistance to phagocytosis and bactericidal faculties of human blood. Acta Path Microbiol Scand, 63 (Suppl): 1-148, 1946.
9. Vahlne G: Serological typing of the colon bacteria. Acta Path Microbiol Scand, 62 (Suppl): 1-127, 1945.
10. Orskov F, Orskov I: Summary of a workshop on the clone concept in the epidemiology, taxonomy and evolution of the Enterobacteriaceae and other bacteria. J Inf Dis, 148: 346-357, 1983.
11. Achtman M, Mercer A, Kusecek B, Pohl A, Heuzenroeder M, Aaronson W, Sutton A, Silver RP: Six widespread clones among Escherichia coli K1 isolates. Infect Immun, 39: 315-335, 1983.
12. Caugant DA, Levin BR, Orskov I, Orskov F, Svanborg-Edén S, Selander RK: Genetic diversity in relation to serotype in Escherichia coli. Infect Immun, 49: 407-413, 1985.
13. Selander RK, Levin BR: Genetic diversity and structure in populations of Escherichia coli. Science, 210: 545-547, 1980.
14. Plos K, Levin BR, Hull R, Hull S, Orskov I, Orskov F, Svanborg-Edén C: The distribution of the pyelonephritis-associated pili (pap) region among E. coli isolates. Evidence for horizontal gene transfer. Infect Immun, 57: 1604-1611, 1989.
15. Väisänen-Rhen V, Elo J, Väisänen E, Siitonen A, Orskov I, Orskov F, Svenson SB, Mäkelä PH, Korhonen TK: P-fimbriated clones among uropathogenic Escherichia coli strains. Infect Immun, 43 (1): 149-155, 1984.
16. Maynard- Smith J, Dowson CG, Sprath BG: Localized sex in bacteria. Nature, 349: 29-31, 1991.
17. Whittham TS, Ochman H, Selander RK: Multilocus genetic structure in natural populations of Escherichia coli. Proc Natl Acad Sci USA, 80: 1751-1755, 1983.
18. Caugant DA, Levin BR, Lidin Janson G, Whittam TS, Svanborg-Edén C, Selander RK: Genetic diversity and relationships among strains of Escherichia coli in the intestine and those causing urinary tract infections. Prog Allergy, 33 (203): 203-27, 1983a. **a?**
19. Caugant DA, Levin BR, Selander RK: Genetic diversity and temporal variation in the E. coli population of a human host. Genetics, 98: 467-90, 1981.

20. Levin BR, Svanborg C: Selection and evolution of virulence in bacteria: an ecumenical excursion and modest suggestion. Parasitology, 100: 103-115, 1990.
21. Svanborg-Edén C, Hull S, Leffler H, Norgren S, Plos K, Wold A: The large intestine as a reservoir for Escherichia coli causing extra-intestinal infections. In: "The regulatory and protective role of the normal microflora" (Eds Grubb R, Mitvedt T, Norin E), 1989, pp 47-58. **Publisher?**
22. Mabeck CE, Orskov F, Orskov I: Escherichia coli serotypes and renal involvement in urinary tract infection. Lancet, I: 1312-1314, 1971**?a?**
23. Mabeck CE, Orskov F, Orskov I: Studies in urinary tract infections. 8. Escherichia coli O:H serotypes in recurrent infections. Acta Med Scand 190: 279-282, 1971**b.?**
24. Lindberg U, Hanson LÅ, Jodal U, Lidin Janson G, Lincoln K, Olling S: Asymptomatic bacteriuria in schoolgirls. II. Differences in Escherichia coli causing asymptomatic bacteriuria. Acta Paediatr Scand 64: 432-436, 1975**b?**.
25. Svanborg-Edén C, de Man P: Bacterial virulence in urinary tract infection. Infect Dis Clin North Am, 1: 731-750, 1987.
26. Duguid JP, Smith IW, Dempster G, Edmunds PN: Non-flaggelar filamentous appendages ("fimbriae") and haemagglutinating activity in Bacterium coli. J Pathol Bacteriol, 70: 335-348, 1955.
27. Brinton CC: The structure, function, synthesis and and genetic control of bacterial pili and a molecular model for DNA and RNA transport in gram negative bacteria. Trans NY Acad Sci, 27: 1003-1054, 1965.
28. Ottow JG: Ecology, physiology and genetics of fimbriae and pili. Annu Rew Microbiol, 29: 79-108, 1975.
29. Orskov I, Orskov F: Serologic classification of fimbriae. Curr Top Microbiol Immun, 151: 71-90, 1990.
30 Svanborg-Edén C, Hansson S, Jodal U, Lidin-Janson G, Lincoln K, Linder H, de Man P, Mårild S, Martinell J, Plos K, Sandberg T, Stenqvist K: Host parasite interaction in the urinary tract. J Infect Dis, 157: 421-426, 1988.
31. Duguid JP, Old DC: Adhesive properties of Enterobacteriaceae. In bacterial adherence, receptors and recognition. (Ed EH Beachey), Chapman and Hall, London, 1980, pp 185-217.
32. Klemm P: Fimbrial adhesins. Rev Infect Dis, 7: 321-340, 1985.
33. Hanson MS, Brinton Cc Jr: Identification and characterization of E. coli type-1 pilus tip adhesion protein. Nature, 332: 265-258, 1988.
34. Hanson MS, Hempel J, Brinton Cc Jr: Purification of the Escherichia coli type 1 pilin and minor pilus proteins and partial characterization of the adhesin protein. J Bacteriol, 170: 3350-3358, 1988.
35 Jann K et al: Isolation and characterization of the a-sialyl-b-2,3 galactosyl- specific adhesin from fimbriated Escherichia coli . PNAS, 84: 3462-3466, 1987.
36. Lund, B, F Lindberg, B-I Marklund, and S Normark: The papG protein is the a-D-galactopyranosyl-(1-4)-b-D-galactopyranose-binding adhesin of uropathogenic Escherichia coli. PNAS, 84: 5898-5902, 1987.
37. Lund B, Lindberg F, Normark S: Structure and antigenic properties of the tip-located P pilus proteins of uropathogenic Escherichia coli. J Bacteriol, 170: 1887-1894, 1988.
38. Hanson M S, Brinton Cc Jr: Identification and characterization of E. coli type-1 pilus tip adhesion protein. Nature, 332: 265-268, 1988.
39. Hacker J: Genetic determinants coding for fimbriae and adhesins of extraintestinal Escherichia coli. Curr Top Microbiol Immun 151: 1-27, 1990.
40. Johnson James R: Virulence factors in Escherichia coli urinary tract infection. Clin Microbial Rev, 4: 80-128, 1991.
41. Leffler H, Svanborg-Edén C: Chemical identification of a glycosphingolipid receptor for Escherichia coli attaching to human urinary tract epithelia cells and agglutinating human erythrocytes. FEMS Microbiol Lett, 8: 127-134, 1980.
42. Källenius G, Möllby R, Svensson SB, Cedergren B: The P^k antigen as receptors for the hemagglutination of pyelonephritic Escherichia coli. FEMS Microbiol Lett, 7: 297-302, 1980.
43. Korhonen T K, Parkkinen J, Hacker J, Finne J, Pere A, Rhen M, Holthofer H: Binding of Escherichia coli S fimbriae to human kidney epithelium. Infect Immun, 54:322-327, 1986.
44. Marre R, Hacker J: Role of S- and common type-1 fimbriae of Escherichia coli in experimental upper and lower urinary tract infection. Microbiol Pat, 2: 223-226, 1987.

45. Parkkinen J, Ristimäki A, Westerlund B: Binding of Escherichia coli S fimbriae to cultured human endothelial cells. Infect Immun, 57: 2256-2259, 1989.
46. Duguid JP, Gillies RR: Fimbriae and adhesive properties in dysenteric bacilli. J Pathol Bacteriol, 74: 397-411, 1957.
47. Ofek I, Mirelman D, Sharon N: Adherence of Escherichia coli to human mucosal cells mediated by mannose receptors. Nature, 265: 623-625, 1977.
48 Duguid JP, Clegg S, Wilson MI: The fimbrial and non fimbrial haemagglutinins of Escherichia coli. J Med Microbiol, 12: 213-227, 1979.
49. Orskov I, Orskov F: Escherichia coli in extraintestinal infections. J Hyg, 95: 551-575, 1985.
50. Orskov F, Orskov I, Jann B, Jann K: Tamm-Horsfall protein or uromucoid is the normal urinary slime that traps type 1 fimbriated Escherichia coli. Lancet, I: 8173, 1980 (Letter).
51. Parkkinen J, Virkola R, Korhonen TK: Identification of factors in human urine that inhibit the binding of Escherichia coli adhesins. Infect Immun, 56: 2623-2630, 1988.
52. Wold AE, Mestecky J, Svanborg Eden C: Agglutination of E. coli by secretory IgA a result of interaction between bacterial mannose-specific adhesins and immunoglobulin carbohydrate. Monogr Allergy, 24: 307-309,1988.
53. Topley N, Steadman R, Mackenzie R, Knowlden JM, Williams JD: Type 1 fimbriated strains from Escherichia coli initiate renal parenchymal scarring. Kidney Int, 36: 609-616, 1989.
54. Hagberg L, Jodal U, Korhonen TK, Lidin-Janson G, Lindberg U, Svanborg-Edén C: Adhesion, hemagglutination, and virulence of Escherichia coli causing urinary tract infections. Infect Immun 31: 564-570, 1981.
55. Marre R, Hacker J, Henkel W, Goebel W: Contribution of cloned virulence factors from uropathogenic Escherichia coli strains to nephropathogenicity in an experimental rat pyelonephritis model. Infect Immun, 54: 761-767, 1986.
56. O'Hanley P, Lark D, Falkow S, Schoolnik G: Molecular basis of Escherichia coli colonization of the upper urinary tract in BALB/c mice. Gal-Gal pili immunization prevents Escherichia coli pyelonephritis in the BALB/c mouse model of human pyelonephritis. J Clin Invest, 75: 347-360, 1985.
57. Hull RA, Gill RE, Hsu P, Minshew BH, Falkow S: Construction and expression of recombinant plasmids encoding type 1 or D- mannose resistant pili from the urinary tract infection Escherichia coli isolate. Infect Immun, 33: 933-938, 1981.
58. Clegg S: Cloning of genes determining the production of mannose-resistant fimbriae in a uropathogenic strain of Escherichia coli belonging to serogroup O6. Infect Immun, 38: 739-744, 1982.
59. Rhen M, Klemm P, Korhonen TK: Identification of two new hemagglutinins of Escherichia coli, N-acetyl-D-glucosamine-specific fimbriae and a blood group M specific agglutinin by cloning the corresponding genes in Escherichia coli K-12. J Bacteriol, 168: 1234-1242, 1986.
60. Hacker J, Ott M, Schmith G, Hull R, Goebel W: Molecular cloning of the F8 fimbrial antigen from Escherichia coli. FEMS Microbiol Lett, 36: 139-144, 1986.
61. van Die I, Bergmans H: Nucleotide sequence of the gene encoding the F72 fimbrial subunit of a uropathogenic Escherichia coli strain. Gene, 32: 83-90, 1984.
62. van Die I, Spierings G, van Megen I, Zuidweg E, Hoekstra W, Bergmans H: Cloning and genetic organization of the gene cluster encoding F7 fimbriae of a uropathogenic Escherichia coli and comparison with the $F7_2$ gene cluster. FEMS Microbiol Lett 28: 329-334, 1985.
63. Lund B, Lindberg FP, Båga M, Normark S: Globoside-specific adhesins of uropathogenic Escherichia coli are encoded by similar trans-complementable gene clusters. J Bacteriol, 162: 1293-1301, 1985.
64. Båga M, Normark S, Hardy J, O'Hanley P, Lark D, Olsson O, Schoolnik G, Falkow S: Nucleotide sequence of the papA gene encoding the pap pilus subunit of human uropathogenic Escherichia coli. J Bacteriol, 157: 330-333, 1984.
65. Lindberg FP, Lund B, Normark S: Genes of pyelonephrithogenic Escherichia coli required for digalactoside specific agglutination of human cells. EMBO J, 3: 1167-1173, 1984.
66. Lindberg F, Lund B, Johansson L, Normark S: Localization of the receptor-binding protein adhesin at the tip of the bacterial pilus. Nature, 328: 84-87, 1987.
67. Hultgren SJ, Porter TN, Schaeffer AJ, Duncan JL: Role of Type 1 pili and effects of phase variation on lower urinary tract infections produced by Escherichia coli. Infect Immun, 50: 370-377, 1985.

68. Lindberg F, Tennent JM, Hultgren SJ, Lund B, Normark S: PapD, a periplasmic transport protein in P-pilus biogenesis. J Bacteriol, 171: 6052-6058, 1989.
69 Norgren M, Båga M, Tennent JM, Normark S: Nucleotide sequence, regulation and functional analysis of the pap C gene required for cell surface localization of Pap pili of uropathogenic Escherichia coli. Mol Microbiol, 1: 169-178, 1987.
70 Båga M, Norgren M, Normark S: Biogenesis of E. coli Pap pili: pap H a minor pilin subunit involved in cell anchoring and length modulation. Cell, 49: 197-206, 1987.
71. Tennent JM, Lindberg F, Normark S: Integrity of Escherichia coli P pili during biogenesis: properties and role of pap J. Mol Microbiol, 4: 747-758, 1990.
72. Tennent JM, Hultgren S, Marklund B-I, Forssman K, Göransson M, Uhlin B-E, Normark S: In Molecular basis of bacterial pathogenesis (Eds BH Iglewski, VL Clark), Academic Press Inc, San Diego, 1990, pp 79-110.
73. Ekbäck C, Mörner S, Lund B, Normark S: Correlation of genes in the pap gene cluster to expression of globoside-specific adhesin by uropathogenic Escherichia coli. FEMS Microbiol Lett, 34: 355-360, 1986.
74. Karr JF, Nowicki B, Truong LD, Hull RA, Hull SI: Purified P-fimbriae from two cloned gene clusters of a single pyelonephritogenic strain adhere to unique structures in the human kidney. Infect Immun, 57: 3594-3600, 1989.
75. Marklund B-I: Structural and functional variation among Gala1-4Gal adhesins of Escherichia coli. Thesis, University of Umeå, Sweden, 1991.
76. Marklund BI, Tennent JM, Garcia E, Hamers A, Båga M, Lindberg F, Gaastra W, Normark S: Horizontal gene transfer of the E. coli pap and prs operons as mechanism for the development of tissue specific adhesive properties (In manuscript).
77. Orndoff PE, Falkow S: Organization and expression of genes responsible for type 1 piliation in Escherichia coli. J Bacteriol, 159: 736-744, 1984.
78. Klemm P: Two regulatory fim genes, fim B and fim E, control the phase variation of type 1 fimbriae in Escherichia coli. EMBO J, 5: 1389-1393, 1986.
79. Klemm P, Christiansen G: Three fim genes required for the regulation of length and mediation of adhesion of Escherichia coli type 1 fimbriae. MGG, 208: 439-445, 1987.
80. Krogfeld KA, Klemm P: Investigation of minor components of Escherichia coli type 1 fimbriae: protein chemical and immunological aspects. Microb Pathogen, 4: 231-238, 1988.
81 Minion FC, Abraham SN, Beachy EH, Goguen JD: The genetic determinant of adhesive function in type 1 fimbriae of Escherichia coli distinct from the gene encoding the fimbrial subunit. J Bacteriol, 165: 1033-1036, 1986.
82. Eisenstein BI: Phase variation of type 1 fimbriae in Escherichia coli is under transcriptional control. Science, 214: 337-338, 1981.
83. Nowicki B, Vuopio Varkila J, Viljanen P, Korhonen TK, Mäkelä PH: Fimbrial phase variation and systemic E. coli infection studied in the mouse peritonitis model. Microb Pathog 1: 335-347, 1986.
84. Rhen M, Mäkelä Ph, Korhonen TK: P-fimbriae of Escherichia coli are subject to phase variation. FEMS Microbiol Lett, 19: 267-271, 1983.
85. Uhlin B-E, Norgren M, Båga M, Normark S: Adhesin to human cells by Escherichia coli lacking the major subunit of a digalactoside-specific pilus-adhesin. Proc Natl Acad Sci, 82: 1800-1804, 1985.
86. Pere A, Nowicki B, Saxén H, Sittonen A, Korhonen TK: Expression of P, type1 and type1C fimbriae of Escherichia coli in the urine of patients with acute urinary tract infection. J Infect Dis, 156: 567-574, 1987.
87. Turck M, Petersdorf RG, Fournier MR: The epidemiology of non-enteric Escherichia coli infections: prevalence of serologic groups. J Clin Invest, 41: 1760-1765, 1962.
88. Gruneberg RN: Relationship of infecting urinary organisms to the faecal flora in patients with symptomatic urinary infections. Lancet, II: 766-768, 1969.
89. Vosti KL, Goldberg LM, Monto AS, Rantz LA: Host parasite interaction in patients with infection due to Escherichia coli. J Clin Invest, 43: 2377, 1964.
90. Lidin-Janson G, Lindberg U: Asymptomatic bacteriuria in schoolgirls. VI. The correlation between urinary and faecal Escherichia coli. Relation to the duration of the bacteriuria and the sampling technique. Acta Paediatr Scand, 66: 349-354, 1977.

91. Lidin-Janson G, Kaijser B, Lincoln K, Olling S, Wedel H: The homogeneity of the fecal coliform flora of normal schoolgirls, characterized by serological and biochemical properties. Med Microbiol Immunol, 164: 247-253, 1978.
92. Lidin-Janson G, Hanson LÅ, Kaijser B, Lincoln K, Lindberg U, Olling S, Wedel H: Comparison of Escherichia coli from bacteriuric patients with those from feces of healthy schoolchildren. J Infect Dis, 136: 346-353, 1977.
93. Wold AE, Caugant DA, Lidin-Janson G, de Man P, Svanborg C: Resident colonic Escherichia. coli strains frequently display uropathogenic characteristics. J Infect Dis, 165: 46-52, 1992.
94. Wold AE, Thorsse'n M, Hull S, Svanborg C: Attachment of Escherichia coli via mannose of Gala1-4Galb containing receptors to human colonic epithelial cells. Infect Immun, 56: 2531-2537, 1988.
95. Plos K, Jodal U, Marklund B-I, Mårild S, Wettergren B, Svanborg C: Intestinal carriage of pap/prs positive strains in infants with and without urinary tract infection. (Submitted for publication).
96. Hagberg L, Hull R, Hull S, Falkow S, Freter R, Svanborg-Edén C: Contribution of adhesion to bacterial persistence in the mouse urinary tract. Infect Immun, 40: 265-272, 1983.
97. Svanborg-Edén C, Hansson LÅ, Jodal U, Lindberg U, Sohl-Åkerlund A: Variable adherence to normal urinary tract epithelial cells of Escherichia coli strains associated with various forms of urinary tract infections. Lancet, II: 490-492, 1976.
98. Svanborg-Edén C, Eriksson B, Hanson LÅ, Jodal U, Kaijser B, Lidin-Janson G, Lindberg U, Olling S: Adhesion to normal human uroepithelial cells of Escherichia coli from children with various forms of urinary tract infection. J Pediatr, 93: 398-403, 1978.
99. Arthur M, Campanelli C, Arbeit RD, Kim C, Steinbach S, Johnson CE, Rubin RH, Goldstein R: Structure and copy number of gene clusters related to the pap P-adhesin operon of uropathogenic Escherichia coli. Infect Immun, 57: 314-321, 1989a.?
100. Arthur M, Johnson CE, Rubin RH, Arbeit C, Campanelli C, Kim C, Steinbach S, Agarwal M, Wilkonson R, Goldstein R: Molecular epidemiology of adhesin and hemolysin virulence factors among uropathogenic Escherichia coli. Infect Immun 57: 303-313, 1989b.?
101. Johansson I-M, Plos K, Marklund B-I, Svanborg C: Pap, papG, prsG DNA sequences in Escherichia coli from the fecal flora and the urinary tract. 1992 (Submitted for publication).
102. Plos K, Lomberg H, Hull S, Johansson I-M, Svanborg-Edén C: Escherichia coli in patients with renal scarring: Genotype and phenotype of Gala1-4 Galb, Forssman and Mannose specific adhesins. Ped Infect Dis, 10: 15-19, 1991.
103. Mårild S, Wettergren B, Hellström M, Jodal U, Lincoln K, Orskov I, Orskov F, Svanborg-Edén C: Bacterial virulence and inflammatory response in infants with febrile urinary tract infection or screening bacteriuria. J Pediatr, 112: 348-354, 1988.
104. Linder H, Engberg I Svanborg-Edén C: Adhesion dependent activation of IL-6 production. Infect Immun, 59:4357-4362, 1991.
105. Hedges S, Svensson M, Svanborg C: Interleukin-6 response of epithelial cells to bacterial stimulation *in vitro*. Infec Immun, 1991 (in press).
106. Plos K, Hull S, Hull R, Svanborg-Edén C: Frequency and organization of pap homologous DNA in relation to clinical origin of uropathogenic Escherichia coli. J Infect Dis, 161: 518-524, 1990.
107. de Man P, Jodal U, Lincoln K, Svanborg-Edén C: Bacterial attachment and inflammation in the urinary tract. J Infect Dis, 158: 29-35, 1988.
108. Hedges S, Andersson P, Lidin-Janson G, de Man P, Svanborg C: Interleukin-6 response to delibirate colonization of the human urinary tract with gram negative bacteria. Infect Immun, 59: 421-427, 1991.
109 Hedges S, Stenqvist K, Lidin-Janson G, Martinell J, Svanborg C: Comparison of urine and serum concentration of interleukin-6 in women with either acute pyelonephritis or asymptomatic bacteriuria. J Infect Dis, 1992 (in press).
110 de Man P, van Kooten C, Aarden L, Engberg I, Svanborg-Edén C: Interleukin-6 induced at mucosal surfaces by gram- negative bacterial infection. Infect Immun, 57: 3383-3388, 1989.
111 Hansson LÅ, Ahlstedt S, Fasth A, Jodal U, Kaijser B, Larsson P, Lindberg U, Sohl-Åkerlund A Svanborg-Edén C: Antigens of Escherichia coli human immune response and the pathogenesis of urinary tract infections. J. Infect Dis, 136 (Suppl): 144-149, 1977.
112 Hagberg L, Briles D, Svanborg-Edén C: Differences in susceptibility to gram negative urinary tract infection between C3H/HeJ and C3H/HeN mice. Infect Immun, 46: 939-844, 1985.
113. Wettergren B, Jodal U, Jonasson G: Epidemiology of bacteriuria during the first year of life. Acta Pediatr Scand, 74: 925-933, 1985.

114. Lomberg H, Jodal U, Svanborg-Eden C, Leffler H, Samuelsson B: P1 blood group and urinary tract infection. Lancet, I: 551-552, 1981 (Letter).

115 Lindstedt R, Baker N, Falk P, Hull R, Hull S, Karr J, Leffler H, Svanborg-Edén C, Larson G: Binding specificities of wild-type and cloned Escherichia coli strains that recognize globo-A. Infect Immun, 57: 3389-3394, 1989.

116. Lindstedt R, Larsson G, Falk P, Jodal U, Leffler H, Svanborg C: The receptor repertoire defines the host range for attaching Escherichia coli strains that recognize globo-A. Infect Immun, 59: 1086-1092, 1991.

117 Winberg J, Anderssen HJ, Bergström T, Jacobsson B, Larsson H, Lincoln K: Epidemiology of symptomatic urinary tract infection in childhood. Acta Pediatr Scand, 252 (Suppl): 1-20, 1974.

118. Lomberg H, Hellström M, Jodal U, Orskov I, Svanborg-Edén C: Properties of Escherichia coli in patients with renal scarring. J Infect Dis, 159: 579-582, 1989.

119. Glauser MP, Meylan P, Billie J: The inflammatory responses and tissue damage. Pediatr Nephrology, 1: 563-565, 1987.

120 Kovatz TG: The role of endotoxin in autoimmune processes. Naturwissenschaften, 49: 572-573, 1961.

121. Holmgren J, Hansson LÅ, Holm SE, Kaijser B: An antigenic relationship between kidney and certain E. coli strains. Int Arch Allergy Appl Immunol, 64: 201-204, 1975.

122. Hodson C, Wilson S: Natural history of chronic pyelonephritic scarring. Britt Med J, 2: 191-194, 1965.

123. Ransley PG, Risdon RA: Reflux nephropathy: Effects of antimicrobiol therapy on the evolution of the early pyelonephritic scar. Kidney Int, 20: 733-742, 1981.

124 Smellie, JM., PG. Ransley, N. Hunter, ICS. Normand and N. Prescod. 1975. Vesicoureteric reflux and renal scarring. Kidney Int 8: 65-72

125 Smellie JM, Ransley PG, Normand ICS, Prescod N, Edwards D: Development of new scars: a collaborative study. Br Med J, 290: 1957-1960, 1985.

126. Winberg J, Bollgren I, Källenius G, Möllby R, Svensson SB: Clinical pyelonephritis and focal renal scarring. A selected review of pathogenesis, prevention and prognosis. Pediatr Clin North Am, 29: 801-814, 1982.

127. Harber MJ, Topley N, Asscher AW: Virulence factors of urinary pathogenes. Clinical Science, 70:531-538, 1986.

128. Lomberg H, Hellström M, Jodal U, Svanborg-Edén C: Renal scarring and non-attaching bacteria. Lancet, II: 1341, 1986.

129. de Man P, Claeson I, Johanson IM, Jodal U, Svanborg-Edén C: Bacterial attachment as a predictor of renal abnormalities in boys with urinary tract infection. J Pediatr, 115: 915-922, 1989.

130. Lomberg H, de Man P, Svanborg-Edén C: Bacterial and host determinants of renal scarring. Apmis, 97: 193-199, 1989.

131. Jann K, Jann B: Cell surface components and virulence: Escherichia coli O and K antigen in relation to virulence and pathogenecity. In "The virulence of Escherichia coli" (Ed M Sussman), Society for general microbiology, 1985, pp 157-176.

THE KIDNEY IN PREGNANCY

Chapter 6

ASPIRIN IN HYPERTENSION OF PREGNANCY

ARIELA BENIGNI, GIUSEPPE REMUZZI

Mario Negri Institute for Pharmacological Research, Bergamo, Division of Nephrology, Ospedali Riuniti, Bergamo, Italy

The question of how to define hypertension in pregnancy is crucial. In normal pregnancy, values of blood pressure are lower than before pregnancy (1). However, the time of the nadir and the degree of decrement of blood pressure in normal pregnancy are still a matter of debate. Thus, MacGillivray and coworkers (2) reported that a decrease in blood pressure occurred at 16-20 weeks and that decrements in systolic and diastolic pressures averaged 8 and 14 mm Hg, respectively. In contrast, Christianson (3) reported nadir values of blood pressure between 20-25 weeks, with systolic and diastolic pressures decreasing only 5 and 6 mm Hg, respectively, while Wilson and coworkers (4) observed maximal decrements at 28 weeks, with a decrease of diastolic levels of 12 mm Hg and no remarkable changes in systolic pressures.

Because of these discrepancies another question is whether in normal pregnancy the upper limits of "normal" blood pressure are different from those of nonpregnant women. Actually, data from 38,636 women indicate a significant increase in perinatal mortality associated with diastolic blood pressure values greater than 84 mm Hg, recorded at any stage of gestation (5). In a similar study, Page and Christianson (6) evaluated 14,833 singleton births and observed an increase in perinatal mortality and intrauterine growth retardation for women with mean arterial pressures exceeding 90 and 95 mm Hg in the second and third trimester, respectively. Together these reports have lead to an empirical consensus that blood pressures of 75 mm Hg in the second and 85 mm Hg in the third trimester are probably upper limits for normal pregnancy.

The frequency of pregnancy-associated hypertension again depends on definitions. An accepted definition of pregnancy-hypertension (7) today is an increase in systolic blood pressure of 30 mm Hg or greater, or an increase in diastolic blood pressure of 15 mm Hg or greater over the average value recorded during the 20 weeks prior to pregnancy. If previous blood pressure values were not known, values of 140/90 mm Hg or greater after 20 weeks of pregnancy are enough to diagnose pregnancy-induced hypertension. Using these criteria hypertension complicates approximately 10% of all pregnancies (7); the frequency increases to 20% if the women are young nulliparas and to 40 to 50% in women carrying multiple fetuses (8). Probably the most concise and practical classification is the one recommended by The National High Blood Pressure Education Program Working Group Report on High Blood Pressure in Pregnancy (7), which identifies four categories of hypertension associated with pregnancy: preeclampsia and eclampsia, chronic hypertension (of whatever cause, but mainly essential), preeclampsia superimposed on chronic hypertension, and transient hypertension (gestational hypertension).

Preeclampsia, particularly when superimposed on chronic hypertension or renal disease, represents the greatest danger for the fetus and is associated with life-threatening maternal syndromes (9, 10).

Most pregnant women with chronic hypertension have a form of essential hypertension (11). These are cases of superimposed preeclampsia. In most of them hypertension is mild and the pregnancy uncomplicated (12).

In contrast, cases of chronic hypertension due to specific causes, such as underlying kidney disease, renal-artery stenosis, connective-tissue disorders and pheochromocytoma, have a poor fetal prognosis (13-15).

Transient hypertension occurs late in pregnancy or in the immediate puerperium (16) and is thought to be forerunner of essential hypertension later in life (17, 18). In such cases the increase in blood pressure is usually mild, and the outcome of pregnancy is not affected appreciably. Preeclampsia, the association of hypertension, proteinuria and edema, accounts for more than 50% of the hypertensive disorders of pregnancy and complicates 5% to 10% of all pregnancies (16). It usually occurs in nullipara and manifests in late pregnancy mostly after 20 weeks or near term (16). It is most likely that preeclampsia is superimposed on underlying chronic hypertension or renal disease when its onset is early during pregnancy, while 'pure' preeclampsia develops before midpregnancy in women with trophoblastic disease such as hydatidiform mole or fetal hydrops (19).

Preeclampsia can lead to two life-threatening complications: [1] a syndrome of microangiopathic hemolytic anemia associated with coagulation abnormalities and signs of liver dysfunction (HELLP syndrome), which has a sudden onset and represents a medical emergency requiring prompt termination of pregnancy (19), and [2] eclampsia, a syndrome of neurological signs and convulsions with high fetal and maternal mortality.

Preeclampsia typically regresses rapidly after delivery, and its signs and symptoms usually abate within 48 hours.

Occasionally, within 10 days after delivery, late postpartum eclampsia, characterized by hypertension, proteinuria and convulsions, may occur (20).

PRESUMED PATHOPHYSIOLOGICAL BASIS OF PREECLAMPSIA

Increased vascular resistance was considered few years ago as a primary finding of preeclampsia (21); however, a more complex hemodynamic profile has emerged from more recent studies which include a relatively high cardiac output, normal filling pressure, and inappropriately high systemic vascular resistance, reported consistently by most investigators (19, 22, 23). High vascular resistance can be detected as early as at 18th week, before the onset of hypertension and proteinuria (24).

Hypertension in preeclampsia may be extremely labile. This may possibly reflect the increased sensitivity of the vasculature to endogenous pressor peptides (24) and reversal of the vascular responsiveness to angiotensin II, characteristic of normal pregnancy. Gant and coworkers (24) showed that pregnant women become somewhat refractory to the pressor effects of infused angiotensin II, while women destined to develop preeclampsia begin to lose this refractoriness weeks before the clinical appearance of hypertension. Plasma renin activity and plasma renin substrate are increased in preeclampsia (25). This is associated with a decreased plasma angiotensinase activity (25) increased platelet angiotensin II binding sites (26) and high plasma angiotensin II levels (27).

Although the cause of altered vascular reactivity in preeclampsia is unknown, a considerable body of data suggests that vasoconstriction is due to decrements in vasodilatory prostaglandins, namely prostacyclin (PGI_2) and PGE_2, and/or increases in vasoconstrictor products, such as thromboxane A_2 (TxA_2). Consistent with this hypothesis are studies showing that umbilical veins from preeclamptic pregnancies synthesize less PGI_2 than normal (28). Furthermore, cross-sectional and longitudinal studies of urinary excretion of PGI_2 metabolites, 6-keto-$PGF_{1\alpha}$ and 2,3-dinor-6-keto-$PGF_{1\alpha}$, demonstrated that gestational increment in excretion in PGI_2 metabolites is diminished in pregnancy-induced hypertension (29).

A reduced PGI_2 biosynthesis may favor platelet activation, with consequent formation of TxA_2 in excessive amounts. TxA_2, beside being a potent platelet aggregatory agent (30), also constricts vascular smooth muscle cells (31) and could therefore contribute to the increased peripheral vascular resistance of preeclampsia. That this may be the case is suggested by findings that analogues of TxA_2 cause constriction in human umbilical artery strips and rise perfusion pressure in the isolated human placental cotyledon (32).

Fitzgerald and coworkers (33) first demonstrated that TxA_2 biosynthesis is higher in normal pregnant than in non pregnant subjects, largely as a result of platelet activation. Subsequently, the same authors showed that urinary excretion of TxA_2 metabolites, of platelet origin, was even significantly higher in patients with pregnancy-induced hypertension than in normotensive pregnant women (34).

TxA_2 metabolite excretion correlates with mean arterial blood pressure, plasma lactate dehydrogenase, and platelet count (34) which are indices of the severity of pregnancy-induced hypertension.

The recent observation that in severe preeclampsia PGI_2 synthetase activity in maternal venous and umbilical endothelium was significantly lower (35), while TxA_2 synthetase activity in maternal platelets higher than normal control values (35), further reinforces the concept that changes in the PGI_2 and TxA_2 synthetic pathway may have a role in the excessive peripheral vasoconstriction of preeclampsia.

BIOCHEMICAL SELECTIVITY OF LOW-DOSE ASPIRIN

PGI_2 and TxA_2 derive from arachidonic acid by the action of the enzyme cyclooxygenase and are main products of endothelial cells and platelets, respectively. Aspirin, by acetylating the hydroxyl group of a single serine residue at position 529 within the polypeptide chain of cyclooxygenase (36), reduces the synthesis of both substances.

When given in sufficiently low-doses, aspirin selectively inhibits platelet versus endothelial cell-derived eicosanoids. This is because aspirin irreversibly inhibits cyclooxygenase and *de novo* synthesis of the enzyme is required in order to restore to normal eicosanoid synthesis. Such a process can easily occur in nucleated cells within few hours, while in platelets, that have no protein synthesis, it is function of cell turnover (37). An alternative explanation for the biochemical selectivity of low-dose aspirin relates to its kinetics. Indeed oral administered aspirin undergoes substantial presystemic hydrolysis in the gut and liver before it enters the systemic bloodstream (38). Thus, platelets in gut capillaries, where aspirin is absorbed, are exposed to high concentrations of the active drug, while endothelial cells of the peripheral circulation may be exposed to aspirin concentrations insufficient to inhibit cyclooxygenase enzymes.

LOW-DOSE ASPIRIN AND VASCULAR REFRACTORINESS

The first study which tried to address this issue (39) was carried out by the group of Gant et al (24) who first proposed an angiotensin II sensitivity test to be used as a screening method for women destined to develop pregnancy-induced hypertension. These authors gave 81 mg daily aspirin for one week beginning from 32 weeks' gestation to women sensitive to angiotensin II and found that the treatment dramatically increased the PGI_2/TxA_2 ratio in the plasma of pregnant women sensitive to angiotensin II and this was associated with partial restoration of angiotensin II pressor refractoriness in 53% of 17 women studied. Subsequently (40), the same group of investigators evaluated the effect of the low-dose aspirin therapy on circulating eicosanoids and angiotensin II pressor responsiveness in angiotensin II-sensitive and non-sensitive women and correlated these responses with subsequent clinical outcome. They observed that low-dose aspirin significantly reduced plasma TxB_2 levels in both angiotensin II-sensitive and non-sensitive women. Furthermore, in women who remained sensitive to angiotensin II after low-dose aspirin, plasma 6-keto-$PGF_{1\alpha}$ and PGE_2 levels significantly decreased (40). In this group, all women had hypertensive complications, they delivered early and neonates had low birth weight. In contrast, patients who were either non sensitive to angiotensin II before aspirin or became refractory after aspirin administration had no changes in circulating 6-keto-$PGF_{1\alpha}$ and PGE_2 levels and had improved clinical outcomes, that is, a lower incidence of pregnancy-induced hypertension and a delivery near term (40). Thus, a failure to induce refractoriness to infused angiotensin II by low-dose aspirin is associated with an inhibition of vasodilatory eicosanoids and with development of hypertension in pregnancy.

The effect of low-dose aspirin on vascular refractoriness in angiotensin II-sensitive women was recently confirmed in a randomized, placebo-controlled, double-blind trial (41). This study demonstrated that vascular refractoriness to angiotensin II was restored in 14 of 17 aspirin treated women, in comparison with 5 to 15 women in the placebo group, suggesting that enhanced vasopressor sensitivity to angiotensin II is a pathophysiologic mechanism in the development of pregnancy-induced hypertensive disorders associated with PGI_2/TxA_2 unbalance. Although the mechanism through which such an unbalance affects vascular reactivity is not fully understood, it may be hypothesized that the vasoconstrictor action of angiotensin II in preeclampsia may be enhanced by a defective antagonizing effect of vasodilatory PGI_2 (29) and by up-regulation of angiotensin II receptors (26). Low-dose aspirin, which selectively inhibits TxA_2 synthesis and thus restores the unbalanced PGI_2/TxA_2 ratio in preeclampsia, may contribute to restore refractoriness to the pressor effects of angiotensin II.

LOW-DOSE ASPIRIN TO PREVENT PREGNANCY-INDUCED HYPERTENSION

Many observations and several controlled trials have indicated that aspirin, administered in relatively low-doses, prevent pregnancy-induced hypertension and preeclampsia and improved fetal outcome. In line with this is the observation of Crandon and Isherwood (42), who reported a reduced incidence of third-trimester hypertension in women with history of regular aspirin ingestion. Subsequently, low-dose aspirin (150 mg/day) in combination with dipyridamole (300 mg/day) was shown to reduce the incidence of preeclampsia and to improve perinatal outcome in women with clinical risks for intrauterine growth retardation and/or preeclampsia (43). Most recently, Wallenburg and coworkers (44) randomized 46 normotensive women who had enhanced pressor responsiveness to angiotensin II and who were judged to be at increased risk to developing preeclampsia; these subjects either received 60 mg of aspirin per day or were given placebo (44). The incidence of preeclampsia and caesarean section was significantly reduced in the treated gravidae. The same authors further reported a reduction in the incidence of fetal growth retardation in multigravidae women with a history of idiopathic growth retardation and placental infarction receiving daily 1.6 mg/kg aspirin and 225 mg dypiridamole from 16 to 34 weeks' gestation (45).

Recently, three randomized, prospective controlled studies have confirmed the beneficial effects of low-dose aspirin in pregnant women at high risk of hypertension. Schiff and coworkers (46) gave aspirin (100 mg/day) or placebo to 65 patients at increased risk of preeclampsia selected by a positive roll-over test. The overall incidence of pregnancy-induced hypertension was significantly lower in the aspirin group. Moreover, mean gestational age and mean birthweight centile were higher in the aspirin as compared with the placebo group (46). The study of Benigni and coworkers (47) was designed to determine whether the possible favorable effect of low-dose aspirin in patients at risk of pregnancy-induced hypertension was associated with selective inhibition of platelet-derived TxA_2. Thirty-three pregnant women at risk of pregnancy-induced hypertension because of chronic hypertension, previous obstetrical history, or early onset of preeclampsia were randomly allocated to receive daily 60 mg aspirin or placebo from 12th week of pregnancy until delivery. Women in the aspirin group had longer pregnancies and babies with higher birthweights as compared with the women receiving placebo (47). Moreover, the mean week of delivery and birthweights were similar in the aspirin-treated patients and in the normal pregnant women. Hypertension did not develop in any of the aspirin-treated patients, whereas three women in the placebo group developed hypertension (47). Low-dose aspirin was associated with a significant reduction in the generation of TxA_2 in maternal platelets and in urinary excretion of stable metabolites of TxA_2, TxB_2 and 2,3-dinor-TxB_2, mainly of platelet origin (48), as compared with pretreatment values. In contrast, urinary excretion of 6-keto-$PGF_{1\alpha}$ was not modified, suggesting that 60 mg/daily aspirin exerted a specific inhibition of platelet TxA_2 biosynthesis without interfering with PGI_2 biosynthesis *in vivo* (47).

In similar studies, McParland and coworkers (49) demonstrated the effectiveness of low-dose aspirin in prevention of pregnancy-induced hypertension in 100 nulliparous women screened within a group of 1,226 women identified to be at risk of developing hypertension in pregnancy by means of Doppler uteroplacental flow-velocity waveforms. In this selected group of women 75 mg daily aspirin determined a numerical but not significant decrease in the frequency of pregnancy-induced hypertension in respect to placebo (49). However, significant differences between aspirin and placebo in proteinuric hypertension and hypertension occurring before 37 weeks' gestation were reported.

Although the early studies are most promising, they are far from conclusive because of the small number of patients. A recent meta-analysis (50) of six randomized trials that included 394 women has been performed to estimate the magnitude of protection of aspirin from pregnancy-induced hypertension, the effect of aspirin on severe low-birth weight infants, caesarean section and perinatal mortality and the risk of adverse effects. Meta-analysis is particularly useful when several trials with low statistical power demonstrate no difference between compared groups. In this case, systematic pooling of the results across trials yields more precise estimates of the treatment effect (51). Despite the presence of differences in aspirin regimens and patients populations, the overall results of the meta-analysis suggested that low-dose aspirin significantly reduced the risks of pregnancy-induced hypertension and severe low-birth weight among newborn infants. There were no effect on fetal and neonatal death and there were no maternal or neonatal adverse effects associated with taking aspirin (50).

Several ongoing multicenter trials will possibly confirm the efficacy and safety of low-dose aspirin in pregnancy-induced hypertension. The first randomized double-blind, placebo-controlled trial is organized in the United Kingdom and called CLASP (Collaborative Low-dose Aspirin Study in Pregnancy): 7,000 women will be enrolled between 12 and 32 weeks of pregnancy and will be given 60 mg aspirin daily. Women are eligible if they are thought to be at higher than average risk of developing severe preeclampsia or intrauterine growth retardation, either because of their previous obstetric or medical history or other risk factors (prophylactic trial) or because of possible early signs or symptoms in the pregnancy under observation (therapeutic trial). The study is designed with the principal end points of assessing the effect of aspirin on proteinuric preeclampsia, the duration of pregnancy and the birthweight, both crude and adjusted for sex and gestational maturity. The study will finish by the end of 1992.

A similar trial called ECPPA (Estudio collaborativo para prevenção da prè-eclâmpsia com aspirina) is ongoing in Brazil. The study adopts the same eligibility criteria and aspirin regimen but is expected to have a lower planned sample size (4,000 women) than CLASP.

Finally, 1300 women have been enrolled by the Italian collaborative study (52) and statistical analysis is being performed. This study was designed to test the effect of low-dose aspirin for the prevention of preeclampsia and intrauterine growth retardation in a large population considered at low-medium risk. Pregnant women between 16th and 32th week of gestation were randomly allocated to receive 50 mg daily aspirin or no treatment up to delivery. Women were selected on the basis of family history of preeclampsia in mother or sister, chronic hypertension defined as diastolic blood pressure between 90 and 110 mm Hg and previous obstetrical history of pregnancy-induced hypertension and intra-uterine growth retardation. The main end points of the study are the reduction in the aspirin versus control group of the incidence of pre-term birth and intrauterine growth retardation and the reduction of the incidence of proteinuric preeclampsia. Adverse aspirin effect on maternal and neonatal bleeding have also been recorded (52).

DOES LOW-DOSE ASPIRIN CURE PREGNANCY-INDUCED HYPERTENSION ?

All the above mentioned studies demonstrated the efficacy of low-dose aspirin to prevent development of preeclampsia in women at high risk. Thus all women were treated very early during pregnancy, before clinical signs of preeclampsia were present. A recent prospective, randomized double blind trial (53) has tried to address the issue of whether aspirin can cure preeclampsia. Despite the successful use of this drug in women at risk of developing preeclampsia, daily aspirin (100 mg) given to women hospitalized at 30-36 weeks' gestation because of mild pregnancy-induced hypertension did not influence the clinical course, up to and including delivery, and did not ameliorate neonatal characteristics (53). It is possible that once preeclampsia is present, the accompanying local changes in the placental and renal vascular beds are irreversible and the selective inhibition of TxA_2 by low-dose aspirin is ineffective in arresting the progression of the disease.

THE RISK OF GIVING ASPIRIN IN PREGNANCY

Despite its potential benefit, the use of aspirin in pregnancy has been criticized because of the potential teratogenicity of the drug and for the risk of bleeding associated with the treatment in the mother, fetus and newborn. A retrospective study conducted by Lewis and Schulman (54) reported a significant increase in the average length of gestation, the mean duration of labor and a greater average blood loss in 103 mothers who took over 3,250 mg of aspirin daily in the last 6 months of pregnancy because of musculoskeletal disease. Furthermore, a survey of 599 children born with oral cleft showed that mothers, whose children suffer from this defect, took three times more salicylates during the first trimester of pregnancy than mothers who gave birth to normal children (55). However, a large multicenter study called the Collaborative Perinatal Project (56), which monitored prospectively 50,282 mother-child pairs, 14,864 of which assuming aspirin during the first trimester, was unable to find any evidence of a teratogenic effect with no differences in neonatal birth weight or perinatal death.

It has recently been suggested that aspirin use may increase the risk of certain cardiac malformations. Cardiac defects arising from deviations in septation of the truncus arteriosus (transposition of the great arteries, tetralogy of Fallot, and truncus arteriosus) have been reported to be associated with aspirin exposure in early pregnancy (57, 58). Moreover since the patency of the ductus arteriosus in utero is in part controlled by prostaglandins of the E series, the inhibition of prostanoid synthesis by aspirin has been shown to favor the closure the ductus arteriosus, leading to postnatal pulmonary hypertension and severe neonatal hypoxemia (59). Data on relative risk of cardiac malformations in newborn following exposure of the mother to aspirin are conflicting. Some authors have reported a tenfold increase in such a risk, while others failed to find more cardiac malformations in newborns whose mothers were aspirin users.

Besides the possible risk of cardiac malformations, the use of aspirin may theoretically expose the mother, the fetus and the newborn to the risk of bleeding. Abnormal results in platelet function tests and clinical bleeding in newborns - including intracranial hemorrhage - have been reported, but only with relatively high aspirin doses that is between 320 mg and 15 g/daily (60-62).

In contrast, in all of the studies demonstrating the efficacy of low-dose aspirin, the treatment was not associated with an increased risk of maternal bleeding at delivery (43, 49). Furthermore, no hemorrhagic complications were observed in any of the infants from mothers receiving low-dose aspirin. The results of the majority of these studies were based on physical examination, only few studies explored the effect of low-dose aspirin on fetal and neonatal platelet TxA_2 generation. The early study of Ylikorkala and coworkers (63) showed that maternal ingestion of a single oral dose of 100 mg of acetylsalicylic acid during labor at term resulted in a reduction of fetal platelet TxA_2 synthesis. Furthermore, Sibai and coworkers (64) studied the serum levels of TxA_2 in 30 neonates whose mothers were treated with three regimens of low-dose aspirin (≤80 mg/day) for two weeks or more. Neither TxA_2 levels nor platelet aggregation were modified by any of the doses used. Furthermore, echographic assessment of a patent ductus arteriosus and noninvasive estimates of pulmonary arterial pressure did not show any difference among the groups of mothers taking aspirin or placebo. No hemorrhagic complications such as cephalohematoma, gastrointestinal bleeding and purpura were recorded. Finally, Benigni and coworkers (47) have measured the extent of inhibition of fetal and neonatal platelet cyclooxygenase after 5 months treatment with low-dose aspirin and found that aspirin treatment was associated with a significant reduction in the generation of TxA_2 by umbilical-cord serum of approximately 60% which was still significant at day 1 after birth and recovered almost completely at day 5. Since at least 90% inhibition of platelet cyclooxygenase is required in humans to inhibit thromboxane-dependent platelet aggregation, they concluded that the inhibition of fetal platelet cyclooxygenase by low-dose aspirin, may still ensure normal hemostatic competence in the fetus.

CONCLUSIONS

Preeclampsia is the major hypertensive disorder of pregnancy characterized by increased vascular responsiveness to pressor peptides, possibly due to a PGI_2/TxA_2 ratio tilted in favor of vasoconstrictor TxA_2. Treatment with low-dose aspirin, which selectively inhibits platelet thromboxane A_2 formation sparing vascular prostacyclin, has been shown to restore vascular refractoriness to angiotensin II. The efficacy of low-dose aspirin in preventing preeclampsia and fetal growth retardation in women at risk of developing hypertension in pregnancy has been demonstrated by several studies.

Although the results of the trials are encouraging, they are far from conclusive, mainly because of the small numbers of patients. A definitive answer will derive from data of the ongoing large clinical trials in United Kingdom, Brazil and Italy. Preliminary studies suggest that low-dose aspirin does not cure preeclampsia when signs of disease are evident.

Despite the efficacy of aspirin administration, the possible teratogenic effect of the drug must be taken into account, particularly when it is taken during the first trimester of pregnancy and the risk of bleeding associated with aspirin administration must be considered. Although the issue of aspirin teratogenicity in pregnancy is controversial, control against the indiscriminate use of aspirin in any dose is urged. Before the data from the ongoing clinical trial become available, systematic clinical evaluation of possible hemorrhagic complications will add precious evidence to our understanding of the safety of aspirin during pregnancy.

REFERENCES

1. Hytten FE, Leitch I: The physiology of human pregnancy. Blackwell Scientific Publications, Oxford, 1971.
2. MacGillivray M, Rose GA, Rowe B: Blood pressure survey in pregnancy. Clin Sci, 37: 395-407, 1969.
3. Christianson RE: Studies on blood pressure during pregnancy. Am J Obstet Gynecol, 125: 509-513, 1976.
4. Wilson M, Morganti AA, Zervoudakis I, Letcher RL, Romney BM, Van-Oeyon P, Papera S, Sealey JE, Laragh JH: Blood pressure, the renin-aldosterone system and sex steroids throughout normal pregnancy. Am J Med, 68: 97-104, 1980.
5. Friedman EA, Neff RK: Pregnancy hypertension: a systematic evaluation of clinical diagnostic criteria. PSG Publishing Co, Littleton, 1977.
6. Page EW, Christianson R: The impact of mean arterial pressure in the middle trimester upon the outcome of pregnancy. Am J Obstet Gynecol, 125: 740-746, 1976.
7. Lenfant C, Gifford RW Jr, Zuspan FP: National high blood pressure education program working group report on high blood pressure in pregnancy. Am J Obstet Gynecol, 163: 1689-1712, 1990.
8. Lindheimer MD, Katz AI: Hypertension in pregnancy. In: "Current Therapy in Nephrology and Hypertension" (Ed RJ Glassock), Marcell Decker, Toronto,1987, pp 320-334.
9. Sibai BM, Mc Cubbin JH, Anderson GA, Lipshitz J, Dilts PVJr: Eclampsia I. Observations from 67 recent cases. Obstet Gynecol, 58: 609-613, 1981.
10. Weinstein L: Syndrome of hemolysis, elevated liver enzymes, and low platelet count: a severe consequence of hypertension in pregnancy. Am J Obstet Gynecol, 142: 159-167, 1982.
11. Davison JM, Lindheimer MD: Hypertension and pregnancy. In: "Diseases of the Kidney" (Eds RW Schrier, CW Gottschalk), Little Brown, Boston, 1988, pp 1653-1686.
12. Sibai BM, Ardella TN, Anderson GD: Pregnancy outcome in 211 patients with mild chronic hypertension. Obstet Gynecol, 61: 571-576, 1983.
13. Lindheimer MD, Katz AI: Renal physiology and disease in pregnancy. In: "The Kidney: Physiology and Pathophysiology" (Eds DW Seldin, G Giebisch), Raven Press, New York, 1992, pp 3371-3431.
14. Ballou SP, Morley JJ, Kushner I: Pregnancy and systemic sclerosis. Arthritis Rheum, 27: 295-298, 1984.
15. Burgess GEIII: Alpha blockade and surgical intervention of pheochromocytoma in pregnancy. Obstet Gynecol, 53: 266-270, 1979.

16. Barron WM, Murphy MB, Lindheimer MD: Management of hypertension during pregnancy. Hypertension, 1809-1823, 1990.
17. Fisher KA, Luger A, Spargo BH, Lindheimer MD: Hypertension in pregnancy: clinical-pathological correlations and remote prognosis. Medicine, 60: 267-276, 1981.
18. Chesley LC: Hypertension in pregnancy: definitions, familial factor, and remote prognosis. Kidney Int, 18: 234-240, 1980.
19. Chesley LC: Hypertensive disorders in pregnancy. Appleton-Century-Crofts, New York, 1978.
20. Sibai BH: Eclampsia. In: "Handbook of Hypertension" Vol. 10 of "Hypertension in Pregnancy" (Ed PC Rubin), Elsevier, Amsterdam, 1988, pp 320-340.
21. Groenendijk R, Trimbos JB, Wallenburg HC: Hemodynamic measurements in preeclampsia: preliminary observations. Am J Obstet Gynecol, 150: 232-236, 1984.
22. Easterling TR, Benedetti TJ: Preeclampsia: A hyperdynamic disease model. Am J Obstet Gynecol, 160: 1447-1453, 1989.
23. Sowers JR, Zemel MB, Bronsteen RA, Zemel PC, Walsh MF, Standley PR, Sokol RJ: Erythrocyte cation metabolism in preeclampsia. Am J Obstet Gynecol, 161: 441-445, 1989.
24. Gant NF, Daley GL, Chand S, Whalley PJ, Mac Donald PC: A Study of angiotensin II pressor response throughout primigravid pregnancy. J Clin Invest, 52: 2682-2689, 1973.
25. Tapia HR, Johnson CE, Strong CE: Renin-angiotensin system in normal and in hypertensive disease of pregnancy. Lancet, II: 847-850, 1972.
26. Baker PN, Broughton Pipkin F, Symonds EM: Platelet angiotensin II binding sites in hypertension in pregnancy. Lancet, II: 1151, 1989.
27. Baker PN, Broughton Pipkin F, Symonds EM: Platelet angiotensin II binding sites in normotensive and hypertensive women. Clin Sci, 98: 436-440, 1990.
28. Remuzzi G, Marchesi D, Zoja C, Muratore D, Mecca G, Misiani R, Rossi E, Barbato M, Capetta P, Donati MB, de Gaetano G: Reduced umbilical and placental vascular prostacyclin in severe preeclampsia. Prostaglandins, 20: 105-110, 1980.
29. Fitzgerald DJ, Entmann SS, Mulloy K, Fitzgerald GA: Decreased prostacyclin biosynthesis preceding the clinical manifestations of pregnancy-induced hypertension. Circulation, 75: 956-963, 1987.
30. Bhagwat SS, Hamann PR, Still WC, Bunting S, Fitzpatrick FA: Synthesis and structure of the platelet aggregation factor thromboxane A_2. Nature, 315: 511-513, 1985.
31. Ellis EF, Oelz O, Roberts LJII, Payne NA, Sweetman BJ, Nies AS, Oates JA: Coronary arterial smooth muscle contraction by a substance released from platelets: evidence that it is thromboxane A_2. Science, 193: 1135-1137, 1976.
32. Tuvemo T, Standberg K, Hamberg M: Contractile action of a stable prostaglandin endoperoxide analogue on the human umbilical artery. Acta Physiol Scand, 102: 495-496, 1978.
33. Fitzgerald DJ, Mayo G, Catella F, Entman SS, Fitzgerald GA: Increased thromboxane biosynthesis in normal pregnancy is mainly derived from platelets. Am J Obstet Gynecol, 157: 325-336, 1987.
34. Fitzgerald DJ, Rocki W, Murray R, Mayo G, Fitzgerald GA: Thromboxane A_2 synthesis in pregnancy-induced hypertension. Lancet, 335: 751-754, 1990.
35. Satoh K, Seki H, Sakamoto H: Role of prostaglandins in pregnancy-induced hypertension. Am J Kidney Dis, 17: 133-138, 1991.
36. Funk CD, Funk LB, Kennedy ME, Pong AS, Fitzgerald GA: Human platelet/erythroleukemia cell prostaglandin G/H synthase: cDNA cloning, expression, and gene chromosomal assignment. FASEB J, 5: 2304-2312, 1991.
37. Patrono C: Aspirin and human platelets: from clinical trials to acetylation of cyclooxygenase and Back. TIPS, 10: 453-458, 1989.
38. Pedersen AK, Fitzgerald GA: Dose-related kinetics of aspirin. Presystemic acetylation of platelet cyclooxygenase. N Engl J Med, 311: 1206-1211, 1984.
39. Spitz B, Magness RR, Cox SM, Brown CEL, Rosenfeld CR, Gant NF: Low-dose aspirin. Effect on angiotensin II pressor responses and blood prostaglandin concentrations in pregnant women sensitive to angiotensin II. Am J Obstet Gynecol, 159: 1035-1043, 1988.
40. Brown CEL, Gant NF, Cox K, Spitz B, Rosenfeld CR, Magness RR: Low-dose aspirin. Relationship of angiotensin II pressor responses, circulating eicosanoids, and pregnancy outcome. Am J Obstet Gynecol, 163: 1853-1861, 1990.
41. Wallenburg HCS, Dekker GA, Makovitz JW, Rotmans N: Effect of Low-dose aspirin on vascular refractoriness in angiotensin-sensitive primigravid women. Am J Obstet Gynecol, 164: 1169-

1173, 1991.
42. Crandon AJ, Isherwood DM: Effect of aspirin on incidence of pre-eclampsia. Lancet, I: 1356, 1979.
43. Beaufils M, Uzan S, Donsimoni R, Colau JC: Prevention of pre-eclampsia by early antiplatelet therapy. Lancet, I: 840-842, 1985.
44. Wallenburg HCS, Dekker GA, Makovitz JW, Rotmans P: Low-dose aspirin prevents pregnancy-induced hypertension and pre-eclampsia in angiotensin-sensitive primigravidae. Lancet, I: 1-3, 1986.
45. Wallenburg HCS, Rotmans N: Prevention of recurrent idiopathic fetal growth retardation by Low-dose aspirin and dipyridamole. Am J Obstet Gynecol, 157: 1230-1235, 1987.
46. Schiff E, Peleg E, Goldenberg M, Rosenthal T, Ruppin E, Tamarkin M, Barkai G, Ben-Baruch G, Yahal I, Blankstein J, Goldman B, Mashiach S: The use of aspirin to prevent pregnancy-induced hypertension and lower the ratio of thromboxane A_2 to prostacyclin in relatively high risk pregnancies. N Engl J Med, 321: 351-356, 1989.
47. Benigni A, Gregorini G, Frusca T, Chiabrando C, Ballerini S, Valcamonico A, Orisio S, Piccinelli A, Pinciroli V, Fanelli R, Gastaldi A, Remuzzi G: Effect of low-dose aspirin on fetal and maternal generation of thromboxane by platelets in women at risk for pregnancy-induced hypertension. N Engl J Med, 321: 357-362, 1989.
48. Fitzgerald GA, Pedersen AK, Patrono C: Analysis of prostacyclin and thromboxane biosynthesis in cardiovascular disease. Circulation, 67: 1174-1177, 1983.
49. McParland P, Pearce JM, Chamberlain GVP: Doppler, ultrasound and aspirin in recognition and prevention of pregnancy-induced hypertension. Lancet, 335: 1552-1555, 1990.
50. Imperiale TF, Petrulis AS: A meta-analysis of low-dose aspirin for the prevention of pregnancy-induced hypertensive disease. JAMA, 266: 261-265, 1991.
51. Sacks HS, Berrier J, Reitman D, Ancona-Berk VA, Chalmers TC: Meta-analyses of randomized controlled trials. N Engl J Med, 316: 450-455, 1987.
52. Italian Collaborative Study: Multicenter randomized Italian study of low-dose aspirin for the prevention of pre-eclampsia and intrauterine growth retardation. J Nephrol, 2: 127-129, 1991.
53. Schiff E, Barkai G, Ben-Baruch G, Mashiach S: Low-dose aspirin does not influence the clinical course of women with mild pregnancy-induced hypertension. Obstet Gynecol, 76: 742-744, 1990.
54. Lewis RB, Schulman JD: Influence of acetylsalicylic acid, an inhibitor of prostaglandin synthesis, on the duration of human gestation and labour. Lancet, II: 1159, 1973.
55. Saxen I: Associations between oral clefts and drugs during pregnancy. Int J Epidemiol, 4: 37, 1975.
56. Slone D, Heinonen OP, Kaufman DW, Siskind V, Monson RR, Shapiro S: Aspirin and congenital malformations. Lancet, I: 1373, 1976.
57. Rothman KJ, Fyler DC, Goldblatt A, Kreidberg MB: Exogenous hormones and other drug exposures of children with congenital heart disease. Am J Epidemiol, 109: 433-439, 1979.
58. Jick H, Holmes LB, Hunter JR, Madsen S, Stergachis A: First-trimester drug use and congenital disorders. JAMA, 246: 343-346, 1981.
59. Perkins RM, Levin DL, Clark R: Serum salicylate levels and right-to-left ductus shunts in newborn infants with persistent pulmonary hypertension. J Pediatr, 96: 721, 1980.
60. Stuart MJ, Gross SJ, Elrad H, Graeber JE: Effects of acetylsalicylic-acid ingestion on maternal and neonatal hemostasis. N Engl J Med, 307: 909-912, 1982.
61. Bleyer WA, Breckenridge RT: Studies on the detection of adverse drug reactions in the newborn. II. The effects of prenatal aspirin on newborn hemostasis. Rev Esp Estomatol, 18: 2049-2053, 1970.
62. Rumack CM, Guggenheim MA, Rumack BH, Peterson RG, Johnson ML, Braithwaite WR: Neonatal intracranial hemorrhage and maternal use of aspirin. Obstet Gynecol, 58: S52-S56, 1981.
63. Ylikorkala O, Makila U-M, Kaapa P, Viinikka L: Maternal ingestion of acetylsalicylic acid inhibits fetal and neonatal prostacyclin and thromboxane in humans. Am J Obstet Gynecol, 155: 345-349, 1986.
64. Sibai BM, Mirro R, Chesney CM, Leffler C: Low-dose aspirin in pregnancy. Obstet Gynecol, 74: 551, 1989.

THE KIDNEY AND DIABETES

Chapter 7

STRATEGIES FOR SLOWING PROGRESSION OF DIABETIC NEPHROPATHY

ANNE MARIE V. MILES AND ELI A. FRIEDMAN

Renal Disease Division, Department of Medicine, State University of New York, Health Science Center at Brooklyn, Brooklyn, New York 11203, USA

THE SCOPE OF THE PROBLEM

Over the past 15 years renal disease attributed to diabetes mellitus has emerged as the leading cause of end-stage renal disease (ESRD) in the United States (Figure 1) (1). ESRD is also the leading cause of death in patients with insulin-dependent diabetes mellitus (IDDM) (2); ESRD registries and death certificates, however, may incorrectly presume that all "insulin-treated" diabetics have IDDM, hence deaths in patients with non-insulin dependent diabetes (NIDDM) may also contribute to this statistic. Indeed, most diabetics in ESRD programs have NIDDM, because of the much higher prevalence of NIDDM over IDDM (1). The health care costs per year incurred by diabetics with ESRD in the United States are 20% greater than non-diabetic ESRD patients (3), and the overall expense of medical care for diabetic ESRD patients exceeds $1 billion per year (4). Data from around the world confirm the dominant importance of diabetes to ESRD programs: The European Dialysis and Transplant Association (EDTA) reports that, in 1972, 0.5% of patients treated for ESRD were diabetics, while, in 1985, the figure had risen to 10.5% (5). In Australia and New Zealand, the annual increase in new diabetic ESRD patients has been less marked: 8% in 1985 versus 14% in 1990 (6); while in Japan, in 1990, diabetes accounted for 26.2% of 16,543 new patients begun on maintenance hemodialysis (7).

Evidence to be reviewed herein suggests that in many diabetic persons, it may be possible to prevent or retard the progression of clinical nephropathy. Knowledge of the pathogenesis of diabetic nephropathy permits the design of strategies to block its development. Major tasks include identification of the large minority of diabetics at risk for nephropathy, determining which prophylactic or therapeutic strategies to employ, and how early during the course of illness to intervene. A discussion of the clinical stages and pathogenesis of nephropathy in IDDM and NIDDM will be followed by a discourse on the current state of knowledge regarding prevention and treatment of diabetic nephropathy.

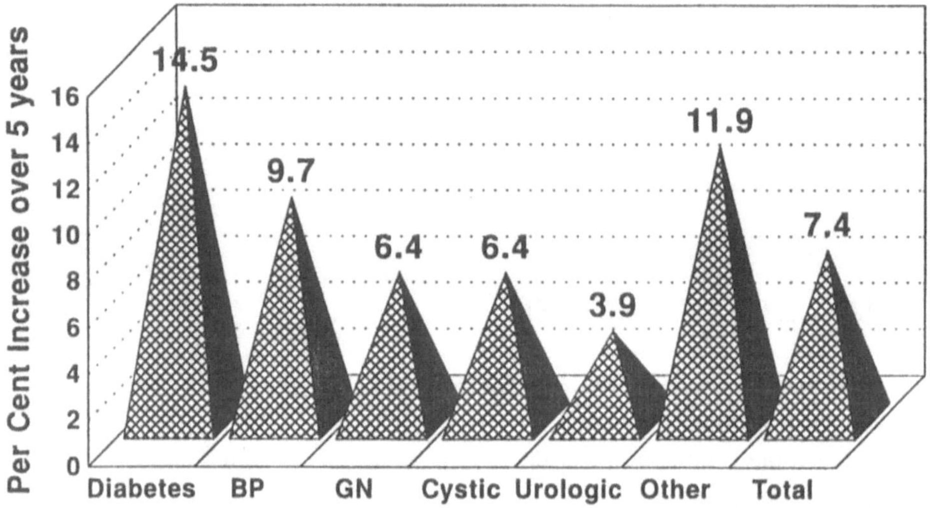

Figure 1. Percent increase in the prevalence of end stage renal disease due to diabetes mellitus and other common renal diseases in the United States between 1985 and 1989.

NEPHROPATHY IN INSULIN-DEPENDENT DIABETES MELLITUS

Since symptoms herald the onset of IDDM within days or weeks, the profile of preclinical and clinical nephropathy in the disease has been well mapped. Five stages have been identified (8):

Stage 1: Glomerular hyperfiltration and renomegaly

Markedly increased inulin clearance in recently diagnosed patients with IDDM was first recognized in the 1930's and 40's (9, 10) and glomerular hyperfiltration was later confirmed by many workers (11-18). Glomerular filtration rates (GFRs) of up to 40% of normal values are seen (15), and, in some studies, the elevation in GFR is positively correlated with serum glucose concentration (19). The precise proportion of newly diagnosed diabetics who have hyperfiltration is not known but it appears to occur in the large majority of patients (20). Both functional and structural abnormalities probably mediate glomerular hyperfiltration (21-23). Possible mediators of hyperfiltration are listed in Table 1.

Table 1. Possible mediators of hyperfiltration in diabetes mellitus.

Hyperglycemia	Blunting of tubuloglomerular feedback
Insulinopenia	Abnormal polyol metabolism
Increased growth hormone/glucagon levels	Abnormal calcium metabolism
Dietary protein	Abnormal kinin metabolism
Increased renal prostaglandins	Increased levels of organic acids: amino acids, ketoacids, lactate
Increased atrial natriuretic protein/ECF volume expansion	Decreased response of renal arterioles to pressor hormones

The closely linked but not necessarily cause and effect relationship between hyperglycemia and hyperfiltration is evidenced by the observation that GFR starts to fall within 8 days of initiation of insulin therapy (24-27), and falls further during 3 months of therapy (24). Even with good or fair glucose control, however, the GFR remains chronically above control levels in 25-40% of patients (8, 20, 28, 29). This subgroup of hyperfiltering patients eventually develop reductions in their GFR (20, 30, 31) and clinical nephropathy at a much greater rate than control diabetics with normal GFR (20, 32, 33), through mechanisms which are almost certainly multifactorial and closely interrelated along the lines shown in Figure 1. Since some diabetics with persistently elevated GFRs show no progression to nephropathy (20), however, glomerular hyperfiltration is probably not an independent risk factor for development of progressive nephropathy (34, 35). Microalbuminuria which is fully reversible upon control of blood glucose is also frequently reported in this first stage (8, 14, 17, 36).

Renal involvement at this stage is probably totally reversible, but since at least 50% of patients will never manifest renal insufficiency, intervention here does not seem warranted until definite prognostic markers for the development of nephropathy are identified, as the side effects of attempting to prevent nephropathy may proffer greater risk of harm than the chance of developing renal failure.

Stage 2: Early glomerular lesions

Mild thickening of the glomerular basement membrane (GBM) begins 18-24 months after onset of IDDM and may be pronounced after 3 1/2-5 years (37, 38). GBM thickening is present even in diabetics who do not go on to develop nephropathy (39). The glomerular mesangial matrix also starts to expand after 2-3 years of disease (40) and increases out of proportion to the increase in glomerular volume. Exercise-induced microalbuminuria is the only clinical evidence of renal involvement during this stage (41), which may extend from 4-5 to 15 years following diagnosis of diabetes. It should be noted that very few studies have explored this stage of IDDM, and those have been exclusively in Caucasians.

Stage 3: Incipient diabetic nephropathy: the microalbuminuric stage

Microalbuminuria is defined as a urinary albumin excretion rate (UAER) of 15-20 to 200-300 μg/min (equivalent to about 20-500 mg/day). It is not detectable on dipstick urinalysis and in its lower ranges is not discovered on routine 24 hour urine protein screening. Quantitation of low concentrations of urinary albumin is performed by radioimmunoassay, nephelometric immunoassay, or enzyme linked immunosorbent assay. A semi-quantitative dipstick test is also available (Micro-Bumintest, Miles, Ellkart, Ind.). Although it may initially be intermittent, microalbuminuria may also be exacerbated or caused by hypertension, hyperglycemia, exercise, urinary tract infections, hypervolemia, and protein loads. Reproducibility of surveys of microalbuminuria may therefore be limited especially when collection periods are shorter than 24 hours. Intrapatient day-to-day variability in urine albumin excretions with coefficients of variation of about 45% have been reported (42-45). For these reasons, at least three measurements of urinary albumin over the course of a year should be made in order to confirm microalbuminuria.

In 25-40% of individuals with IDDM, fixed microalbuminuria develops after 5-15 years of onset of diabetes (46, 47). The majority of these persons will follow a progressive downhill course without intervention (20, 48-51). Typically, albumin excretion increases by about 25 μg/min/yr while GFR remains normal or elevated (14). At levels of microalbuminuria above 70 μg/min however, GFR may begin to fall (20). There is considerable variation amongst patients in the rate of progression of nephropathy. An increase in blood pressure to values higher than usually found in non-albuminuric patients, but not in the range usually diagnostic of hypertension, is also characteristic of this stage. About 40% of persons with IDDM have persistent hypertension (>140-160/90 mm Hg) along with microalbuminuria (52), presumably related to the development of nephropathy (53), though renal biopsy confirmation is lacking.

Glomerular morphology may be normal or abnormal at this stage (54). If there is associated hypertension or decreased creatinine clearance however, morphological changes viz: GBM thickness, mesangial expansion, are always present (54). Renal involvement in stages 2 and 3 can probably be arrested, or significantly retarded (*vide infra*).

Stage 4: Clinical nephropathy: macroalbuminuria, falling GFR

30-40% of individuals with IDDM evolve to this stage which is characterized by proteinuria >200-300 μg/min (300-500 mg/day). The incidence of macroalbuminuria peaks in patients who have had diabetes for 15-20 years (8). The macroalbuminuric stage is observed in those diabetics who have evolved through the preceding stages (20). Without intervention, GFR in macroalbuminuric patients with IDDM falls relentlessly at about 1 ml/min/month (55); and UAER increases by about 2500 μg/min/year with great inter-patient variation (8). The nephrotic syndrome is common, and edema often occurs at values of serum albumin much higher than that seen in other causes of nephrosis, perhaps because of its conversion to glycated albumin.

The histological picture in macroalbuminuric type 1 diabetics is that of well established diffuse glomerulosclerosis (56, 57), the typical Kimmelstiel-Wilson lesions of nodular glomerulosclerosis are seen in only about 50% of cases (58).

As will be discussed, the course of nephropathy during this stage may be slowed by some therapeutic interventions, but the slide to ESRD may be inevitable.

Stage 5: End stage renal disease

ESRD and its multiple complications and co-morbid conditions occurs after 20-30 years of diabetes in 30-40% of patients with IDDM (6). Uremic symptoms and signs are manifested at creatinine clearances which are higher than that in non-diabetics, and renal replacement therapy (RRT) is usually needed within 2-3 years of the onset of the nephrotic syndrome. The need for initiation of RRT may be postponed for months to years with dietary and fluid restrictions, and use of erythropoietin in those patients who have symptoms largely related to anemia.

RENAL INVOLVEMENT IN NIDDM

Much less is known about the natural history of nephropathy in NIDDM than in IDDM, because the precise time of onset of NIDDM is often not known due to many years of asymptomatic disease: 50% of patients with NIDDM do not know they have the disease (59). In addition, prospective studies are lacking.

The prevalence of clinical nephropathy or ESRD in NIDDM is reported as between 2.5-10% (60-63). Recent studies, however, indicate that nephropathy in NIDDM in certain populations may occur at rates which are similar to the IDDM population. Such equivalence in attack rates has been reported in American Pima Indians (64-69), Blacks (61, 70), and Hispanics (61, 70, 71). The interval between manifestation of NIDDM and onset of ESRD varies from 5-10 years; the older the patient at diagnosis of diabetes, the more rapid the progression to ESRD (72).

Hyperfiltration is inconstantly documented in NIDDM. Some studies have reported no elevation in GFR in patients with NIDDM (62, 63, 73-78). This suggests that glomerular injury may be pathogenetically different from that in IDDM. Recently however, there have been reports of moderate to marked increases in GFR in type 2 diabetes in Pima Indians (79), Black Americans (80-82), and whites (83-85). The discrepancy between these and previous reports may be related to differences in the ethnic groups studied, variation in the method of GFR estimation, and/or to the fact that patients may not be studied at equivalent points during the course of their disease. In addition, patients with NIDDM are often elderly at diagnosis of their disease and hence the effect of age itself (86-88) or associated hypertensive and atherosclerotic renal disease (86, 89) may contribute to GFR reduction at the time of study.

Fixed microalbuminuria is found in 20-37% of patients with newly diagnosed NIDDM (62, 63, 90, 91). The high prevalence of microalbuminuria in those recently diagnosed as having NIDDM may reflect a longer period of unrecognized disease, or the presence of other factors known to cause microalbuminuria such as hypertension, urinary tract infection, or non-diabetic glomerulopathy (92). Microalbuminuria in NIDDM was associated with a 4 times increased risk of progression to macroalbuminuria in a prospective study of 76 Danish non-insulin dependent diabetics followed for 9 years (93). A normal urinary albumin concentration may be present despite NIDDM of long duration however (94, 95).

The predictive value of microalbuminuria for subsequent ESRD in NIDDM is not well established: there is no documented increased risk of progression to renal failure or death from renal failure in microalbuminuric type 2 diabetics. GFR may remain stable over many years of micro- (94), or macroalbuminuria (63, 96, 97), and the GFR does not differ in normoalbuminuric and microalbuminuric patients with NIDDM (78). Microalbuminuria does, however, predict increased cardiovascular mortality in NIDDM (93, 98-100), as it does in the non-diabetic population (98).

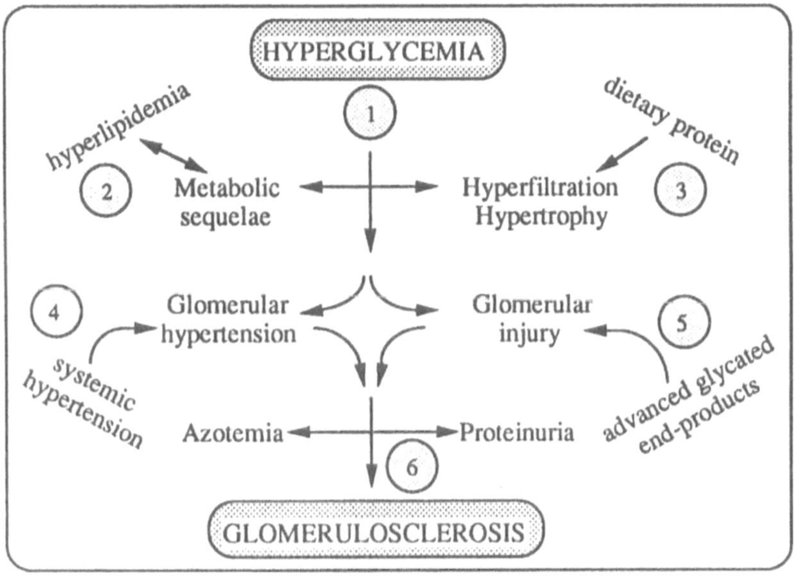

Figure 2. Interplay of factors in the pathogenesis of diabetic nephropathy and possible sites of intervention: 1, 3, 4 useful in retarding short and/or long-term sequela; 2, 5 and 6 currently unproven.

Though hypertension is common in NIDDM, a positive correlation between progressive elevation of blood pressure and worsening proteinuria and renal function has not been found in short term studies (101-105).

Firstly, hypertension is often present at diagnosis of NIDDM [in up to 50-70% of cases (106-108)]; often occurs in the absence of renal disease; and is more closely related to the presence of obesity, advancing age and hyperinsulinism (109).

In NIDDM those who develop clinical diabetic nephropathy do, however, manifest a higher prevalence of hypertension than that in patients without renal involvement (110, 111).

SLOWING DIABETIC NEPHROPATHY

Three main areas of intervention have been found to be of use in retarding the progress of diabetic nephropathy.

Figure 2 illustrates several points in the pathogenesis of diabetic glomerulopathy which may be vulnerable to interruption. Most studies of the efficacy of these regimens have been performed in IDDM. Recognizing that the overwhelming majority of ESRD patients with diabetic nephropathy have NIDDM, the therapeutic approaches found of value in IDDM are now also used in NIDDM.

1. Blood pressure control

The single most important treatment component in diabetic nephropathy is blood pressure reduction. As diastolic blood pressure rises during the stage of incipient diabetic nephropathy, microalbuminuria worsens (112, 113), and GFR falls (114). The deleterious effect of systemic hypertension is thought to occur because the dilated afferent glomerular arterioles of the diabetic kidney (related to hyperglycemia and other metabolic and hormonal factors) allows transmission of systemic blood pressure to the glomeruli, further increasing glomerular capillary hypertension already present due to hyperfiltration and/or glomerular hypertrophy (22, 35, 115-117). Morphologic evidence of the importance of hypertension to the progression of diabetic nephropathy comes from hypertensive diabetics with unilateral renal artery stenosis, where the kidney with arterial stenosis, protected from the effect of systemic blood pressure, exhibits minimal if any morphologic changes of diabetes; while the contralateral side with a patent artery, shows typical changes of diabetic nephropathy (118).

Blood pressure and risk of nephropathy form a continuum (29), raising the questions of what level of blood pressure to start treatment and the optimum value at which to maintain the blood pressure. The Working Group on Hypertension in Diabetes (119) suggest that blood pressure be lowered to at least 140/90 mm Hg, however it may be prudent to lower blood pressure to levels present before development of microalbuminuria or, if these values are not known, to between 120-130/80-85 mm Hg.

Several long term studies show that blood pressure control is the most important intervention to slow progression of diabetic renal disease (8, 55, 120-123). Treatment of hypertension in the microalbuminuric stage significantly slows or arrests progression (124); while once macroalbuminuria ensues, the rate of deterioration can only be slowed (55, 121, 122). In a pioneer Danish trial of blood pressure reduction in IDDM, 6 hypertensive adults with nephrotic-range proteinuria were treated with metoprolol, hydralazine and furosemide for 28-86 months resulting in a reduction in mean blood pressure from 162/103 to 144/95 mm Hg, a 60% reduction in the rate of fall of GFR from 1.23 to 0.49 ml/min/mo (using the patients pretreatment course as a control), and a slowing of the increase in albumin excretion by 5 to 10% per year (55). In a later study using a similar antihypertensive regimen (122), 10 hypertensive patients with IDDM followed for 32 to 91 months had mean blood pressure decreased from 143/96 to 129/84 mm Hg. This was associated with a 75% reduction in the rate of decline of GFR from 0.89 to 0.22 ml/min/mo. With antihypertensive therapy, survival for > 8 yrs in persons with IDDM and clinical or advanced nephropathy is improved from 48 to 87% (125). The improvement in survival is related to postponement of uremia and reduction of cardiac disease and not to earlier use of dialysis or renal transplantation.

An interesting link between hypertension and nephropathy in diabetes, which may hold hope as a possible marker for nephropathy, has emerged in the past decade. Diabetics who have a family history of essential hypertension have a higher incidence of nephropathy (126-128). Since essential hypertension is associated with increased activity of red cell sodium-lithium countertransport system (129) and diabetics who hyperfilter have increased activity of this membrane transport system (130), a genetic or familial tendency to hypertension may increase the risk of phenotypic expression of hypertension and/or nephropathy in the diabetic. This theory has been challenged (131), however, particularly since the mechanism of increased sodium-lithium countertransport activity in hypertension and in diabetes is different (132).

In NIDDM information on the effect of antihypertensive therapy on the progression of nephropathy is sparse. Treatment of micro- or macroalbuminuric persons with NIDDM may or may not reduce albuminuria (133-137) and the effect on GFR is not pronounced (136). A report from French workers, however, document, over a 5 yr period, a reduction in the incidence of renal failure from 80 to 25% in macroalbuminuric patients with both NIDDM and IDDM (138). Control of hypertension in NIDDM has most impact in reducing elevated cardiovascular mortality (107).

ANGIOTENSIN CONVERTING ENZYME INHIBITORS: A SPECIFIC ROLE IN DIABETIC NEPHROPATHY?

Observations in experimental diabetes and other models of progressive renal disease suggest that all anti-hypertensive agents may not be equally efficacious in reducing proteinuria and slowing glomerular injury. In animal models of diabetic and other types of nephropathy, there is a selective effect of angiotensin converting enzyme inhibitors (ACEIs) in decreasing glomerular pressure and single nephron GFR (SNGFR) and in retarding or abolishing glomerular injury (139-144). In addition to its effect in decreasing systemic blood pressure, the beneficial hemodynamic effect of ACEIs is thought to be due to the abolition of the angiotensin II-mediated constriction of the efferent arteriole which contributes to glomerular hypertension (139). Since, however, enalapril can improve renal function and histology in five-sixth nephrectomized rats in the presence of continued elevation of glomerular capillary pressure (145), ACEIs may act by other than hemodynamic mechanisms. Inhibition of mesangial cell proliferation and matrix production (145), possibly by enhancement of the cyclooxygenase pathway (146) with increased prostaglandin production (147), has been suggested. In addition, in human studies ACEIs have been shown to decrease the passage of large molecular weight dextrans and albumin through the GBM. An ACEI-induced change in the barrier function of the GBM with reduction in the size distribution of glomerular pores has been postulated (148). Other advantages of ACEIs include their favorable effect on lipid metabolism (149), their improvement of insulin sensitivity (150), and the infrequency of side effects such as fluid retention and orthostasis. Table 2 shows the results of selected clinical trials of ACEIs in microalbuminuric normotensive and hypertensive, and macroalbuminuric diabetics with or without azotemia.

Table 2. ACE inhibition in diabetic nephropathy.

Study (Ref. No.)	N.	Time (Months)	BP (mm Hg)		UAER (μg/min)		GFR (ml/min)		Controlled
			Pre	Post	Pre	Post	Pre	Post	
151^	16	3	149±11/94±6	135±13/86±7	1589	1075	9±20	93±25	No
152^	10	6	100*	90*	90	30	130±23	141±24	Yes
153^	18	24	146±3/93±1	↓	982±1.25	390±1.1	98±5	↓ rate of all	Yes
154^	8	1.5	131±6/78±3	122±4/74±2	86±37	51±19	149±13	140±10	Yes
155^	15	12	128/78	122/77	378	↓by 11%	111	↓ rate of all	Yes
156^	18	3	126±3/74±2	124±3/72±2	59.1±0.15	27.7±13.9		71±5	Crossover
157°	10	2	151±10/83±5	149±8/82±4	10.6±2.2°°	↓ by 50%	-	-	No
158°	14	24	163±13/97±6	155±14/94±6	2.9±2°°	2.8±1.9°°	-	↓ rate	No
136°	12	6	162±17/103±5	139±26/89±10	4.5±3.1°°	3.4±2.3°°	57±17	51±19	No
159°	12	<1	110±1*	102±3*	1343±337	879±299	-	→	Crossover
160°	22	2	118±2*	107±1*	2.3°°	1.2°°	-	-	

^ normo- or microalbuminuric patients;
° macroalbuminuric or azotemic patients;
* mean arterial pressure;
°° g/day

Studies in normotensive patients with microalbuminuria (152, 154-156) have all been short term, so that it is still unclear whether ACEIs should be exhibited at this stage. In hypertensive patients with incipient nephropathy, ACEIs decrease the rate of fall of GFR by about 50% after 1-2 yrs follow up (152, 155); however, control of blood pressure using other antihypertensive agents produces similar or better effects (124). While reduction in proteinuria may be more marked during ACEI therapy and can sometimes occur in the absence of significant reductions in systemic blood pressure (157), there is no evidence that ACEIs decrease the risk of, or time to evolution to ESRD above other antihypertensive drug combinations. Long term, controlled, prospective trials of ACEIs in microalbuminuric, hypertensive diabetics are needed. In hypertensive diabetics with overt nephropathy, less marked reductions in proteinuria and the rate of decline in GFR are seen with ACEI therapy (157, 158, 160).

In view of their efficacy, lack of side effects and good metabolic profile, ACEIs are recommended as first line treatment for hypertensive diabetics (119).

Antihypertensive drug combinations are often needed in the treatment of hypertension in diabetes. The best choices are those agents which have the greatest efficacy and least adverse effects. Calcium channel blockers are often used as first or second line therapy. While diuretics may have adverse effects on glucose control and the lipid profile, they are often essential in attaining blood pressure control in patients with falling GFRs. Beta blockers, central α_2-agonists (eg: clonidine), or peripheral vasodilators (prazosin, hydralazine, minoxidil) may also be valuable adjuncts. Weight loss and physical training should also be recommended in obese persons with NIDDM to enhance insulin sensitivity and ameliorate the lipid profile (161, 162).

2. Dietary protein restriction

A final determination of the value of dietary protein restriction in early diabetic nephropathy is still pending; in advanced nephropathy however, the value of a protein-restricted diet is somewhat more established.

As in normal patients (163, 164), dietary protein intake modulates renal hemodynamics in diabetic patients (165). The cumulative risk of diabetic nephropathy may be increased in individuals with IDDM who ingest a high protein diet (166). In 12 adults with IDDM of <10 years duration and <200 mg/day proteinuria, increasing dietary protein intake from a baseline 2.17 g/kg/day to 3.5 g/kg/day and then restricting intake to 1.5 g/kg/day resulted in GFR increasing from 124±17 ml/min to 149±26 ml/min and then falling to 119±16 ml/min (165). In addition, hyperglycemia and amino acid loading are synergistic in increasing GFR (167). Dietary protein raises SNGFR and glomerular blood flow by producing afferent arteriolar vasodilatation, an effect which has been demonstrated in streptozotocin-diabetic rats (115, 168). Moderate and severe protein restriction early in the course of diabetes normalizes glomerular hypertension and SNGFR in this model (115, 168, 169). Total proteinuria, albuminuria and morphologic glomerular injury are also retarded (115). The reduction in albuminuria has been shown, in human studies, to be due to decreased fractional clearance of albumin (112, 170) and immunoglobulin G (170); hence, protein restriction may also alter the sieving characteristics of the GBM.

Though challenged in the past (171, 172), a role for dietary protein restriction in IDDM has emerged, as it has in non-diabetic renal disease where 2 to 10 fold reductions in the rate of progression of renal failure have been reported (173-175). In newly diagnosed normo- (176) or microalbuminuric patients with IDDM, short-term protein restriction (to 0.6 g/kg/day) lowers GFR-UAER in patients with normal (177, 178) or supranormal (112, 177) GFRs.

In a prospective, randomized, controlled study, one of the most well constructed to date (179), 20 subjects with IDDM and clinical proteinuria (mean 3144±417 mg/day) or renal impairment (iothalamate clearance 46±4.8 ml/min/1.73 m^2) were given a 0.6 g/kg/day protein diet over a mean follow up of 34.7 months. At the end of the study, there was a 4 fold decrease in the rate of fall of GFR compared to that in 15 controls. After 3 months, compared to baseline values, mean protein excretion had fallen by 24% (760 mg) in the study group, and risen by 22% (928 mg) in the controls. At the conclusion of the study, the reduction in proteinuria in the study population was only 6% (196 mg), however, while the controls had had a 24% (1024 mg) increase. Other studies of protein restriction in patients with IDDM and advanced nephropathy or renal failure performed over 17-37 month periods have reported 2-4 to 46 fold reductions in the rate of fall of GFR (178, 180-185) and significant falls in proteinuria as well. Proteinuria in nephrotic diabetics may also be reduced by dietary protein restriction (186-188).

Few studies address the effect of a protein-restricted diet in persons with NIDDM and clinical nephropathy. Available information, however, is not as encouraging as that in IDDM. For example of 13 patients with NIDDM, renal insufficiency and proteinuria who were treated for 12.2±12.9 months with a 30 g protein, 350 mg phosphorus diet, only 2 evinced a slowing in the rate of fall of 1/creatinine (189). An initial negative nitrogen balance was followed after 4 weeks by neutral or positive nitrogen balance.

Neither the point in the course of diabetic nephropathy to start protein restriction, nor the optimal level of protein intake is established. We recommend a 0.6-0.8 g/kg/day protein diet in both IDDM and NIDDM once macroalbuminuria and/or a falling GFR is noted providing that overall nutritional status is satisfactory. The American Diabetes Association recommends a 0.8 g/kg/day protein diet in "diabetics who have or are at risk for nephropathy" (190). In diabetics with normoalbuminuria or microalbuminuria, a normal protein diet is recommended at present until long-term studies prove whether protein restriction is beneficial to this group. Difficulty with compliance and the risk of malnutrition are the two main drawbacks to sustained dietary protein restriction. In Zeller et al's study (179), however, no significant change occurred in any measured nutritional index in diabetics given 0.6 g protein /kg/day for up to 5 years, showing that if a low protein diet remains isocaloric, with high quality protein, nutritional status can be well maintained.

3. Glycemic control

Hyperglycemia plays a significant role in initiating and propagating the functional and morphologic changes of diabetic nephropathy. In streptozotocin-diabetic rats, basement membrane thickening increases proportional to the severity of hyperglycemia (191) and histopathological changes of nephropathy are reversed by insulin therapy, islets of Langerhans transplants (192), and transplantation of affected kidneys into non-diabetic, isogeneic recipients (193, 194). In humans, the prevalence of microalbuminuria (29, 42, 67, 120) and late diabetic complications has been associated with poor glycemic control in many studies (195-198). Longitudinal studies show that poor metabolic control, with glycosylated hemoglobin (HbA_{1c}) levels of ≥7.5%, is common in patients with fixed microalbuminuria and increased GFRs (191). The time from the onset of diabetes to the start of clinical proteinuria is shortened by poor glycemic control (197), and the risk of developing macroalbuminuria is 4 to 5 times greater in patients with poor control (199, 200).

Insulin requirements tend to be higher in patients in whom nephropathy develops than in those whose renal function remains normal (110, 198), also suggesting that higher levels of glycemia may predispose to nephropathy. As in the rat model, a case report of transplantation of kidneys with diabetic glomerulopathy into non-diabetic patients documented marked regression of the diabetic lesions, though sampling error may have been contributory (201, 202).

The important role which factors beside hyperglycemia must play, however, is attested to by the fact that many patients with poor glycemic control never go on to develop nephropathy (198).

In normoalbuminuric hyperfiltering patients with IDDM, insulin pump therapy for 1 or 2 years significantly reduces or normalizes GFR (27, 203, 204), though the kidneys may remain enlarged (27). Strict glycemic control for 3 weeks decreases GFR and kidney volume and abolishes the deleterious effect of i.v. amino acids in further elevating the GFR seen in patients on conventional therapy (167). No long-term studies of the effect of euglycemia on normoalbuminuric patients with IDDM are available, and it is therefore not known if intervention at this early stage is warranted. At the other extreme, once macroalbuminuria develops, strict glycemic control is ineffective in reversing or retarding nephropathy (110, 164, 205-209).

Studies to determine whether tight glucose control [keeping HbA_{1c} levels ≤7.5% using continuous subcutaneous insulin infusion (CSII) via an insulin pump, or multiple daily insulin injections (MDI)] initiated at the microalbuminuric stage will retard the development of overt nephropathy are in progress.

Efforts to attain strict glucose control in the 8 month Kroc study (210), the 2 year Steno study (211), the 3 year Dallas study (212), and the 4 year Oslo study (213) all resulted in significant reductions in microalbuminuria in patients with IDDM. MDI appears to be as effective as CSII in lowering HbA_{1c} levels and decreasing proteinuria (211, 213).

In the Steno study (211), 18 patients were allocated to optimized glucose control and 18 to conventional therapy; 5 patients in the latter group developed clinical proteinuria (defined as >300 mg/day), while none managed by optimized glucose control became macroalbuminuric. Patients on conventional therapy had a greater tendency towards hypertension and often needed initiation of antihypertensive therapy. Because reduction in blood pressure itself may decrease proteinuria, the study was curtailed after 2 years.

An update from the Steno Group (214), expanded to include 36 patients (18 on CSII and 16 on conventional therapy) who had been enrolled in an independent study 3 years earlier to assess the progress of retinopathy and neuropathy (215), was recently published giving 5 to 8 years of follow up. The total number of patients progressing to clinical nephropathy was higher in the conventional treatment group, but not significantly different than in the optimized control group. However, of 19 subjects with microalbuminuria in the range 100 to 300 mg/day, 9 received CSII and 2 of the nine developed clinical nephropathy, while all 10 subjects who received conventional therapy progressed to clinical nephropathy (214). No progression was observed among 32 patients with low-range microalbuminuria (30-99 mg/day) on either treatment protocol. In the 19 patients with high-range microalbuminuria, average GFR declined with conventional treatment (from 110±23 ml/min/1.73 m^2 at entry, to 87±24 ml/min/1.73 m^2 after 5-8 years); but remained stable in those on CSII (113±23 ml/min/1.73 m^2 versus 100±26 ml/min/1.73 m^2). In patients with UAE in the range 30-99 mg/day, GFR and the degree of microalbuminuria remained stable in both the optimized control group and the conventional therapy group. These data suggest that it is the subset of microalbuminuric diabetics with UAE in the higher range (>100 mg/day) who stand to benefit most from optimized glucose control.

Another recent report on the effect of glycemic control on the microalbuminuria of IDDM comes from the Stockholm Diabetes Intervention Study (SDIS) group (216), where 96 patients (44 on MDI therapy and 52 on conventional insulin therapy) have been followed for 5 years. In the MDI group, (where mean HbA_{1c} levels decreased from 9.5±0.2% to 7.2±0.1%) mean GFR at entry was 122±3 mls/min and 112±3 mls/min after 5 years. Similar values of 126±3 mls/min versus 115±4 mls/min were seen in the conventional treatment group (where mean HbA_{1c} levels had fallen from 9.4±0.2% to 8.7±0.1%). However, while 5 patients on conventional therapy had a GFR of <90 mls/min after 5 years, only 1 patient on intensified (MDI) therapy had a GFR <90 mls/min. In the MDI group, UAER fell from 55.7±26.7 to 46.0±26.1 µg/min; while in the conventional treatment group, there was a 3 fold rise in the UAER from 74.3±31.0 to 239.9±129.7 µg/min.

The progress of microalbuminuria in IDDM is therefore significantly retarded by tight metabolic control; the possibility that overt nephropathy and renal failure may be decreased awaits the results of more prolonged follow up. A huge, multicenter study is underway in the United States (217, 218) designed to assess the outcome in MDI- and CSII-treated subjects with IDDM with <40 mg/day proteinuria, compared with conventional insulin therapy. Weight gain and a tendency to serious hypoglycemia have been reported as adverse consequences of tight metabolic control in IDDM in a preliminary report (217).

In NIDDM, poor glucose control is associated with development of clinical proteinuria (219), and also correlates with the degree of structural renal damage (220), and possibly the prevalence of uremia (221).

Information on the effect of tight glucose control on prevention or regression of microvascular or macrovascular complications are almost entirely lacking. In one study, a hypocaloric diet over 6 months in 24 microalbuminuric subjects with NIDDM decreased fasting blood glucose from 10.9±0.8 to 5.7±0.3 mmol/l and reduced the urinary clearance of albumin by >50% (222).

While attainment of the best possible level of metabolic control is advised for both patients with IDDM and NIDDM, it must be appreciated that the case for blocking organ damage, especially nephropathy, is unproven.

The authors speculation as to the cumulative of induction of normotension, euglycemia, and dietary protein restriction in slowing the course of diabetic nephropathy is depicted in Figure 3.

Other interventions

Many other prophylactic or therapeutic modalities have been tried in experimental or human diabetic nephropathy and, though promising in animal models, have yet to be established as beneficial in clinical diabetes.

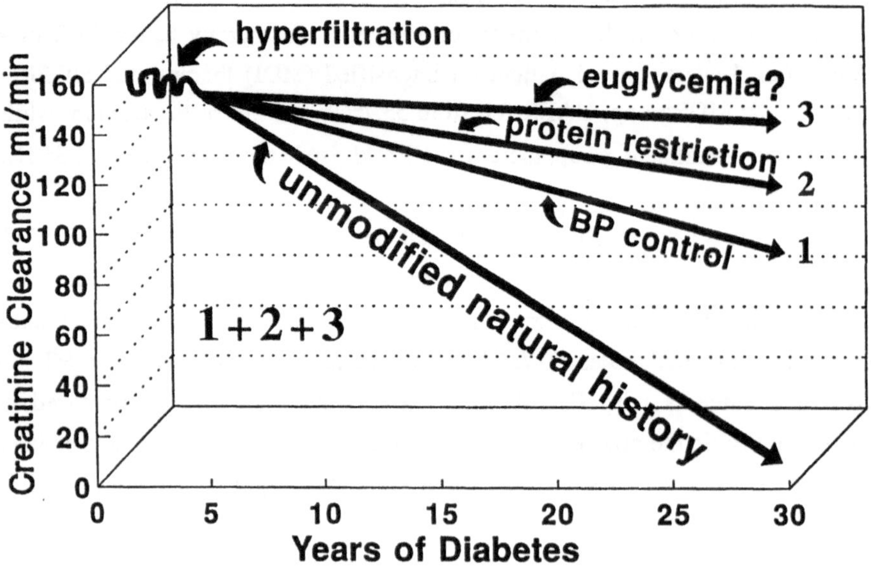

Figure 3. The probable impact of the three main strategies in slowing progression of diabetic nephropathy.

ALDOSE REDUCTASE INHIBITORS

These enzyme blocking chemicals have been tried mainly in experimental diabetes on the rationale that inhibition of the production of sorbitol by the enzyme aldose reductase and the concurrent repletion of cellular stores of myoinositol and phosphatidylinositol may retard glomerulopathy. Glomeruli from diabetic rats have been shown to have increased sorbitol content which is decreased by inhibition of aldose reductase (223). Sorbinil or dietary myoinositol supplementation decreases the elevated GFR in diabetic rats despite persistent hyperglycemia and in the absence of blood pressure reduction (223-228). Aldose reductase inhibitors also reduce urinary albumin excretion in association with a decrease in the elevated glomerular prostaglandin levels seen in experimental diabetes (229). Mogensen et al (204) reported a significant drop in GFR in 20 recently diagnosed patients with IDDM who were treated for 6 months with an aldose reductase inhibitor, but no decrease in UAER or renal blood flow occurred. Other workers were unable to confirm a fall in GFR in subjects with IDDM treated with aldose reductase inhibition (230). Despite the promise of results in streptozotocin-diabetic rats, no role for aldose reductase inhibitors has been defined in human diabetes.

AMINOGUANIDINE

Nonenzymatic glycosylation of tissue and plasma proteins with formation of advanced glycosylation end products (AGEs) may alter vascular wall structure and function (231); and the chronic glycosylation of protein within cells and in the extracellular matrix has been postulated to be at the root of most diabetic complications (231). High levels of AGEs have been found in arterial-wall collagen samples from patients with diabetes, especially in those with advancing nephropathy (232). Aminoguanidine is a nucleophilic hydrazine compound which inhibits the AGE-mediated cross-linking of soluble proteins to matrix proteins (233). Preliminary data in animals show a beneficial effect of aminoguanidine in inhibiting diabetes-induced GBM thickening (233), and in reducing albuminuria (234-236). There are no human data on the use of the drug in the prevention of diabetic nephropathy.

PROSTAGLANDIN SYNTHETASE INHIBITORS

Imbalance between the production of vasodilator prostaglandins and thromboxane has been implicated in the pathogenesis of diabetic nephropathy (237-239). Some studies report significant reduction of glomerular hyperfiltration in experimental models of diabetic nephropathy when prostaglandin synthetase inhibitors are used (240, 241). The results of short-term prostaglandin synthetase inhibitor studies in humans are inconsistent in reducing hyperfiltration and albuminuria (242-245). There is currently no established role for the use of these agents in the prevention or treatment of diabetic nephropathy.

LIPID LOWERING AGENTS

Hyperlipidemia may be an independent risk factor in the progression of renal disease (246). Some 40% of type 1 diabetics have hyperlipidemia (247), and the decline in GFR in type 1 diabetics with clinical nephropathy is much more rapid in patients who have hyperlipidemia (248). Treatment of hyperlipidemia in animal models of progressive renal disease ameliorates renal damage (249, 250), and cholesterol-rich diets produce accelerated glomerulosclerosis in unilaterally nephrectomized rats (251). There are, however, no human studies assessing the impact of lipid lowering agents on the progression of diabetic nephropathy.

SOMATOSTATIN ANALOGUES

Growth hormone and glucagon have been linked to the pathogenesis of diabetic hyperfiltration (23). However, a short-term trial of the somatostatin analogue Octreotide (which inhibits pancreatic release of glucagon as well as central growth hormone release) in 10 normotensive, normoalbuminuric subjects with IDDM resulted in only a 5% reduction in GFR despite a significant fall in serum glucagon levels and normalization of elevated growth hormone levels (204). Somatostatin analogues are not indicated in the prevention or treatment of diabetic nephropathy at present.

PENTOXIFYLLINE

Hemorheologic factors including decreased red cell deformability may also play a role in the pathogenesis of the microvascular and renal complications of diabetes (252, 253). The xanthine derivative pentoxifylline has been used in a small number of clinical trials in the hope of reducing glomerular hypertension and albuminuria in nephropathic diabetics: 6-24 month studies have reported decreased total proteinuria and fractional clearance of albumin in the microalbuminuria of both IDDM and NIDDM (254, 255). There are no long term studies, hence pentoxifylline has not been shown to reduce the risk of clinical proteinuria or azotemia.

ERYTHROPOIETIN

The reduction in exertional dyspnea and improved physical performance which accompanies the correction of anemia by administration of human recombinant erythropoietin to dialysis patients may also be of great benefit in the pre-dialytic azotemic diabetic; and while not retarding the course of the underlying renal disease may prolong, by months, the need for initiation of RRT. Potential concerns are worsening of blood pressure control, and worsening of renal failure related to the decreased plasma volume and increased whole blood viscosity accompanying the expansion in red cell mass. Blood pressure should be well controlled before initiating therapy, and no acceleration in the rate of decline of renal function has been observed in 5 diabetics with mean serum creatinine 3.5±0.28 mg/dl treated with erythropoietin for a 1 yr period (256).

No controlled, prospective trial of erythropoietin in pre-dialysis diabetics has been reported.

PANCREATIC/ISLET CELL TRANSPLANTATION

Islet cell transplantation in experimental diabetes can prevent or cause regression of nephropathic changes (257). Success in performance of whole organ pancreatic transplantation is more advanced than islet grafting at this time, however; and results in diabetics who have received combined pancreas and kidney transplants indicate that glomerulopathy may be attenuated in the renal allograft (258). Correction of hyperglycemia with pancreas transplantation normalizes many of the hormonal and metabolic perturbations in IDDM, affording a path to prevention or abrogation of nephropathy and other diabetic complications. It should be kept in mind however, that the majority of diabetic ESRD patients have NIDDM (1), for which pancreas or islet transplants are valueless.

CONCLUSIONS

In 1992 the diabetic with renal disease may be offered three treatment modalities which are widely accepted to be of use in slowing progression of their nephropathy (Figure 3). Aggressive blood pressure control slows the development of diabetic nephropathy at all stages of disease. Angiotensin converting enzyme inhibitors and calcium blockers are good first line choices, especially in view of the evidence in rat models that ACEIs prevent glomerular hypertension and injury. Any drug or combination of drugs with least side effects which keeps blood pressure below 140/90 mm Hg may be of equal advantage, however (259, 260). It may be beneficial to treat any increase in blood pressure which is above normal for the patients age even if not in the range usually diagnostic of hypertension. For example, the target blood pressure in a 27 year old woman with IDDM should be closer to 120/70 mm Hg than to 140/90 mm Hg. There is currently not enough evidence to justify treatment of normotensive, normoalbuminuric patients with IDDM with ACEIs.

Strict glucose control has not been shown to slow the progression to ESRD in patients who manifest clinical proteinuria or impaired renal function. In normo- or microalbuminuric patients, optimized glucose control with maintenance of HbA_{1c} levels

<7.5% decreases the rate of increase in UAE and there is hope that in the long term it may also reduce the incidence of clinical proteinuria and ESRD. Multiple daily doses of insulin seem to be as efficacious as the insulin pump in attaining this goal. After about 5 years of disease, individuals with IDDM should therefore be screened annually for the presence of microalbuminuria, and glucose control tightened (if necessary with CSII or MDI) upon its discovery.

In short term studies, dietary protein restriction in normo- or microalbuminuric IDDM patients reduces their high and almost certainly deleterious GFR. Long term studies are needed, however, in order to justify initiation of dietary restriction at this stage. In macroalbuminuric or azotemic diabetic patients, a 0.6 g/kg/day protein-restricted diet produces a 4 fold reduction in the rate of fall of GFR and significantly reduces proteinuria. Protein restriction to 0.6-0.8 g/kg/day is therefore recommended at present, only in diabetics with clinical proteinuria or renal impairment, as long as their nutritional status is adequate.

Application of the measures described above has revolutionized the natural history of diabetic microvasculopathy. When managed in collaboration with an aggressive ophthalmologist, the pre-ESRD functional life of individuals with IDDM and NIDDM has been extended remarkably. It is reasonable to anticipate that additional advances, especially treatment with aminoguanidine, will further extend the interval of symptom-free life in those destined to develop diabetic nephropathy.

REFERENCES

1. United States Renal Data System: USRDS 1991 Annual Data Report. The National Institutes of Health, National Institute of Diabetes and Digestive Diseases. Bethesda, MD, August 1991.
2. Borch-Johnsen K: Incidence of nephropathy in insulin dependent diabetes as related to mortality. In: "The kidney and hypertension in diabetes mellitus" (Ed CE Mogensen), Topics in Renal Medicine (Series Ed VE Andreucci), Martinus Nijhoff, Boston, pp 33-40.
3. Smith DG, Harlan LC, Hawthorne VM: The charges for ESRD treatments of diabetics. J Clin Epidemiol, 42: 111-118, 1989.
4. Eggers PW: Effect of transplantation on the Medicare end-stage renal disease program. N Engl J Med, 318: 223-229, 1988.
5. Brunner FP: End stage renal disease due to diabetic nephropathy: data from the EDTA Registry. J Diab Compl, 3: 127-135, 1989. ANZDATA Report 1991. Australia and New Zealand Dialysis and Transplant Registry. Editor: Disney APS. Adelaide, South Australia.
6. Balodimus MC: Diabetic nephropathy. In: "Joslin's Diabetes" (Eds A Marble, P White, RF Bradley, LP Krall), Lea & Febiger, Philadelphia, 1971, pp 526-561.
7. Agishi T: Annual Statistical Report, 1991. Japanese Society for Dialysis Therapy.
8. Mogensen CE, Christensen CK, Vittinghus E: The stages in diabetic renal disease with emphasis on the stage of incipient diabetic nephropathy. Diabetes, 32 (Suppl 2): 64-78, 1983.
9. Cambier P: Application de la theorie de Rehberg a l'etude clinique des affections rénales et du diabetes. Ann Med, 35: 273-299, 1934.
10. Spuhler O: Zur Physio-Pathologie der Niere. Hans Huber, Bern, 1946, pp 45.

11. Fiaschi E, Grassi B, Andres G: La funzione renale nel diabete mellito. Rassegna di fisiopatologia clinica e terapeutica, 24: 372, 1952.
12. Stalder G, Schmid R: Severe functional disorders of glomerular capillaries and renal hemodynamics in treated diabetes mellitus in childhood. Ann Pediatr, 193: 129-138, 1959.
13. Ditzel J, Schwartz M: Abnormally increased glomerular filtration rate in short-term insulin-treated diabetic subjects. Diabetes, 16: 264-267, 1967.
14. Mogensen CE: Kidney function and glomerular permeability to macromolecules in early juvenile diabetes. Scand J Clin Lab Invest, 28: 79-90,1971.
15. Mogensen CE: Glomerular filtration rate and renal plasma flow in short term and long term juvenile diabetes. Scand J Clin Lab Invest, 28: 91-100, 1971.
16. Ditzel J, Junker K: Abnormal glomerular filtration rate, renal plasma flow, and renal protein excretion in recent and short term diabetics. Br Med J, 2: 13-19, 1972.
17. Mogensen CE: Kidney function and glomerular permeability to macromolecules in juvenile diabetes. Dan Med Bull, 19 (Suppl 3): 24, 1972.
18. Hannedouche TP, Delgado AG, Gnionsahe DA, Boitard C, Lacour B, Grunfeld JP: Renal hemodynamics and segmental tubular reabsorption in early type 1 diabetes. Kidney Int, 37: 1126-1133,1990.
19. Wiseman MJ, Viberti GC, Keen H: Threshold effect of plasma glucose in the glomerular hyperfiltration of diabetes. Nephron, 38: 257-260, 1984.
20. Mogensen CE, Christensen CK: Predicting diabetic nephropathy in insulin-dependent patients. N Engl J Med, 311: 89-93, 1984.
21. Christiansen JS: On the pathogenesis of the increased glomerular filtration rate in short-term insulin-dependent diabetes. Dan Med Bull, 31: 349-361, 1984.
22. Castellino P, Shohat J, DeFronzo RA: Hyperfiltration and diabetic nephropathy: Is it the beginning? Or is it the end? Sem Nephrol, 10: 228-241,1990.
23. Bank N: Mechanisms of diabetic hyperfiltration. Kidney Int, 40: 792-908, 1991.
24. Mogensen CE, Andersen MJF: Increased kidney size and glomerular filtration rate in untreated juvenile diabetes: Normalization by insulin treatment. Diabetologia, 11: 221-224, 1975.
25. Christiansen JS, Gammelgaard J, Tronier B, Svendsen PA, Parving H-H: Kidney function and size in diabetics before and during insulin treatment. Kidney Int, 21: 683-688, 1982.
26. Christiansen JS, Frandsen M, Parving H-H: The effect of intravenous insulin infusion on kidney function in insulin-dependent diabetes mellitus. Diabetologia, 20: 199-204, 1981.
27. Wiseman MJ, Saunders AJ, Keen H, Viberti GC: Effect of blood glucose control on increased glomerular filtration rate and kidney size in insulin-dependent diabetes. N Engl J Med, 312: 617-621, 1985.
28. Mogensen CE, Steffes MW, Deckert T, Christiansen JS: Functional and morphological renal manifestations in diabetes mellitus. Diabetologia, 21: 89-93, 1981.
29. Wiseman M, Viberti G, Mackintosh D, Jarrett RJ, Keen H: Glycemia, arterial pressure and microalbuminuria in type 1 (insulin-dependent) diabetes mellitus. Diabetologia, 26: 401-405, 1984.
30. Jones SL, Wiseman MJ, Viberti GC: Glomerular hyperfiltration as a risk factor for diabetic nephropathy: Five year report of a prospective study. Diabetologia, 34: 59-60, 1991 (Letter).
31. Azevedo MJ, Gross JL: Follow up of glomerular hyperfiltration in normoalbuminuric type 1 (insulin-dependent) diabetic patients. Diabetologia, 34: 611, 1991 (Letter).
32. Mogensen CE: Early glomerular hyperfiltration in insulin-dependent diabetics and late nephropathy. Scand J Clin Lab Invest, 46: 201-206, 1986.
33. Mogensen CE, Christensen CK Christiansesn JS, Boye N, Pedersen MM, Schmitz A: Early hyperfiltration and late, renal damage in insulin-dependent diabetes. Ped Adolesc Endocrinol, 17: 197-205,1988.
34. Messent J, Jones S, Wiseman M, Viberti GC: Glomerular hyperfiltration and albuminuria A 8 year prospective study. Diabetologia (Suppl 2), 34: AI, 1991 (Abstract).
35. Lafferty HM, Brenner BM: Are glomerular hypertension and "hypertrophy" independent risk factors for progression of renal disease? Sem Nephrol, 3: 294-304, 1990.
36. Viberti GC, Pickup JC, Jarrett RJ, Keen H: Effect of control of blood glucose on urinary excretion of albumin and b2 microglobulin in insulin-dependent diabetics. N Engl J Med, 300: 638-641, 1979.
37. Østerby R, Gundersen HJG: Glomerular size and structure in diabetes mellitus: 1. Early abnormalities. Diabetologia, 11: 225-229, 1975.

38. Østerby R: Early phases in the development of diabetic glomerulopathy: Quantitative electron microscopic study. Acta Med Scand, S574 (Suppl): 3-82, 1974.
39. Østerby R: Basement membrane morphology in diabetes mellitus.In: "Diabetes Mellitus: theory and practice" (Eds M Ellenberg, H Rigkin), Medical Examination Publishing, New York, 1983, pp 323-341.
40. Østerby R: A quantitative electron microscopic study of mesangial regions in glomeruli from patients with short term juvenile diabetes mellitus. Lab Invest, 29: 99-110, 1973.
41. Vittinghus E, Mogensen CE: Albumin excretion and renal hemodynamic response to physical exercise in normal and diabetic man. Scand J Clin Lab Invest, 41: 627-632, 1981.
42. Gatling W, Knight C, Mullee MA, Hill RD: Microalbuminuria in diabetes: a population study of the prevalence and assessment of three screening tests. Diabetic Med, 5: 343-347, 1988.
43. Rowe DJF, Bagga H, Betts PB: Normal variations in rate of albumin excretion and albumin to creatinine ratios in overnight and daytime urine collections in non-diabetic children. Br Med J, 291: 693-694,1985.
44. Chachati A, von Frenckell R, Foidart-Willems J, Godon JP, Lefèbvre PJ. Variability of albumin excretion in insulin-dependent diabetics, Diabetic Med, 4: 437-440, 1987.
45. Cohen DL, Close CF, Viberti GC: The variability of overnight urinary albumin excretion in insulin-dependent diabetic and normal subjects. Diabetic Med, 4: 437-440, 1987.
46. Parving H-H, Hommel E, Mathiesen E, Skøtt P, Edsberg B, Bahnsen M, Lauritzen M, Hougaard P, Lauritzen E: Prevalence of microalbuminuria, arterial hypertension, retinopathy and neuropathy in patients with insulin-dependent diabetes. Br Med J, 296: 156-160,1988.
47. Viberti G, Keen H: The patterns of proteinuria in diabetes mellitus: relevance to pathogenesis and prevention of diabetic nephropathy. Diabetes, 33: 686-692, 1984.
48. Mogensen CE: Microalbuminuria as a predictor of clinical diabetic nephropathy. Kidney Int, 31: 673-689, 1987.
49. Parving H, Øxenbøll B, Svendsen PA, Christiansen JS, Andersen AR: Early detection of patients at risk of developing diabetic nephropathy: a longitudinal study of urinary albumin excretion. Acta Endocrinol (Copenhagen), 100: 550-555, 1982.
50. Mathiesen ER, Øxenbøll B, Johansen K, Svendsen PA, Deckert T. Incipient nephropathy in type 1 (insulin-dependent) diabetes. Diabetologia, 26: 406-410, 1984.
51. Viberti GC, Hill RD, Jarrett RJ, Argyropoulous A, Mahmud U, Keen H: Microalbuminuria as a predictor of clinical nephropathy in insulin-dependent diabetes mellitus. Lancet, I: 1430-1432, 1982.
52. Borch-Johnsen K: Incidence of nephropathy in insulin-dependent diabetes as related to mortality. In: "The kidney and hypertension in diabetes mellitus" (Ed CE Mogensen), Topics in Renal Medicine (Series Ed VE Andreucci), Martinus Nijhoff, Boston, 1988, pp 33-40.
53. Nørgaard K, Feldt-Rasmussen B, Borch-Johnsen K, Saelan H, Deckert T: Prevalence of hypertension in type 1 (insulin-dependent) diabetes mellitus. Diabetologia, 33: 407-410, 1990.
54. Chavers BM, Bilous RW, Ellis EN, Steffes MW, Mauer SM: Glomerular lesions and urinary albumin excretion in type 1 diabetes without overt proteinuria. N Engl J Med, 320: 966-970, 1989.
55. Mogensen CE: Long term anti-hypertensive treatment inhibiting progression of diabetic nephropathy. Br Med J, 285: 685-688, 1982.
56. Mauer SM, Steffes MW, Ellis EN, Sutherland DE, Brown DM, Goetz FC: Structural-functional relationships in diabetic nephropathy. J Clin Invest, 74: 1143-1155, 1984.
57. Steffes MW, Østerby R, Chavers B, Mauer SM: Mesangial expansion as a central mechanism for loss of kidney function in diabetic patients. Diabetes, 38: 1077-1081, 1989.
58. Gellman DD, Pirani CL, Soothill JF, Muehrcke RC, Maduros W, Kark RM: Structure and function in diabetic nephropathy. The importance of diffuse glomerulosclerosis. Diabetes, 8: 251-256, 1959.
59. Harris MI, Hadden WC, Knowles WC, Bennett PH: Prevalence of diabetes and impaired glucose tolerance and plasma glucose levels in the United States population aged 20-74 years. Diabetes, 36: 523-534, 1987.
60. Marks HH: Longevity and mortality of diabetics. Am J Public Health, 55: 416-422, 1965.
61. Herman WH, Teutsch SM: Kidney disease associated with diabetes. Diabetes in America. Washington DC, US Govt Printing Office, pp 1-31, 1985 (NIH publication no. 85-1468).
62. Damsgaard EM, Mogensen CE: Microalbuminuria in elderly hyperglycemic patients and controls. Diabetic Med, 3: 430-435, 1986.

63. Fabre J, Balant LP, Dayer PG, Fox HM, Vernet AT: The kidney in maturity onset diabetes: a clinical study of 510 patients. Kidney Int, 21: 730-738, 1982.
64. Hasslacher CH, Ritz E, Wahl P: Similar risks of nephropathy in patients with type I or type II diabetes mellitus. Nephrol Dial Transplant, 4: 859-863, 1989.
65. Kunzelman CL, Knowles WC, Pettit DJ, Bennett PH: Incidence of proteinuria in type 2 diabetes in the Pima Indians. Kidney Int, 35: 681-687, 1989.
66. Knowles WC, Bennett PH, Hamman RF, Miller M: Diabetes incidence and prevalence in Pima Indians: a 19-fold greater incidence than in Rochester, Minnesota: Am J Epidemiol, 108: 497-505, 1978.
67. Nelson RG, Kunzelman CL, Pettit DJ, Saad MF, Bennett PH, Knowles WC: Albuminuria in type 2 (non-insulin dependent) diabetes mellitus and impaired glucose tolerance in Pima Indians. Diabetologia, 32: 870-876, 1989.
68. Nelson RG, Newman JM, Knowles WC, Sievers ML, Kunzelman CL, Pettit DJ, Moffet CD, Teutsch SM, Bennett PH: Incidence of end-stage renal disease in type 2 (non-insulin dependent) diabetes mellitus in Pima Indians. Diabetologia, 31: 730-736, 1988.
69. Ritz E, Nowack D, Fliser D, Koch M, Tschope W: Type II diabetes mellitus: Is the renal risk adequately appreciated? Nephrol Dial Transplant, 6: 679-682,1991.
70. Cowie CC, Port FK, Wolfe RA, Savage PJ, Moll PP, Hawthorne VM: Disparities in incidence of diabetic end stage renal disease according to race and type of diabetes. N Engl J Med, 321: 1074-1079, 1989.
71. Pugh JA, Stern MP, Haffner SM, Eifler CW, Zapata M: Excess incidence of end stage renal disease in Mexican Americans. Am J Epidemiol, 127: 135-144, 1988.
72. Nolph KD, Lundblad AS, Novak JW: Current concepts: Continuous ambulatory peritoneal dialysis. N Engl J Med, 318: 1595-1600, 1988.
73. Friedman EA: Diabetic nephropathy. Strategies in prevention and management. Kidney Int, 21: 780-791, 1982.
74. Mogensen CE: Comparative renal pathophysiology relevant to IDDM and NIDDM patients. Diab Metab Rev, 4: 453-483, 1988.
75. Friedman EA: No supranormal GFR in type II diabetes. Kidney Int, 31: 179, 1988 (Abstract).
76. Schmitz A, Hvid-Hansen H, Christensen T: Kidney function in newly diagnosed type 2 (non-insulin dependent) diabetes before and after treatment. Diabetologia, 32: 434-439, 1989.
77. Schmitz AH, Christensen T, Taagehoej, Jenson F: Glomerular filtration rate and kidney volume in normoalbuminuric non-insulin dependent diabetes: lack of glomerular hyperfiltration and renal hypertrophy in uncomplicated NIDDM. Scand J Clin Lab Invest, 49: 103-108, 1989.
78. Schmitz A, Christensen T, Møller A, Mogensen CE: Kidney function and cardiovascular risk factors in non-insulin dependent diabetics (NIDDM) with microalbuminuria. J Int Med, 228: 347-352, 1990.
79. Myers BD, Nelson RG, Williams GW, Bennett PH, Hardy SA, Berg RL, Loon NL, Knowler WC, Mitch WE: Glomerular function in Pima Indians with non-insulin dependent diabetes mellitus of recent onset. J Clin Invest, 88: 524-530, 1991.
80. Lebovitz HE, Palmisano J: Cross-sectional analysis of renal function in black Americans with non-insulin dependent diabetes mellitus. Diabetes Care, 13 (Suppl 4): 1186-90, 1990.
81. Palmisano JJ, Lebovitz HE: Renal function in black Americans with type II diabetes. J Diabetic Complications, 3: 40-44, 1989.
82. Palmisano J, Sachmechi I: Renal function in type 2 diabetes. Diabetes, 36 (Suppl 2): 206A, 1987 (Abstract).
83. Bérionade V: Creatinine clearance in non-insulin dependent diabetes mellitus. Kidney Int, 31: 179, 1986 (Abstract).
84. Bruton BL, Perusek MC, Lancaster JL, Kopp DT, Tuttle KR: Effects of glycemia on basal and amino-acid stimulated (AA-S) renal hemodynamics and kidney size in non-insulin dependent diabetes (NIDD). JASN, 1: 623, 1990 (Abstract).
85. Nowack R, Raum E, Blum W, Ritz E: Renal hemodynamics in recent onset type II diabetes. Am J Kid Dis (in press).
86. Davies DF, Shock NW: Age changes in glomerular filtration rate, effective renal plasma flow, and tubular excretory capacity in adult males. J Clin Invest, 29: 496-502, 1950.
87. Rowe JW, Andres R, Tobin JD, Norris AH, Shock NW: The effect of age on creatinine clearance in men: a cross-sectional and longitudinal study. J Gerontol, 31: 155-163, 1976.

88. Lindeman RD, Tobin JD, Shock NW: Longitudinal studies on the rate of decline in renal function with age. J Am Geriat Soc, 33: 278-285, 1985.
89. Takazakura E, Wasabu N, Handa A, Takada A, Shinoda A, Takeuchi J: Intrarenal vascular changes with age and disease. Kidney Int, 2: 224-230, 1972.
90. Uusitupa M, Siitonen O, Penttila I, Aro A, Pyörälä K: Proteinuria in newly diagnosed type II diabetic patients. Diabetes Care, 10: 191-194, 1987.
91. Gall MA, Rossing p, Skøtt P, Damsbo P, Vaag A, Bech K, Dejgaard A, Lauritzen M, Lauritzen E, Hougaard P, Beck-Nielsen H, Parving H-H: Prevalence of micro- and macroalbuminuria, arterial hypertension, retinopathy and large vessel disease in European type 2 (non-insulin dependent) diabetic patients. Diabetologia, 34: 655-661, 1991.
92. Parving H-H, Gall M-A, Skøtt P, Jørgensen HE, Jørgensen F, Larsen S: Prevalence and causes of albuminuria in non-insulin dependent diabetic (NIDDM) patients Kidney Int, 37: 243, 1990 (Abstract).
93. Mogensen CE: Microalbuminuria predicts clinical proteinuria and early mortality in maturity-onset diabetes. N Engl J Med, 310: 356-360, 1984.
94. Mogensen CE: A complete screening of urinary albumin concentration in an unselected diabetic outpatient clinic population (1082 patients). Diabetic Nephropathy, 2: 11-18, 1983.
95. Jerums G, Cooper ME, Seeman E, Murray RML, McNeil J: Spectrum of proteinuria in type I and type II diabetes. Diabetes Care, 10: 419-427, 1987.
96. Freidman R, Gross JL: Evolution of glomerular filtration rate in proteinuric NIDDM patients. Diabetes Care, 14: 355-359, 1991.
97. Stein ACR: Estudio comparativo e evolutivo de pacientes diabéticos com diferentes graus de proteinuria. In: "Curso de Pos-Gradua-çao em Medicina: Nefrologia". Universidade Federal de Rio Grande do Sul, Porto Alegre, Brasil, 1984, pp 85-90.
98. Yudkin JS, Forrest FD, Jackson CA: Microalbuminuria as a predictor of vascular disease in non-diabetic subjects. Lancet, I: 530-533, 1988.
99. Schmitz A, Vaeth M: Microalbuminuria- a major risk factor in non-insulin dependent diabetes. A 10 year follow-up study of 503 patients. Diabetic Med, 5: 126-134, 1988.
100. Jarrett RJ, Viberti GC, Argyropoulos A, Hill RD, Mahmud U, Murrells TJ: Microalbuminuria predicts mortality in non-insulin dependent diabetes. Diabetic Med, 1: 17-19, 1984.
101. Douglas JG: Hypertension and diabetes in blacks. Diabetes Care, 13 (Suppl 4): 1191-1195, 1990.
102. Reubi FC, Franz KA, Horber F: Hypertension as related to renal function in diabetes mellitus. Hypertension, 7 (Suppl II): 21-28, 1985.
103. Jerums G, Cooper ME, Seeman E, Murray RM, McNeil JJ: Comparison of early renal dysfunction in type I and type II diabetes: differing associations with blood pressure and glycemic control. Diab Res Clin Prac, 4: 133-141, 1988.
104. Jarrett RJ: Hypertension in diabetic patients and differences between insulin-dependent diabetes mellitus and non-insulin dependent diabetes mellitus. Am J Kid Dis, 13: 14-16, 1989.
105. Jarrett RJ: Hypertension in glucose intolerance and diabetes. J Int Med, 229 (Suppl 2): 85-88, 1991.
106. Standl E, Steigler H, Roth R, Shultz K, Lemacher K: On the impact of hypertension on the prognosis of NIDDM. Results of the Schwabing-GP program. Diab Metabol, 15: 352-358, 1989.
107. Panzram G: Mortality and survival in type 2 (non-insulin dependent) diabetes mellitus. Diabetologia, 30: 123-131, 1987.
108. Ritz E, Hasslacher C, Beutel G: Hypertension and diabetic nephropathy. J Nephrol, 1: 11-15, 1991.
109. DeFronzo RJ, Ferranini E: Insulin resistance: A multi-faceted syndrome responsible for NIDDM, obesity, hypertension, dyslipidemia and atherosclerotic cardiovascular disease. Diabetes Care, 14: 173-194, 1991.
110. Viberti GC, Walker JD: Diabetic nephropathy: Etiology and prevention. Diab/Metab Rev, 4: 147-162, 1988.
111. Weidmann P, Beretta-Piccoli C, Trost BN: Pressure factors and responsiveness in hypertension accompanying diabetes mellitus. Hypertension, 7 (Suppl 2): 33-42, 1985.
112. Cohen D, Dodds R, Viberti GC: Effect of protein restriction in insulin-dependent diabetics at risk of nephropathy. Br Med J, 294: 795-798, 1987.
113. Christensen CK, Mogensen CE: The course of incipient diabetic nephropathy: studies of albumin excretion and blood pressure. Diabetic Med, 2: 97-102, 1985.

114. Parving H-H, Smidt UM, Friisberg B, Bonnevie-Nielsen V, Andersen AR: A prospective study of glomerular filtration rate and arterial blood pressure in insulin-dependent diabetics with diabetic nephropathy. Diabetologia, 20: 457-461, 1981.
115. Zatz R, Meyer TW, Rennke HG, Brenner BM: Predominance of hemodynamic rather than metabolic factors in the pathogenesis of diabetic nephropathy. Proc Nat Acad Sci USA, 82: 5963-5967, 1985.
116. Hostetter TH, Troy JL, Brenner BM: Glomerular hemodynamics in experimental diabetes. Kidney Int, 19: 410-415, 1981.
117. Hostetter TH: Pathogenesis of diabetic glomerulopathy: Hemodynamic considerations. Sem Nephrol, 10: 219-227, 1990.
118. Bérionade VC, Lefèbvre R, Falardeau P: Unilateral nodular diabetic glomerulosclerosis: Recurrence of an experiment of nature. Am J Nephrol, 7: 55-59, 1987.
119. Working Group on Hypertension in Diabetes. Statement on hypertension in diabetes mellitus. Final report. Arch Int Med, 147: 830-842, 1987.
120. Mogensen CE: Renal function changes in diabetes. Diabetes, 25: 872-879, 1976.
121. Parving H-H, Andersen AR, Smidt UM, Svendsen PAA: Early aggressive anti-hypertensive therapy reduces rate of decline in kidney function in diabetic nephropathy. Lancet, II: 1175-1179, 1983.
122. Parving H-H, Andersen AR, Smidt UM, Hommel E, Mathiesen ER, Svendsen PA: Effect of antihypertensive treatment on kidney function in diabetic nephropathy. Br Med J, 294: 1443-1447, 1987.
123. Parving H-H, Andersen AR, Hommel E, Smidt U: Effects of long term antihypertensive treatment on kidney function in diabetic nephropathy. Hypertension, 7 (Suppl II): 114-117, 1985.
124. Christensen CK, Mogensen CE: Acute and long term effect of antihypertensive treatment on exercise-induced albuminuria in incipient diabetic nephropathy. Scand J Clin Lab Invest, 46: 553-559,1986.
125. Mathiesen ER, Borch-Johnsen K, Jensen DV, Deckert T: Improved survival in patients with diabetic nephropathy. Diabetologia, 32: 884-886, 1989.
126. Krolewski AS, Canessa M, Warren JH, Laffel LMB, Christlieb AR, Knowles WC, Rand LI: Predisposition to hypertension and susceptibility to renal disease in insulin-dependent diabetes mellitus. N Engl J Med, 318: 140-145, 1988.
127. Mangili R, Bending JJ, Scott G, Li LK, Gupta A, Viberti G: Increased sodium-lithium countertransport activity on red cells of patients with insulin-dependent diabetes and nephropathy. N Engl J Med, 318: 146-150, 1988.
128. Viberti G, Keen H, Wiseman MJ: Raised arterial pressure in parents of proteinuric insulin-dependent diabetics. Br Med J, 295: 515-519, 1987.
129. Ibsen KK, Jensen HA, Wieth JC, Funder J: Essential hypertension: Sodium-lithium countertransport in erythrocytes from patients and from children having one hypertensive parent. Hypertension, 4: 703-709, 1982.
130. Carr S, Mbanya JC, Thomas T, Keavey P, Taylor R, Alberti KGMM, Wilkinson R. Increase in glomerular filtration rate in patients with insulin-dependent diabetes and elevated erythrocyte Na-Li countertransport. N Engl J Med, 322: 500-505, 1990.
131. Jensen JJ, Mathiesen ER, Norgaard K, Hommel E, Borch-Johnsen K, Funder J, Brahm J, Parving H-H, Deckert T: Increased blood pressure and sodium-lithium countertransport activity are not inherited in diabetic nephropathy. Diabetologia, 33: 619-624, 1990.
132. Rutherford PA, Thomas TH, Wilkinson R: The mechanism of raised sodium-lithium countertransport in Type I diabetes mellitus is different from that in essential hypertension. Diabetic Med, 7 (Suppl 2): 1A, 1990 (Abstract).
133. Baba T, Tomiyama T, Murabayashi S, Takebe K: Renal effects of nicardipine, a calcium antagonist, in hypertensive type 2 (non-insulin dependent) diabetic patients with and without nephropathy. Eur J Clin Pharmacol, 38: 425-429, 1990.
134. D'Angelo A, Giannini S, Benetollo P, Castrignano R, Lodetti MG, Malvasi L, Pati T, Crepaldi G: Efficacy of captopril in hypertensive diabetic patients. Am J Med, 84 (Suppl 3A): 155-158, 1988.
135. Romero I, Salinas I, Teixidó J, Lucas A, Felip A, Sanmarti A: Long term follow up of the effect captopril on severe proteinuria in hypertensive diabetic patients. J Human Hypertension, 4: 671-675, 1990.

136. Valvo F, Bedogna V, Casagrande P, Antiga L, Zamboui M, Bonmartini F, Oldrizzi L, Rugin C, Maschio G: Captopril in patients with type 2 diabetes and renal insufficiency: systemic and renal hemodynamic alterations. Am J Med, 85: 344-348, 1988.
137. Cheng IKP, Ma JTC, Yeh GR, Chan MK: Comparison of captopril and enalapril in the treatment of hypertension in patients with non-insulin dependent diabetes mellitus and nephropathy. Int Urol Nephrol, 22: 295- 303, 1990.
138. Hasslacher CH, Borgholtz G, Ritz E, Wahl P: Impact of hypertension on prognosis in insulin-dependent diabetes mellitus. Diab Métab (Paris), 15: 338-342, 1989.
139. Zatz R, Dunn BR, Meyer TW, Andersen S, Rennke HG, Brenner BM: Prevention of diabetic glomerulopathy by pharmacological amelioration of glomerular capillary hypertension. J Clin Invest, 77: 1925-1930, 1986.
140. Fujihara CK, Padilha RM, Zatz R: Glomerular abnormalities in long term experimental diabetes. Role of hemodynamic and non-hemodynamic factors and effect of antihypertensive therapy. Diabetes, 41: 286-293, 1992.
141. Bank N, Klose R, Aynedjian HS, Nguyen D, Sablay LB: Evidence against increased glomerular pressure initiating diabetic nephropathy. Kidney Int, 31: 898-905, 1987.
142. Rabkin R, Petersen J, Kitaji J, Marck B, Murphy W, Muirhead EE: Effect of antihypertensive therapy on the kidney in spontaneously hypertensive rats with diabetes. Kidney Int, 25: 205, 1984 (Abstract).
143. Fujihara CK, Padilha RM, Santos MM, Zatz K: Role of glomerular hypertension, glomerular hypertrophy and lipid deposition in the genesis of glomerulosclerosis of experimental diabetes. Kidney Int, 37: 506, 1990 (Abstract).
144. Andersen S, Rennke HG, Garcia DL, Brenner BM: Short- and long-term effects of antihypertensive therapy in the diabetic rat. Kidney Int, 36: 526-536, 1989.
145. Fogo A, Yoshida Y, Ichikawa I: Angiotensin converting enzyme inhibition (CEI) suppresses accelerated growth of glomerular cells *in vivo* and *vitro*. Kidney Int, 33, 296, 1986 (Abstract).
146. Galler M, Backenroth R, Folkert VW, Schlondorff D: Effect of converting enzyme inhibitors on prostaglandin synthesis by isolated glomerular and aortic strips from rats. J Pharmacol Exp Ther, 220: 23-28, 1982.
147. Homma T, Ichikawa I, Hoover RL: Prostaglandins of mesangium origin inhibit mesangial cell proliferation and matrix synthesis. Kidney Int, 33: 268, 1988 (Abstract).
148. Morelli E, Loon N, Meyer T, Peters W, Myers BD: Effects of converting-enzyme inhibition on barrier function in diabetic glomerulopathy. Diabetes, 39: 76-82, 1990.
149. Pollare T, Lithell H Berne C: A comparison of the effect of hydrochlorothiazide and captopril on glucose and lipid metabolism in patients with hypertension. N Engl J Med, 321: 868-873, 1989.
150. Rett K, Jauch KW, Wicklmayr M, Dietze G, Fink E, Mehnert H: Angiotensin converting enzyme inhibitors in diabetes: Experimental and human experience. Postgrad Med J, 62 (Suppl 2): 59-64, 1986.
151. Hommel E, Parving H-H, Mathiesen E, Edsberg B, Damkjæ Nielsen M, Giese J: Effect of captopril on kidney function in insulin-dependent diabetics with nephropathy, Br Med J, 293: 467-470, 1986.
152. Marre M, Leblanc H, Suarez l, Thanh-Tam G, Menard J, Possa P: Converting enzyme inhibition and kidney function in normotensive diabetic patients with persistent microalbuminuria. Br Med J, 294: 1448-1452, 1987.
153. Parving H-H, Hommel E, Smidt UM: Protection of kidney function and decrease in albuminuria by captopril in insulin dependent diabetics with nephropathy. Br Med J, 297: 1086-1091, 1988.
154. Mimran A, Insua A, Ribstein J, Monnier L, Bringer J, Mirouze J: Contrasting effects of captopril and nifedipine in normotensive patients with incipient diabetic nephropathy. J Hypertension, 6: 919-923, 1988.
155. Parving H-H, Hommel E, Nielsen MD, Giese J: Effect of captopril on blood pressure and kidney function in normotensive insulin-dependent diabetics with nephropathy. Br Med J, 299: 533-536, 1989.
156. Weigmann TB, Herron KG, Chonko AM, MacDougall ML, Moore WV: Effect of angiotensin-converting enzyme inhibition on renal function and albuminuria in normotensive type 1 diabetic patients. Diabetes, 41: 62-67, 1992.
157. Taguma Y, Kitamoto Y, Futaki G, Ueda H, Monma H, Ishizaki M, Takahashi H, Sekino H, Sasaki Y: Effect of captopril on heavy proteinuria in azotemic diabetics. N Engl J Med, 313: 1617-1620, 1985.

158. Bjorck S, Nyberg G, Mulec H, Goran G, Herletz H, Aurell M: Beneficial effect of angiotensin converting enzyme inhibition on renal function in patients with diabetic nephropathy. Br Med J, 293: 471-474, 1986.
159. Holdaas H, Hartmann A, Lien MG, Nilsen L, Fauchal P, Jervell J, Berg KJ: Lisinopril, but not nifedipine, reduces urinary albumin excretion in diabetic nephropathy. Kidney Int, 37: 239, 1990 (Abstract).
160. Bjorck S, Mulec H, Johnsen SA, Nyberg G, Aurell M: Enalapril but not metoprolol reduces proteinuria in diabetic nephropathy. Kidney Int, 37: 236, 1990 (Abstract).
161 Henry RR, Wallace P, Olefsky JM: Effects of weight loss on mechanisms of hyperglycemia in obese non-insulin dependent diabetes mellitus. Diabetes, 35: 990-998, 1986.
162. Schneider SH, Vitug A, Ruderman SV: Atherosclerosis and physical activity. Diab/Metab Rev, 1: 513-553, 1986.
163. Maschio G, Oldrizi L, Rugiu C: The effects of dietary protein restriction on the course of early chronic failure. In: "The progressive nature of renal disease". Contemporary issues in Nephrology, vol 14 (Eds Mitch WE, Brenner BM, Stein JH), Churchill-Livingstone, New York, 1986, pp 203-210.
164. Bosch JP, Sacaggi A, Lauer A, Ronco C, Belledonne M, Glabman S: Renal functional reserve in humans. Am J Med, 75: 943-950, 1983.
165. Kupin WL, Cortes P, Dumler S, Feldcamp CS, Kilates MC, Levin NW: Effect on renal function on change from high to moderate protein intake in type 1 diabetic patients. Diabetes, 36: 73-79, 1987.
166. Krolewski AS, Warram JH, Christlieb AR, Busick EJ, Kahn CR: The changing natural history of nephropathy in type 1 diabetes. Am J Med, 78: 785-794, 1985.
167. Tuttle KR, Bruton L, Perusek MC, Lancaster JL, Kopp DT, DeFronzo R: Effect of strict glycemic control on renal hemodynamic response to amino acids and renal enlargement in insulin-dependent in insulin-dependent diabetes mellitus. N Engl J Med, 324: 1626-1632, 1991.
168. Wen S-F, Huang T-P, Moorthy AV: Effects of low-protein diet on experimental diabetic nephropathy in the rat. J Lab Clin Med, 106: 589-597, 1985.
169. Rennke HG, Sandstrom D, Zatz R, Meyer TW, Cowan RS, Brenner BM. The role of dietary protein in the development of glomerular structural abnormalities in long term experimental diabetes mellitus. Kidney Int, 29: 289, 1986 (Abstract).
170. Bending JJ, Dodds RA, Keen H, Viberti GC: Renal response to restricted protein intake in diabetic nephropathy. Diabetes, 37: 1641-1646, 1988.
171. Zeller KR, Jacobsen H: Reducing dietary protein intake to retard progression of diabetic nephropathy. Am J Kid Dis, 13: 17-19, 1989.
172. El Nahas AM, Coles GA: Dietary treatment of chronic renal failure: ten unanswered questions. Lancet, I: 597-600, 1986.
173. Barsotti G, Morelli E, Gianonni A, Guiducci A, Lupetti S, Giovanetti S: Restricted phosphorus and nitrogen intake to slow the progression of chronic renal failure: A controlled trial. Kidney Int, 16 (Suppl): S278-S284, 1983.
174. Mitch WE, Walser M, Steinman TI, Hill S, Zeger S, Tungsanga K: The effects of a keto-amino acid supplement to a restricted diet on the progression of chronic renal failure. N Engl J Med, 311: 623-629, 1984.
175. Rosman JB, ter Wee PM, Meijer S, Piers-Becht TPM, Sluiter WJ, Donker AJM: Prospective randomised trial of early dietary protein restriction in chronic renal failure. Lancet, II: 1291-1296, 1984.
176. Azevedo MJ, Padilha LM, Gross JL: A short-term low-protein diet reduces glomerular filtration rate in insulin-dependent diabetes mellitus patients. Brazilian J Med Biol Res, 23: 647-654, 1990.
177. Rudberg S, Dalquist G, Aperia A, Persson B: Reduction of protein intake decreases glomerular filtration rate in young type 1 (insulin-dependent) diabetic patients mainly in hyperfiltering patients. Diabetologia, 31: 878-883, 1988.
178. Pedersen MM, Mogensen CE, Jørgensen SF, Møller B, Lykhe G, Pederson O: Renal effects from limitation of high dietary protein in normoalbuminuric diabetic patients. Kidney Int, Suppl 27: S115-S121, 1989.
179. Zeller, Whittaker E, Sullivan L, Raskin P, Jacobsen HR: Effect of restricting dietary protein on the progression of renal failure in patients with insulin-dependent diabetes mellitus. N Engl Med, 324: 78-84, 1991.

180. Evanoff G, Thompson C, Brown J, Weinman E: Prolonged dietary protein restriction in diabetic nephropathy. Arch Int Med, 149: 1129-1133, 1989.
181. Walker JD, Bending JJ, Dodds RA, Mattock MB, Murrells TJ, Keen H, Viberti GC: Restriction of dietary protein and progression of renal failure in diabetic nephropathy. Lancet, II: 1411-1414, 1989.
182. Viberti GC, Dodds RA, Bending JJ: Non-glycemic intervention in diabetic nephropathy: The role of dietary protein intake. In: "The kidney and hypertension in diabetes" (Ed CE Mogensen), Topics in Renal Medicine (Series Ed VE Andreucci), Martinus Nijhoff, Boston, 1988, pp 205-215.
183. Evanoff GV, Thompson CS, Brown J, Weinman EJ: The effect of dietary protein restriction on the progression of diabetic nephropathy: a 12 month follow-up. Arch Int Med, 147: 492-495, 1987.
184. Wiseman MJ, Bognetti E, Dodds R, Keen H, Viberti GC: Changes in renal function in response to protein restricted diet in type 1 (insulin-dependent) diabetic subjects. Diabetologia, 30 154-159, 1987.
185. Barsotti G, Ciardella F, Morelli E, Cupisti A, Mantovanelli A, Giovanetti S: Nutritional treatment of renal failure in type 1 diabetes. Clin Nephrol, 29: 280-287, 1988.
186. Anderson S: Low protein diets and diabetic nephropathy. Sem Nephrol, 3: 287-293, 1990.
187. Kaysen G, Gambertoglio J, Jiminez I, Jones H, Huthchinson FN: Effects of dietary protein intake on albumin homeostasis in nephrotic patients. Kidney Int, 29: 572-577, 1986.
188. El Nahas AM, Masters-Thomas A, Brady SA, Farrington K, Wilkinson V, Hilson AJW, Varghese Z, Moorhead JF: Selective effects of low protein diets in renal diseases. Br Med J, 289: 1337-1341, 1984.
189. Shichiri M, Nishio Y, Ogura M, Marumo F: Effect of low-protein, very-low-phosphorus diet on diabetic renal insufficiency with proteinuria. Am J Kid Dis, 18: 26-32, 1991.
190. Wylie-Rosett J: Evaluation of protein in dietary management of diabetes mellitus. Diabetes Care, 11: 143-148, 1988.
191. Fox CJ, Darby SC, Ireland JT, Sönksen PH: Blood glucose control and glomerular capillary basement membrane thickening in experimental diabetes. Br Med J, 2: 605-607, 1977.
192. Mauer SF, Steffes MW, Sutherland D, Najarian J, Michael AF, Brown DM: Studies of the rate of regression of the glomerular lesions in diabetic rats treated with pancreatic islet transplantation. Diabetes, 24: 280-285, 1975.
193. Weil R, Nozawara M, Koss M, Weber C, Reemtsma K, McIntosh RM: Pancreatic transplantation in diabetic rats: renal function, morphology, ultrastructure and immunohistology. Surgery, 78: 142-148, 1975.
194. Mauer SM, Steffes MW, Brown DM: Animal models of diabetic nephropathy. Adv Nephrol, 8: 280-285, 1975.
195. Skyler JS: Complications of diabetes mellitus: relationship to metabolic dysfunction. Diabetes Care, 2: 499-509, 1979.
196. Rosenstock J, Friberg T, Raskin P: Effect of glycemic control on microvascular complications in patients with type I diabetes mellitus. Am J Med, 81: 1012-1018, 1986.
197. Hasslacher C, Ritz E: Effect of control of diabetes mellitus on progression of renal failure. Kidney Int, 32 (Suppl 22): 53-56, 1987.
198. Mathiesen ER, Ronn B, Jensen T, Storm B, Deckert T: Microalbuminaria is prior to elevation of blood pressure in diabetic nephropathy. In: "First Workshop on Blood Pressure and Diabetic Nephropathy: Pathogenesis and treatment". EDNSG, Pisa, 1989 (Abstract).
199. Mauer SM, Steffes MW, Brown DM: The kidney in diabetes. Am J Med, 70: 603-612, 1981.
200. Nyberg G, Bhlomé G, Nordén G: Input of metabolic control on progression of clinical diabetic nephropathy. Diabetologia, 30: 82-86, 1987.
201. Abouna GM, Al-Adnani MS, Kremer GD, Kumar SA, Daddah SK, Kusma G: Reversal of diabetic nephropathy in human cadaveric kidneys after transplantation into non-diabetic recipients. Lancet, II: 1274-1276, 1983.
202. Abouna G, Adnani MS, Kumar MS, Samhan SA: Fate of transplanted kidneys with diabetic nephropathy. Lancet, I: 622-624, 1986.
203. Christensen CK, Christiansen JS, Schmitz A, Christensen T, Hermansen K, Mogensen CE: Effect of continuous subcutaneous insulin infusion on kidney function and size in IDDM patients. A 2 year controlled study. J Diab Compl, 1: 91-95, 1987.
204. Beck-Nielsen H, Richelsen B, Mogensen CE, Olsen T, Ehlers N, Nielsen CB, Charles P: Effect of insulin pump treatment for one year on renal function and retinal morphology in patients with IDDM. Diabetes Care, 85: 585-589, 1984.

205. Mogensen CE: Prevention and treatment of renal disease in insulin-dependent diabetes mellitus. Sem Nephrol, 10: 260-273, 1990.
206. Drury PL, Watkins PJ, Viberti GC, Walker JD: Diabetic nephropathy. Br Med Bull, 45: 127-147,1989.
207. Tamborlane WV, Puklin JE, Bergman M, Verdonck C, Rudolf MC, Felig P, Genel L, Sherwin R: Long term improvement of metabolic control with the insulin pump does not reverse diabetic microangiopathy. Diabetes Care, 5: 58-64, 1982.
208. Viberti GC, Bilous RW, Mackintosh B, Bending JJ, Keen H: Long term correction of hyperglycemia and progression of renal failure in insulin dependent diabetes. Br Med J, 286: 598-602,1983.
209. Bending JJ, Viberti GC, Watkins PJ, Keen H: Intermittent clinical proteinuria and renal function in diabetes: Evolution and the effect of glycemic control. Br Med J, 292: 83-86, 1986.
210. The Kroc Collaboration Study Group: Blood glucose control and the evolution of diabetic retinopathy and albuminuria. A preliminary multicenter trial. N Engl J Med, 311: 365-372, 1984.
211. Feldt-Rasmussen B, Mathiesen E, Deckert T: Effect of two years of strict metabolic control on the progression of incipient nephropathy in insulin-dependent diabetes. Lancet, II: 1300-1304, 1986.
212. Rosenstock J, Raskin P: The effect of glycemic control on urinary excretion rate (AER) in type I diabetes mellitus. Diabetes, 36: 425, 1987 (Abstract).
213. Dahl-Jorgensen K, Hanssen KF, Kierulf P, Bjøro T, Sandvik L, Aagenaes O: Reduction of urinary albumin excretion after 4 years of continuous subcutaneous insulin infusion in insulin-dependent diabetes mellitus. Acta Endocrinol, 117: 19-25, 1988.
214. Feldt-Rasmussen B, Mathiesen ER, Jensen T, Lauritzen T, Deckert T: Effect of improved metabolic control on kidney function in type I (insulin-dependent) diabetic patients: an update of the Steno studies. Diabetologia, 34: 164-170, 1991.
215. Lauritzen T, Frost-Larsen K, Larsen HW, Deckert T: Steno Study Group. 2 years experience with continuous subcutaneous insulin infusion in relation to retinopathy and neuropathy. Diabetes, 34 (Suppl 3): 74-79, 1985.
216. Reichard P, Berglund B, Britz A, Cars I, Nilsson BY, Rosenqvist U: Intensified conventional insulin treatment retards the microvascular complications of insulin-dependent diabetes mellitus (IDDM): the Stockholm Diabetes Intervention Study (SDIS) after 5 years. J Int Med, 230: 101-108, 1991.
217. The DCCT Research Group: The Diabetes Control and Complications Trial (DCCT): design and methodologic considerations for the feasibility phase. Diabetes, 35: 530-545, 1986.
218. The DCCT Research Group: Weight gain associated with intensive therapy in the Diabetes Control and Complications Trial. Diabetes Care, 11: 567-573, 1988.
219. Ballard DJ, Humphrey LL, Melton LJ 3d, Frohnert PP, Chu PC, O'Fallon WM, Palumbo PJ Epidemiology of persistent proteinuria in type II diabetes mellitus. Diabetes, 37: 405-412, 1988.
220. Takazakura E, Nakamoto Y, Hayakawa H, Kawai H, Muramoto S, Yoshida K, Shimizu M, Shinoda A, Takeuchi J: Onset and progression of diabetic glomerulosclerosis: a prospective study based on serial renal biopsies. Diabetes, 24: 1-9, 1975.
221. Cahill GF Jr: Will euglycemia prevent vasculopathy? In: "The Diabetic Renal-Retinal Syndrome. Prevention and Management" (Eds EA Friedman, FA L'Esperance Jr), Grune and Stratton, New York, 1982, pp 529-535.
222. Vasquez B, Flock EV, Savage PJ, Nagulesparan EA, Bennion LJ, Baitd HR, Bennett PH: Sustained reduction of proteinuria in Type 2 (non-insulin dependent) diabetes following diet-induced reduction of hyperglycemia. Diabetologia, 26: 127-133, 1984.
223. Beyer-Mears A, Ku L, Cohen MP: Glomerular polyol accumulation in diabetes and its prevention by oral sorbinil. Diabetes, 33: 604-606, 1984.
224. Cohen MP, Dasmahapatra A, Shapiro E: Reduced glomerular Na-K triphosphatase activity in acute streptozotocin diabetes and its prevention by sorbinil. Diabetes, 34: 1071-1075, 1985.
225. Craven P, DeRubertis FR: Sorbinil suppresses glomerular prostaglandin production and reduces hyperfiltration in the streptozotocin-diabetic rat. Clin Research, 36: 517a, 1988.
226. Goldfarb S, Simmons DA, Kerns EFO: Amelioration of glomerular hyperfiltration in acute experimental diabetes mellitus by dietary myo-inositol supplementation and aldose reductase inhibition> Trans Assoc Am Phys, 99: 67-72, 1986.
227. Mower P, Wildes B, Bank N: Sorbinil correction of diabetic hyperfiltration unassociated with changes in AII receptors. Kidney Int, 33: 380, 1988 (Abstract).

228. Tilton RG, Chang K, Pugliese G, Kilo C, Williamson JR: Inhibitors of aldose reductase block diabetes-induced increases in blood flow and glomerular filtration rate and markedly reduce 24 hour urinary albumin excretion in the rat. Diabetes, 36 (Suppl 1): 43, 1987 (Abstract).
229. Chang WP, Dimitriadis E, Allen T, Dunlop ME, Cooper M, Larkins RG: The effect of aldose reductase inhibitors on glomerular prostaglandin production and urinary albumin excretion in experimental diabetes mellitus. Diabetologia, 34: 225-231, 1991.
230. Pedersen MM: Renal effects of an aldose reductase inhibitor (statil) during 6 months of treatment in type I (insulin-dependent diabetic patients. Diabetologia, 32: 516A, 1989 (Abstract).
231. Brownlee M: Glycosylation of proteins and microangiopathy. Hosp Pract, 27: 46-50, 1992.
232. Makita Z, Radoff F, Rayfield EJ,Yang Z, Skolnik E, Delaney V, Friedman EA, Cerami A, Vlassara H: Advanced glycosylation end-products in patients with diabetic nephropathy. N Engl J Med, 325: 836-842, 1991.
233. Brownlee M, Cerami A, Vlassara H: Advanced glycosylation end products in tissue: Biochemical basis for a new therapeutic approach to the complications of diabetes. N Engl J Med, 318: 1315-1321, 1988.
234. Soulis-Liparota T, Cooper M, Papazoglou D, Clarke B, Jerums G: Retardation by aminoguanidine of development of albuminuria, mesangial expansion, and tissue fluorescence in streptozotocin-induced diabetic rat. Diabetes, 40: 1328-1332, 1991.
235. Yamin MA, Brownlee M, Cerami A, Vlassara H: Nonenzymatic glycosylation of matrix and the pathogenesis of diabetic angiopathy. J Nephrol, 1: 23-26, 1991.
236. Edelstein BD, Brownlee M: Aminoguanidine ameliorates albuminuria in diabetic hypertensive rats. Diabetologia, 35: 96-97, 1992.
237. Craven PA, Caines MA, DeRubertis FR: Sequential alterations in glomerular prostaglandin and thromboxane synthesis in diabetic rats: Relationship to the hyperfiltration of early diabetes. Metabolism, 36: 95-103, 1987.
238. Gambardello S, Andreani D, Cancelli A: Renal hemodynamics and urinary excretion of 6-keto-prostaglandin F1a and thromboxane b_2 in newly diagnosed type I diabetic patients. Diabetes, 37: 1044-1048, 1988.
239. Trevisan R, Fioretto P, Giorato C, Sacerdoti D, Borsato M, Mantero F, Crepaldi G, Tiengo A, Nosadini R: Determinants of glomerular hyperfiltration in type 1 (insulin-dependent) diabetes. Diabetologia, 34: A62, 1991 (Abstract).
240. Craven PA, DeRubertis FR: Role for local prostaglandin and thromboxane production in the regulation of glomerular filtration rate in the rat with streptozotocin-induced diabetes. J Lab Clin Med, 113: 674-681, 1989.
241. Jensen PK, Steven K, Blaehr H, Christiansen JS, Parving H-H: Effects of indomethacin on glomerular hemodynamics in experimental diabetes. Kidney Int, 29: 490-495, 1986.
242. Tagiri Y, Inoguchi T, Umeda F, Nawata H: Reduction of urinary albumin excretion by thromboxane synthetase inhibitor, OKY-046, through modulating renal prostaglandins in patients with diabetic nephropathy. Diab Res Clin Pract, 10: 231-239, 1990.
243. Christiansen JS, Feldt-Rasmussen B, Parving H-H: Short term inhibition of prostaglandin synthesis has no effect on the elevated glomerular filtration rate of early insulin-dependent diabetes. Diabetic Med, 2: 17-20, 1985.
244. Esmatjes E, Fernandez MR, Halperin I, Camps J, Gaya J, Arroyo V, Rivera F, Figuerola D: Renal hemodynamic abnormalities in patients with short-term insulin dependent diabetes mellitus: role of renal prostaglandins. J Clin Endocrinol Metab, 60: 1231-1236,1985.
245. Hommel E, Mathiesen E, Arnold-Larsen S, Edsberg B, Olsen UB, Parving H-H: Effects of indomethacin on kidney function in type I (insulin-dependent) diabetic patients with nephropathy. Diabetologia, 30: 78-83, 1987.
246. Kasiske BL, O'Donnell MP, Schmitz PG, Keane WF: The role of lipid abnormalities in the pathogenesis of chronic, progressive renal disease. Adv Nephrol Necker Hosp, 20: 109-125, 1991.
247. Winocour PH, Durrington PN, Ishola M, Hillier VF, Anderson DC: The prevalence of hyperlipidemia and related clinical features in insulin-dependent diabetes mellitus. Q J Med, 70: 265-276, 1989.
248. Mulec H, Johnson S-A, Björck S: Relation between serum cholesterol and diabetic nephropathy. Lancet, 335: 1537-1538, 1990 (Letter).
249. Kasiske BL, O'Donnell MP, Cleary MP, Keane WF: Treatment of hyperlipidemia reduces glomerular injury in obese Zucker rats. Kidney Int, 33: 667-672, 1988.

250. Kasiske BL, O'Donnell MP, Garvis WJ, Keane WF: Pharmacologic treatment of hyperlipidemia reduces glomerular injury in rat 5/6 nephrectomy model of chronic renal failure. Circ Res, 62: 367-374, 1988.
251. Kasiske BL, O'Donnell MP, Schmitz PG, Kim Y, Keane WF, Phillips F, Daniels F, Holden G: Renal injury of diet-induced hypercholesterolemia in rats. Kidney Int, 37: 880-891, 1990.
252. Simpson LO: A hypothesis proposing increased blood viscosity as a cause of proteinuria and increased vascular permeability. Nephron, 31: 89-93, 1982.
253. Simpson LO, Shand BI, Olds RJ: A reappraisal of the influence of blood rheology on glomerular filtration and its role in the pathogenesis of diabetic nephropathy. J Diabetic Compl, 1: 137-144, 1987.
254. Solerte SB, Ferrari E: Diabetic retinal vascular complications, erythrocyte filtrability and pentoxifylline. Results of a 2 year follow-up study. Pharmatherapeutica, 4: 341-346 1985.
255. Solerte BF, Fioravante M, Bozzetti A, Schifino N, Patti AL, Fedele P, Viola C, Ferrari E: Pentoxifylline, albumin excretion rate and proteinuria in type I and type II diabetic patients with microproteinuria. Results of a short-term randomised study. Acta Diabetol Lat, 23: 171-177,1986.
256. Brown CD, Friedman EA: Clinical and blood rheologic stability in erythropoietin-treated predialysis patients. Am J Nephrol, 10 (Suppl 2): 29-33, 1990
257. Mauer SM, Sutherland DER, Steffes MW, Leonard RJ, Najarian JS, Michael AF, Brown DM: Pancreatic islet transplantation. Effects on the glomerular lesions of experimental diabetes in the rat. Diabetes, 23: 748-753, 1974.
258. Bilous RW, Mauer SM, Sutherland DER, Najarian JS, Goetz FC, Steffes MW: The effects of pancreas transplantation on the glomerular structure of renal allografts in patients with insulin dependent diabetes. N Engl J Med, 321: 80-85, 1989.
259. Sawicki PT, Heinemann L, Muhlhauser I: Enalapril and metoprolol in diabetic nephropathy. Br Med J, 300: 1446-1448, 1990.
260. Sawicki PT, Muhlhauser I, Baba T, Berger M: Do angiotensin converting enzyme inhibitors represent a progress in hypertensive care in diabetes mellitus? Diabetologia, 33: 121-124, 1990.

HEREDITARY RENAL DISEASES

Chapter 8

ALPORT'S SYNDROME

MARTIN C. GREGORY

Divisions of Internal Medicine and Nephrology, Department of Medicine, University of Utah School of Medicine, Salt Lake City, Utah, 84132, USA

INTRODUCTION

Every nephrologist knows what Alport's syndrome is, but no one can define it to the satisfaction of all. Cecil Alport emphasized the association of deafness with nephritis in the family he studied (1). In deference to his contribution, Alport's syndrome commonly denotes hereditary hematuric nephritis with deafness. This simple definition has several drawbacks. Firstly, true deafness, defined as inability to hear and understand speech even with amplification (2), is rarely found in Alport patients; hearing loss is a more precise term. Secondly, families with and others without appreciable hearing loss have clinically, histologically, ultrastructurally, and immunochemically indistinguishable renal disease (3). Thirdly, mutations in COL4A5*, the gene responsible for many or most cases of Alport's syndrome, have been found in families with (4, 5) and without (6-8) hearing loss. Hearing loss is best regarded as one of the features shown by some kindreds but not others: ocular abnormalities, abnormalities of the formed elements of the blood, and esophageal, tracheobronchial and genital leiomyomatosis fall into the same category.

DEFINITION

In this chapter, Alport's syndrome will be defined as progressive nonimmune hereditary hematuric glomerulonephritis characterized ultrastructurally by irregular

* Abbreviations used in the text: cDNA, complementary deoxyribonucleic acid; COL4A5, the gene near Xq22 coding for the a5 chain of type IV collagen; EBM epidermal basement membrane; ESRD, end-stage renal disease; FNS1, familial nephritis serum; GBM, glomerular basement membrane; PCR, polymerase chain reaction; RFLP, restriction fragment length polymorphic marker

thickening, thinning, and lamellation of the glomerular basement membrane (GBM) (3). Nonrenal features may or may not be present. This definition deliberately ignores two features apparently central to the etiology and pathogenesis of the condition: nonreactivity of GBM and epidermal basement membranes (EBM) with familial nephritis serum (FNS1) (9), and mutations in the COL4A5 gene (4-7, 10-12). At present neither of these apparently fundamental features has been shown in all families that are widely accepted as variants of Alport's syndrome. In the present state of knowledge, finding either a mutation in COL4A5 or a lack of basement membrane reactivity with FNS1 is sufficient but not necessary to make a diagnosis of Alport's syndrome. Until an etiologic or pathogenetic definition is agreed by all workers it is desirable to preserve the concept of a "syndrome" with varying causes and heterogeneous clinical presentations.

PREVALENCE

The prevalence of Alport's syndrome is not well established. Including kindreds with and without hearing loss, the estimated Alport's syndrome gene frequency is 1:5,000 in the Intermountain West of the United States (3).

Alport's syndrome has been widely reported and is probably not restricted to particular races or areas.

ETIOLOGY AND PATHOGENESIS

Collagen chemistry and immunochemistry

Arguing from the disorganized ultrastructure of the GBM (13-16), Spear (15) hypothesized in 1973 that a genetic defect of collagen lay at the basis of Alport's syndrome. This prescient suggestion could be taken no further until more sophisticated methods in collagen immunochemistry and genetics became available (17).

Glomerular basement membrane appears ultrastructurally as a featureless sheet 150 nm thick.

The main structural protein is type IV collagen, with lesser quantities of heparan sulphate proteoglycan, laminin, nidogen, and entactin. Type IV collagen is composed principally of triple helical heterotrimers of two a1(IV) chains and one a2(IV) chain. At the carboxyl end of each chain there is a noncollagenous (NC) globular region whose structure has been highly conserved from Drosophila to man. The NC region of each heterotrimer assembles "head to head" with the NC region of another heterotrimer. The terminus of the collagenous region assembles "tail to tail" with three other heterotrimers. This supramolecular assembly produces an extensive flexible sheet. In addition to the a1(IV) and a2(IV) chains, two other chains, a3(IV) and a4(IV) were found in bovine GBM. Analogs of a3(IV) and a4(IV), recognizable by cross-reactive antibodies exist in human tissues (17, 18).

When several patients with Alport's syndrome developed anti-glomerular basement nephritis after transplantation, it was suspected that the newly-transplanted kidney had presented the recipient with a previously unseen chain of collagen.

This sparked a fruitful line of research which has led to the concept that several chains of type IV collagen (perhaps a3, a4, and a5) are lacking from the GBM in Alport's syndrome (19). One of these is the Goodpasture antigen, but the non-collagenous monomer which is recognized by FNS1 is better described as the Alport antigen because this antigen is not that which is recognized by all anti-GBM sera. This topic has been extensively reviewed recently by Kashtan (19).

The presence of a fifth a chain, central to the pathogenesis of Alport's syndrome, has been deduced from the discovery and sequencing of its gene, COL4A5 (5, 20, 21). A disulfide bonded heterodimer of a3(IV) and the 26 kD type IV collagen NC monomer recognized as the Alport antigen has been shown by immunoprecipitation (22). Demonstration of this heterodimer lends strength to the conjecture that a5(IV) may form a heterotrimer with a3(IV) and perhaps another a chain.

Classical genetics and linkage studies

In all kindreds that have been studied adequately the inheritance pattern has been dominant (3): X-linkage is the rule, but cases of male to male transmission have established autosomal transmission in some kindreds, particularly those with accompanying platelet abnormalities (23-25).

Protracted confusion about the mode of inheritance of Alport's syndrome was settled by rigorous likelihood analyses that proved X-linkage in large pedigrees in Utah (26, 27). This conclusion was soon buttressed by several linkage studies using restriction fragment length polymorphic markers (RFLPs) (28-35) that placed the Alport's syndrome locus near Xq22, in the mid-long arm of the X-chromosome. This is a region of relatively low recombination, so that even extremely tight linkage (Lod scores exceeding 20 at zero recombination for several markers in the region Xq21.2-22.1) (29) only confines the gene within a physical distance of around a million base pairs.

Molecular genetics

The genes for the a1 and a2 chains of type IV collagen lie on chromosome 13 (36), and those for the a3 and a4 chains on chromosome 2 (37) yet Alport's syndrome is an X-linked condition in most cases. Moreover, the gene coding for the a3 chain (the presumed Goodpasture antigen) is present in both normals and in those with Alport's syndrome (38).

This impasse was broken when Tryggvason's group (20) screened a placental cDNA library with synthetic oligonucleotides coding for conserved sequences in type IV collagen a chains. Clones that did not hybridize with a1 or a2 cDNA were sequenced. They coded for a novel type IV collagen-like a chain, which was termed a5(IV) (20). The gene for a5(IV), COL4A5, has been located near Xq22 (20), the same area as the gene for Alport's syndrome. The existence of a5(IV) was rapidly confirmed (21). The new chain was called a5 because a3 and a4 chains had been previously isolated from bovine basement membranes and shown to share antigenic determinants with the putative Goodpasture antigen (18). The entire sequence of the expressed portions of COL4A5 is now known (5, 20, 39).

Mutations in COL4A5

Shortly after the discovery of COL4A5, screening of DNA restriction endonuclease digests from members of 18 kindreds with Alport's syndrome revealed mutations in three of them (4).

One was a deletion of exons 5 through 10, one was a small mutation generating a new Pst1 site, and one was an uncharacterized abnormality. The Pst1 abnormality occurred in the large and well characterized Utah kindred P with X-linked adult type nephritis with hearing loss. It was subsequently shown to be a point mutation in exon 3 resulting in the alteration of conserved cysteine residue 1564 to serine (40). Since this time, the number of described mutations has increased rapidly, such that by the beginning of 1992 about 30 had been reported in full or in abstract form (4-7, 10, 41). Despite this rapid progress, at present mutations can be found in only a minority of kindreds. This may reflect the relative crudeness of the methods available, or it may imply that a second gene is involved.

CLINICAL FEATURES

Renal

Persistent microscopic hematuria in all affected males is the central feature (3). Only very exceptionally do affected males fail to show hematuria: we have found one man with intermittent hematuria and a proven mutation in COL4A5. Penetrance of hematuria in gene carrying females was 93% in adult type kindreds (29): our experience is that hematuria in females may be less frequent in juvenile type kindreds. Red cell casts accompany the hematuria in both males and females; they provide more specific but less sensitive evidence of nephritis. Proteinuria is highly variable; heavy proteinuria may portend rapid progression to renal failure (42). ESRD is inevitable in all males (3). Although ESRD occurs at a fairly consistent age within each family, it occurs at widely disparate ages in different families. Families can be grouped into "juvenile" types, whose males develop ESRD below a mean age of 31 years, and "adult" types with ESRD in males after the age of 31. ESRD supervenes in only about 25% of females, usually above the age of 50 years (3), although it can occur at any age.

Auditory

Sensorineural hearing loss is slowly progressive and variable in audiologic contour. Audiograms generally reveal a gently sloping high tone loss or loss most marked in the 2 to 6 kHz range (43, 44).

A noise-induced notch at 4 kHz is commonly superimposed, particularly in older people. The insidious progression of hearing loss permits time for adaptation and many patients are unaware of the severity or even the existence of a hearing deficit. Dynamic compression of the auditory range, marked at around 2 kHz (43), may limit the benefit obtained from hearing aids.

Tinnitus is a distressing complaint for some patients. Hearing loss may eventually become profound, amounting to true deafness, but loss of 40 to 60 dB is more typical. Hearing loss seems to be a feature of nearly all juvenile kindreds, but is present in only perhaps 50% of adult kindreds: the largest known kindred with Alport's syndrome has negligible hearing loss (6, 44).

Ocular

Although present in a minority of kindreds, anterior lenticonus is well recognized as being virtually pathognomonic of Alport's syndrome (45-53). Anterior lenticonus eventually causes severe visual impairment whereas the other highly characteristic ocular manifestation, macular and midperipheral retinal flecks (47, 49, 50, 54-56), has no effect on vision. Posterior polymorphous corneal dystrophy (51, 57, 58) and corneal erosions have also been reported (59, 60)

Hematologic

Thrombocytopenia with giant platelets and a moderate bleeding tendency characterizes kindreds with Epstein's syndrome (23, 61-66) also known as type V Alport's syndrome (3). In some of these families, granulocytes display characteristic inclusion bodies (Fechtner inclusions) (24, 25, 67, 68). This form of Alport's syndrome appears to be transmitted by an autosomal dominant mechanism (23-25) and no mutations in COL4A5 have yet been described.

Dermatologic

No clinical abnormalities of the skin are recognized in Alport's syndrome, but there is a striking immunological abnormality of EBM collagen. "Familial nephritis serum" (FNS1) is an anti-GBM serum obtained from a male Alport's syndrome patient who developed anti-GBM nephritis after renal transplantation (9). This serum stains normal GBM and EBM in a strong continuous fashion. These basement membranes from Alport's syndrome males fail to stain, and in female Alport's syndrome carriers, they stain in an interrupted fashion, as would be expected from tissue mosaicism caused by random inactivation of the X-chromosome (9, 69).

Leiomyomatosis

Initially thought to be a curiosity, the association of nephritis with esophageal, tracheobronchial, and genital leiomyomatosis has now been found in a number of isolated cases (70, 71) and in several families with indisputable Alport's syndrome (53, 72-76). Mutations of COL4A5 have been shown in families with nephritis and leiomyomatosis (10).

DIAGNOSIS

In a kindred with known Alport's syndrome, the keystone of diagnosis is the demonstration of persistent microscopic hematuria with dysmorphic erythrocytes in an individual on the line of descent. Other plausible causes of hematuria should be excluded, although it is rarely necessary to proceed beyond a careful history, physical examination and personal urinalysis. Confirmation by examination of the ultrastructure of a renal biopsy is then necessary only if there is appreciable doubt about the diagnosis.

Frequently, a renal biopsy performed on account of hematuria will disclose a basement membrane nephropathy. If there are advanced and unmistakable changes of Alport's syndrome, the diagnosis can be accepted and the family history pursued, specifically seeking hematuria, and a history of ESRD in the proband's mother's male relatives. In early cases of Alport's syndrome, the changes on the biopsy may be difficult to distinguish from the thin basement membranes of benign familial hematuria. In these circumstances, the family history is critical. Clear instances of male to male transmission and survival of numerous hematuric males to old age cement the diagnosis of benign familial hematuria; lack of male to male transmission and ESRD in adolescent or middle aged males is strong evidence for Alport's syndrome. Failure of GBM of affected males to stain with anti-GBM serum or FNS1, or of EBM to stain with FNS1 (69) is strong evidence for Alport's syndrome. Normal staining will be found in normals, those with thin GBM disease, and in a minority of kindreds with Alport's syndrome. Unfortunately, reliable standardized sera for these purposes are not widely available.

GENETIC DIAGNOSIS

In families in which a mutation has been defined, precise genetic diagnosis is now possible. For example in Utah kindred P, polymerase chain reaction primers flanking the region of the single base change (4) are available. The amplified segment of DNA is cut with the restriction endonuclease Pst1 and the scission products separated on gels and identified by Southern blotting and labelling with radioactive oligonucleotide probes. There is a clear difference between the unsplit wild type DNA and the two bands given by the mutant DNA. For other kindreds like Utah "Super IV" the mutation is defined (6), but suitable PCR primers have not yet been developed, so a clinically useful test for mutations is not yet available. In yet other cases, such as kindred EP, where a large portion of the gene has been deleted (4), affected males and carrier females can easily be detected on southern blots after cutting native DNA with restriction enzymes.

Linkage analysis yields highly reliable diagnoses in families without a defined mutation if a sufficient number of informative meioses can be studied. Currently available markers, including VNTR (variable number of tandem repeats) markers are highly polymorphic and tightly linked (even intragenic) (77) so it is almost always possible to find informative markers. The weak points of diagnosis by linkage to markers are firstly the assumption of X-linkage, which may not be valid (78), and secondly the need for rigorous diagnoses in the other family members included; misdiagnosis of even a single affected or unaffected family member can invalidate the entire analysis.

Linkage is useful for diagnosis in a large family in which X-linked inheritance is likely by classical analysis provided that blood can be obtained from the subject at risk and from several known affected and known unaffected close relatives. If the pedigree is not extensive enough to decide with reasonable certainty that transmission is X-linked, a minimum of seven informative meioses will be required to establish this by linkage analysis with highly polymorphic markers. In a very small family linkage studies can be attempted if both parents are available, but there is a chance of erroneous conclusions if nephritis is not linked to COL4A5 in this family.

NATURAL HISTORY

Although merciless progression to renal failure occurs in all affected males and a few females, the age of renal failure is heterogeneous. In some families males develop ESRD in childhood or adolescence and in others ESRD is delayed until middle age. While it has been convenient for purposes of classification to group kindreds into "juvenile" with mean age of ESRD in males below the age of 31, and "adult" with mean age of ESRD above that age, it is likely that the kinetics of renal deterioration will depend on the specific mutation in each kindred. Moreover, lifestyle factors, diet, and control of hypertension will all likely modulate the speed of approach to renal failure.

Hearing loss also proceeds at widely varying rates: as a generalization it tends to be more severe in those with juvenile forms of nephritis. It is only in the adult forms that normal hearing has been documented (3, 6, 44).

MYTHS

New knowledge has cast out two entrenched errors. Hyperprolinemia and prolinuria are often quoted as accompaniments of Alport's syndrome. Scriver, who contributed to the first description of Alport's syndrome and type I hyperprolinemia in the same individual, has pointed out that in this pedigree the former condition was dominant and the latter recessive (79). Type I hyperprolinemia is a benign metabolic condition without specific associated conditions (79).

Spherophakia, the first ocular problem described in hereditary nephritis (80), proved to be a misdiagnosis of anterior lenticonus (81) and has not been described subsequently.

THERAPY

No specific therapy has been shown to retard progression of renal damage in Alport's syndrome, but two recent developments offer some hope. On general grounds treatment of hypertension, specifically with angiotensin converting enzyme inhibitors, and dietary protein restriction have been advocated. Dietary restriction of protein, lipid, calcium, and phosphorus delayed progression of hereditary nephritis in affected male and carrier female Samoyed dogs (82). Treatment of 8 patients with juvenile type Alport's syndrome for 8 months with 5 mg/kg/day of cyclosporine A reduced proteinuria remarkably without altering creatinine clearance (42). An alteration of intrarenal hemodynamics was a possible mechanism suggested for this salutary effect and the authors were careful to point out that reduction in proteinuria did not prove a lasting therapeutic benefit of cyclosporine.

Hearing aids are helpful for hearing loss, but no useful therapy for tinnitus is available. Lensectomy and intra-ocular lens replacement has been used successfully to correct the refractive error of lenticonus (53, 83).

BENIGN FAMILIAL HEMATURIA (FAMILIAL THIN GBM DISEASE)

Several families have been described with dominant familial hematuria, normal hearing, and a benign prognosis (84-88). Male to male transmission attests to autosomal inheritance in some kindreds (85, 86). Immunofluorescence microscopy gives normal findings. The GBM stains with naturally occurring or monoclonal (89, 90) anti-GBM antibodies, in contrast to most cases of Alport's syndrome. Ultrastructural examination of the GBM shows uniform attenuation to about half the normal thickness (87, 88, 91, 92), although the specificity of this finding has been challenged (93).

The nomenclature of this condition is also not settled. Some dispute the term "benign familial hematuria" as too broad, encompassing other conditions such as familial IgA nephropathy (94). Others point out that "thin basement membrane" does not define a single specific entity (93).

There is emerging evidence for intermediate forms between Alport's syndrome and "benign familial hematuria". Several members of one family with autosomal dominant inheritance of hematuria had normal EBM reactivity with FNS and a biopsy in a collateral member of the kindred was ultrastructurally typical of thin GBM disease. Nevertheless, there were family members with severe hearing loss and renal failure. Linkage to COL4A5 was excluded by segregation analysis with highly polymorphic RFLP and VNTR markers (78). It seems wise to give a guarded prognosis in cases of apparent "benign familial hematuria" unless several affected members of the family have maintained normal renal function to a ripe old age.

CONCLUSION

The last few years have been a period of remarkable progress in Alport's syndrome. Careful segregation studies have proven X-linkage in nearly all well studied families. The gene responsible was localized to Xq22 and then shown to be COL4A5. Mutations have been shown in an increasing number of families, permitting unequivocal noninvasive diagnoses in these families. Linkage analysis also permits highly reliable diagnoses in large families. Avenues of treatment have been suggested and are amenable to controlled study.

ACKNOWLEDGEMENTS

This work was supported by grants from the Hereditary Nephritis Foundation and the National Institutes of Health (PHS MO1-RR00064 and DK39497).

REFERENCES

1. Alport AC: Hereditary familial congenital haemorrhagic nephritis. Br Med J, 1: 504-506, 1927.
2. Schein JD, Delk MT: The deaf population of the United States. National Association of the Deaf, Silver Springs, MD, 1974.

3. Gregory MC, Atkin CL: Alport syndrome. In: "Diseases of the Kidney" (Eds RW Schrier, CE Gottschalk), 5th Edition, Little Brown & Co, Boston, 1992, pp 571-591.
4. Barker DF, Hostikka SL, Zhou J, Chow LT, Oliphant AR, Gerken SC, Gregory MC, Skolnick MH, Atkin CL, Tryggvason K: Identification of mutations in the COL4A5 collagen gene in Alport syndrome. Science, 248: 1224-1227, 1990.
5. Zhou J, Hertz JM, Leinonen A, Tryggvason K: Complete amino acid sequence of the human a5(IV) collagen chain and identification of a single base mutation on exon 23 converting glycine-521 in the collagenous domain to cysteine in an Alport syndrome patient. J. Biol. Chem, 1992 (in press).
6. Gregory MC, Skinner B, Atkin CL, Barker DF: A novel mutation in COL4A5 relates three families with type IV Alport syndrome. J Amer Soc Nephrol, 2: 254, 1991.
7. Smeets HJM, Melenhorst JJ, Lemmink HH, Schröder CH, Nelen MR, Zhou J, Hostikka SL, Tryggvason K, Ropers HH, Jansweijer MCE, Monnens LAH, Brunner HG, van Oost BA: Kidney International, 1992 (in press).
8. Zhou J, Hertz JM, Tryggvason K: Amer J Hum Genetics, 1992 (in press).
9. Kashtan C, Fish AJ, Kleppel M, Yoshioka K, Michael AF: Nephritogenic antigen determinants in epidermal and renal basement membranes of kindreds with Alport-type familial nephritis. J Clin Invest, 78: 1035-1044, 1986.
10. Antignac C, Dechenes G, Gros F, Knebelmann B, Tryggvason K, Gubler MC: Mutations in the COL4A5 gene in Alport syndrome. J Amer Soc Nephrol, 2: 249, 1991.
11. Kashtan CE, Michael AF, Kleppel MM: Alport syndrome: association of deletions in the COL4A5 gene with post-transplant anti-GBM nephritis. J Amer Soc Nephrol, 2: 256, 1991.
12. Netzer K, Renders L, Pullig O, Tryggvason K, Weber M: Mutations in the COL4A5 gene in X-linked Alport syndrome. J Amer Soc Nephrol, 2: 257, 1991.
13. Spear GS, Slusser RJ: Alport's syndrome. Emphasizing electron microscopic studies of the glomerulus. Am J Pathol, 69: 213-224, 1972.
14. Hinglais N, Grünfeld JP, Bois E: Characteristic ultrastructural lesion of the glomerular basement membrane in progressive hereditary nephritis (Alport's syndrome). Lab Invest, 27: 473-487, 1972.
15. Spear GS: Editorial: Alport's syndrome: a consideration of pathogenesis. Clin Nephrol, 1: 336-337, 1973.
16. Churg J, Sherman RL: Pathologic characteristics of hereditary nephritis. Arch Pathol, 95: 374-379, 1973.
17. Kleppel MM, Kashtan C, Santi PA, Wieslander J, Michael AF: Distribution of familial nephritis antigen in normal tissue and renal basement membranes of patients with homozygous and heterozygous Alport familial nephritis. Relationship of familial nephritis and Goodpasture antigens to novel collagen chains and type IV collagen. Lab Invest, 61: 278-89, 1989.
18. Butkowski R, Langeveld J, Wieslander J, Hamilton J, Hudson BG: Localization of the Goodpasture epitope to a novel chain of basement membrane collagen. J Biol Chem, 262: 7874, 1987.
19. Kashtan CE, Kleppel MM, Butkowski RJ, Michael AF, Fish AJ: Alport syndrome, basement membranes and collagen. Pediatr Nephrol, 4: 523-532, 1990.
20. Hostikka SL, Eddy RL, Byers MG, Hoyhtya M, Shows TB, Tryggvason K: Identification of a distinct type IV collagen alpha chain with restricted kidney distribution and assignment of its gene to the locus of X chromosome-linked Alport syndrome. Proc Natl Acad Sci U S A, 87: 1606-10, 1990.
21. Myers JC, Jones TA, Pohjolainen ER, Kadri AS, Goddard AD, Sheer D, Solomon E, Pihlajaniemi T: Molecular cloning of alpha 5(IV) collagen and assignment of the gene to the region of the X chromosome containing the Alport syndrome locus. Am J Hum Genet, 46: 1024-1033, 1990.
22. Cheong HI, Michael AF, Kleppel MM: Characterization of the Alport antigen: Molecular association with novel basement membrane collagen chains. J Amer Soc Nephrol, 2: 251-251, 1991.
23. Parsa KP, Lee DB, Zamboni L, Glassock RJ: Hereditary nephritis, deafness and abnormal thrombopoiesis. Study of a new kindred. Am J Med, 60: 665-72, 1976.
24. Peterson LC, Rao KV, Crosson JT, White JG: Fechtner syndrome--a variant of Alport's syndrome with leukocyte inclusions and macrothrombocytopenia. Blood, 65: 397-406, 1985.
25. Gershoni-Baruch R, Baruch Y, Viener A, Lichtig C: Fechtner syndrome: clinical and genetic aspects. Am J Med Genet, 31: 357-367, 1988.

26. Hasstedt SJ, Atkin CL: X-linked inheritance of Alport syndrome: family P revisited. Am J Hum Genet, 35: 1241-1251, 1983.
27. Hasstedt SJ, Atkin CL, San Juan ACJ: Genetic heterogeneity among kindreds with Alport syndrome. Am J Hum Genet, 38: 940-953, 1986.
28. Atkin CL, Hasstedt SJ, Menlove L, Cannon L, Kirschner N, Schwartz C, Nguyen K, Skolnick M: Mapping of Alport syndrome to the long arm of the X chromosome. Am J Hum Genet, 42: 249-255, 1988.
29. Barker DF, Fain PR, Goldgar DE, Dietz-Band JN, Turco AE, Kashtan CE, Gregory MC, Tryggvason K, Skolnick MH, Atkin CL: High-density genetic and physical mapping of DNA markers near the X-linked Alport syndrome locus: definition and use of flanking polymorphic markers. Hum Genet, 88: 189-194, 1991.
30. Brunner H, Schröder C, van Oost BC, Lambermon E, Tuerlings J, Menzel D, Olbing H, Monnens L, Wieringa B, Ropers HH: Localization of the gene for X-linked Alport's syndrome. Kidney Int, 34: 507-510, 1988.
31. Flinter FA, Abbs S, Bobrow M: Localization of the gene for classic Alport syndrome. Genomics, 4: 335-338, 1989.
32. Kashtan CE, Rich SS, Michael AF, de Martinville B: Gene mapping in Alport families with different basement membrane antigenic phenotypes. Kidney Int, 38: 925-930, 1990.
33. Szpiro-Tapia S, Bobrie G, Guilloud BM, Heuertz S, Julier C, Frezal J, Grünfeld JP, Hors CMC: Linkage studies in X-linked Alport's syndrome. Hum Genet, 81: 85-87, 1988.
34. Hertz JM, Kruse TA, Thomsen A, Spencer ES: Multipoint linkage analysis in X-linked Alport syndrome. Hum Genet, 88: 157-161, 1991.
35. Vetrie D, Flinter F, Bobrow M, Harris A: Long-range mapping of the gene for the human alpha 5(IV) collagen chain at Xq22-q23. Genomics, 12: 130-138, 1992.
36. Pihlajaniemi T, Tryggvason K, Myers J, Kurkinen M, Lebo R, Cheung M, Prockop DJ, Boyd CD: cDNA clones coding for the pro-a1(IV) chain of human type IV procollagen reveal an unusual homology of amino acid sequences in two halves of the carboxy-terminal domain. J Biol Chem, 260: 7681-7687, 1985.
37. Morrison KE, Mariyama M, Yang-Feng TL, Reeders ST: Sequence and localization of a partial cDNA encoding the human a3 chain of type IV collagen. Am J Hum Genet, 49: 545-554, 1991.
38. Savige JA: The gene corresponding to the putative Goodpasture antigen is present in Alport's syndrome. Clin exp Immunol, 85: 236-239, 1991.
39. Zhou J, Hostikka SL, Chow LT, Tryggvason K: Characterization of the 3' half of the human type IV collagen alpha 5 gene that is affected in the Alport syndrome. Genomics, 9: 1-9, 1991.
40. Zhou J, Barker DF, Hostikka SL, Gregory MC, Atkin CL, Tryggvason K: Single base mutation in alpha 5(IV) collagen chain gene converting a conserved cysteine to serine in Alport syndrome. Genomics, 9: 10-18, 1991.
41. Boye E, Vetrie D, Flinter F, Buckle B, Pihlajaniemi T, Hamamainen E, Myers JC, Bobrow M, Harris A: Major rearrangements in the a5(IV) collagen gene in three patients with Alport syndrome. Genomics, 11: 1125-1132, 1991.
42. Callís L, Vila A, Nieto J, Fortuny G: Effect of cyclosporin A on proteinuria in patients with Alport's syndrome. Pediatr Nephrol, 6: 140-144, 1992.
43. Gleeson MJ: Alport's syndrome: audiological manifestations and implications. J Laryngol Otol, 98: 449-465, 1984.
44. Wester DC. A clinical study of auditory phenotypes in X-linked Alport syndrome using routine and ultra-high frequency audiometry [Dissertation]. Salt Lake City, UT: University of Utah, 1990.
45. Brownell RD, Wolter JR: Anterior lenticonus in familial hemorrhagic nephritis. Arch. Ophthalmol, 71: 481-483, 1964.
46. Arnott EJ, Crawfurd MD, Toghill PJ: Anterior lenticonus and Alport's syndrome. Br J Ophthalmol, 50: 390-403, 1966.
47. Nielsen CE: Lenticonus anterior and Alport's syndrome. Acta Ophthalmol (Copenh), 56: 518-530, 1978.
48. Kapoor S, Dasgupta J: Chromosomal anomaly in a female patient with anterior lenticonus. Ophthalmologica, 179: 271-275, 1979.
49. Perrin D, Jungers P, Grünfeld JP, Delons S, Noel LH, Zenatti C: Perimacular changes in Alport's syndrome. Clin Nephrol, 13: 163-167, 1980.
50. Govan JA: Ocular manifestations of Alport's syndrome: a hereditary disorder of basement membranes? Br J Ophthalmol, 67: 493-503, 1983.

51. Sabates R, Krachmer JH, Weingeist TA: Ocular findings in Alport's syndrome. Ophthalmologica, 186: 204-210, 1983.
52. Streeten BW, Robinson MR, Wallace R, Jones DB: Lens capsule abnormalities in Alport's syndrome. Arch Ophthalmol, 105: 1693-1697, 1987.
53. McCartney PJ, McGuinness R: Alport's syndrome and the eye. Aust N Z J Ophthalmol, 17: 165-168, 1989.
54. Purriel P, Drets M, Pascale E, Sanchez CR, Borras A, Ferreira WA, de LA, Fernandez L: Familial hereditary nephropathy (Alport's syndrome). Am J Med, 49: 753-773, 1970.
55. Gubler M, Levy M, Broyer M, Naizot C, Gonzales G, Perrin D, Habib R: Alport's syndrome. A report of 58 cases and a review of the literature. Am J Med, 70: 493-505, 1981.
56. Gelisken O, Hendrikse F, Schröder CH, Berden JH: Retinal abnormalities in Alport's syndrome. Acta Ophthalmol (Copenh), 66: 713-717, 1988.
57. Thompson SM, Deady JP, Willshaw HE, White RH: Ocular signs in Alport's syndrome. Eye, 1: 146-153, 1987.
58. Teekhasaenee C, Nimmanit S, Wutthiphan S, Vareesangthip K, Laohapand T, Malasitr P, Ritch R: Posterior polymorphous dystrophy and Alport syndrome. Ophthalmology, 98: 1207-1215, 1991.
59. Huismans H: Alport's syndrome (author's transl). Klin Monatsbl Augenheilkd, 172: 775-778, 1978.
60. Burke JP, Clearkin LG, Talbot JF: Recurrent corneal epithelial erosions in Alport's syndrome. Acta Ophthalmol (Copenh), 69: 555-557, 1991.
61. Epstein C. J, Sahud MA, Piel CF, Goodman JR, Bernfield MR, Ablin AR: Hereditary macrothrombocytopathia, nephritis and deafness. Am J Med, 52: 299-310, 1972.
62. Eckstein JD, Filip DJ, Watts JC: Hereditary thrombocytopenia, deafness, and renal disease. Ann. Intern. Med, 82: 639-645, 1975.
63. Bernheim J, Dechavanne M, Bryon PA, Lagarde M, Colon S, Pozet N, Traeger J: Thrombocytopenia, macrothrombocytopathia, nephritis and deafness. Am J Med, 61: 145-150, 1976.
64. Hansen MS, Behnke O, Pedersen N. T, Videbaek A: Megathrombocytopenia associated with glomerulonephritis, deafness, and aortic cystic medianecrosis. Scand J Haematol, 21: 197-205, 1978.
65. Clare NM, Montiel MM, Lifschitz MD, Bannayan GA: Alport's syndrome associated with macrothrombopathic thrombocytopenia. Am J Clin Pathol, 72: 111-117, 1979.
66. Thomas HS, Bauer JH: Hereditary nephritis, deafness and thrombocytopenia. Case report and review. Mo Med, 81: 305-311, 1984.
67. Brivet F, Girot R, Barbanel C, Gazengel C, Maier M, Crosnier J: Hereditary nephritis associated with May-Hegglin anomaly. Nephron, 29: 59-62, 1981.
68. Heynen MJ, Blockmans D, Verwilghen RL, Vermylen J: Congenital macrothrombocytopenia, leucocyte inclusions, deafness and proteinuria: functional and electron microscopic observations on platelets and megakaryocytes. Br J Haematol, 70: 441-448, 1988.
69. Kashtan CE, Atkin CL, Gregory MC, Michael AF: Identification of variant Alport phenotypes using an Alport-specific antibody probe. Kidney Int, 36: 669-674, 1989.
70. Legius E, Proesmans W, Van DB, Geboes K, Lerut T, Eggermont E: Muscular hypertrophy of the oesophagus and "Alport-like" glomerular lesions in a boy. Eur J Pediatr, 149: 623-627, 1990.
71. Rabushka LS, Fishman EK, Kuhlman JE, Hruban RH: Diffuse esophageal leiomyomatosis in a patient with Alport syndrome: CT demonstration. Radiology, 179: 176-178, 1991.
72. Garcia-Torres R, Guarner V: Leiomyomatosis del esóphago, traqueo-bronchial y genital associada con nephropatía hereditaria tipo Alport: un nuevo síndrome. Rev Gastroenterol Mex, 48: 163-170, 1983.
73. Roussel B, Birembaut P, Gaillard D, Puchelle JC, D'Albignac G, Pennaforte F, Fandre M: Léiomyomatose oesophagienne familiale associée à un syndrome d'Alport chez un garçon de 9 ans. Helv Paediatr Acta, 41: 359-368, 1986.
74. Cochat P, Guibaud P, Garcia TR, Roussel B, Guarner V, Larbre F: Diffuse leiomyomatosis in Alport syndrome. J Pediatr, 113: 339-343, 1988.
75. Leborgne J, Le Neel JC, Heloury Y, Audoin AF, David A, Babut JM, Lenne Y: La léiomyomatose oesophagienne diffuse. A propos de 5 observations dont 2 cas familiaux. Chirurgie, 115: 277-286, 1989.

76. Wittig BM, Treichel U, Kohler H, Rumpelt HJ, Meyer zBK: Leiomyomatosis of the gastrointestinal and urogenital tract in combination with hereditary nephritis. Med Klin, 85 Suppl 1, 1990.
77. Barker DF, Cleverly J, Fain PR: Two CA-dinucleotide polymorphisms at the COL4A5 (Alport syndrome) gene in Xq22. Nucleic Acids Research, 20: 929, 1992.
78. Gregory MC, Fain PN, Donaldson C, Barker DF, Atkin CL: Small-kindred linkage analysis reveals genetic heterogeneity in Alport syndrome. J Amer Soc Nephrol, 2: 253, 1991.
79. Phang JM, Scriver CR: Disorders of Proline and Hydroxyproline Metabolism. In: "The Metabolic Basis of Inherited Disease" (Ed CR Scriver, AL Beaudet, WS Sly, D Valle), 6th Edition, McGraw-Hill, New York, 1990, pp 582-583.
80. Sohar E: Renal disease, inner ear deafness, and ocular changes. Arch. Int. Med, 97: 627-630, 1956.
81. Arenberg IK, Dodson VN, Falls HF, Stern SD: Alport's syndrome: Reevaluation of the associated ocular abnormalities and report of a family study. J Ped Ophthalmol, 4: 21-32, 1967.
82. Valli VEO, Baumal R, Thorner P, Jacobs R, Marrano P, Davies C, Qizilbash B, Clarke H: Dietary modification reduces splitting of glomerular basement membranes and delays death due to renal failure in canine X-linked hereditary nephritis. Lab Invest, 65: 67-73, 1991.
83. Grondalski SJ, Bennett GR: Alport's syndrome: review and case report. Optom Vis Sci, 66: 396-398, 1989.
84. Rogers PW, Kurtzman NA, Bunn SM,, White MG: Familial benign essential hematuria. Arch. Intern. Med, 131: 257-262, 1973.
85. Peterson AS, Schubert JJ: Benign hereditary nephritis. J Fam Pract, 4: 437-441, 1977.
86. Eisenstein B, Stark H, Goodman RM: Benign familial haematuria in children from the Jewish communities of Israel: clinical and genetic studies. J Med Genet, 16: 369-372, 1979.
87. Tiebosch AT, Frederik PM, van Breda Vriesman PJ, Mooy JM, van Rie H, van de Wiel TW, Wolters J, Zeppenfeldt E: Thin-basement-membrane nephropathy in adults with persistent hematuria. N Engl J Med, 320: 14-18, 1989.
88. Lang S, Stevenson B, Risdon RA: Thin basement membrane nephropathy as a cause of recurrent hematuria in childhood. Histopathology, 16: 331-337, 1990.
89. Dische FE, Brooke IP, Cashman SJ, Severn A, Taube D, Parsons V, Kershaw M, Reed A, Pusey CD: Reactivity of monoclonal antibody P1 with glomerular basement membrane in thin-membrane nephropathy. Nephrol Dial Transplant, 4: 611-617, 1989.
90. Pettersson E, Törnroth T, Wieslander J: Abnormally thin glomerular basement membrane and the Goodpasture epitope. Clin Nephrol, 33: 105-109, 1990.
91. Tina L, Jenis E, Jose P, Medani C, Papadopoulou Z, Calcagno P: The glomerular basement membrane in benign familial hematuria. Clin Nephrol, 17: 1-4, 1982.
92. Basta-Jovanovic G, Venkataseshan VS, Gil J, Kim DU, Dikman SH, Churg J: Morphometric analysis of glomerular basement membranes (GBM) in thin basement membrane disease (TBMD). Clin Nephrol, 33: 110-114, 1990.
93. Dische FE, Anderson VE, Keane SJ, Taube D, Bewick M, Parsons V: Incidence of thin membrane nephropathy: morphometric investigation of a population sample. J Clin Pathol, 43: 457-460, 1990.
94. Julian BA, Quiggins PA, Thompson JS, Woodford SY, Gleason K, Wyatt RJ: Familial IgA nephropathy. N Engl J Med, 312: 202-208, 1985.

PEDIATRIC NEPHROLOGY

Chapter 9

THE USE OF RECOMBINANT HUMAN GROWTH HORMONE IN CHILDREN WITH CHRONIC RENAL FAILURE

RICHARD N. FINE

Department of Pediatrics, State University of New York at Stony Brook, Stony Brook, NY 11794-8111, USA

INTRODUCTION

Growth retardation is one of the serious clinical manifestations associated with irreversible renal insufficiency in infants, children and adolescents. Although the relationship was first noted at the end of the last century (1), the availability of dialysis and renal transplantation, which could prolong the lives of children who developed end-stage renal disease (ESRD), focused attention on the medical and psychosocial consequences of the growth retardation that accompanies chronic renal failure (CRF) (2, 3).

Despite extensive investigative efforts which were detailed in four international conferences beginning in 1977 (4-7), the precise cause of the growth retardation in children with CRF remains unknown. Multiple factors have been implicated (8): [1] age at onset of CRF; [2] concomitant acidosis; [3] progressive renal osteodystrophy; [4] inadequate caloric intake; and [5] perturbations of various growth factors. In addition, repetitive episodes of electrolyte imbalance in infants with dysplastic kidneys also have been identified as contributing to the growth retardation in these children (9).

Correction of acidosis, prevention and/or treatment of renal osteodystrophy, provision of adequate caloric intake, and correction of any electrolyte abnormalities have not uniformly achieved optimal linear growth in children with CRF. That growth retardation persists despite the presumed correction of these untoward factors is indicated by the recent report of the North American Pediatric Renal Transplant Cooperative Study (NAPRTCS) (10). Of more than 1500 pediatric recipients of renal allografts, who received a renal transplant since January 1987, the majority manifested significant growth retardation at the time of transplantation [<5th percentile on the Growth Curve and/or a

Standard Deviation Score (SDS) more negative than minus 2.00]. Moreover, 25% of these patients had not previously received prior dialysis (pre-emptive transplantation).

From these observations, investigators suggested that perturbations of the various growth factors and their end-organ effects could be likely candidates to explain the growth retardation. Growth hormone (GH) levels are elevated in children with CRF (11). Measurement of somatomedin-C (insulin-like growth factor, IGF) by bioassay revealed low levels both in adults and children with CRF (12, 13), whereas results from radioimmunoassay revealed elevated levels of IGF in children with CRF (14). This discrepancy led Phillips et al to conclude that an inhibitor of somatomedin-C activity is present in uremia (15). Utilizing newer techniques (radioimmunoassay and radioreceptor assay following acid chromatography), Powell and coworkers demonstrated normal IGF-I levels, slightly elevated IGF-II levels, and elevated IGF binding protein (IGF-BP) levels in children with CRF (16). A theoretical possibility is that IGF-BP binds circulating free IGF-I levels and functions as uremic inhibitor. The presence of elevated GH levels in growth-retarded children with CRF dampened interest in the potential therapeutic efficacy of exogenous GH in reversing the defect.

Human GH is a single-chain polypeptide composed of 191 amino acids with a molecular mass of 22 kDa which is synthesized in the anterior lobe of the pituitary gland (17). The GH gene is present on the long arm of chromosome 17 (17). Secretion of GH is regulated by the hypothalamic growth hormone releasing hormone (GHRH). Circulating GH exerts a negative feedback control by both inhibiting GHRH and stimulating somatostatin release. GH is secreted by the pituitary in surges, with the major peak occurring shortly after the onset of deep sleep. Other physiologic stimuli of GH release are physical exercise, hypoglycemia, and ingestion of a high-protein meal (18).

Circulating GH acts both directly on sensitive cells and/or by stimulation of insulin-like growth factor (IGF) production. Regulation of glucose metabolism is a direct effect, whereas stimulation of somatic growth is indirect (19).

IGF-I and IGF-II are single-chain insulin-like polypeptides composed of 70 and 67 amino acids, respectively. Both substances are bound tightly to carrier proteins, resulting in virtually no free IGF-I or IGF-II being measurable in the serum (18).

Growth hormone provides the major stimulus for IGF-I production in the liver, kidney, and other tissues, whereas IGF-II is produced in a number of tissues but is less GH dependent (18). The IGF may exert their effect on the cells producing them (autocrine growth factor) or on adjacent cells (paracrine growth factor); therefore, tissue rather than circulating levels of the IGF may be of physiologic significance (20).

Receptors for IGF-I are present in glomerular mesangial cells, and receptors for IGF-I and IGF-II have been identified in glomeruli and proximal tubular cells. Receptors for GH are also present in proximal tubular cells (21). IGF-I is synthesized by mesangial cells, which are GH independent, and by collecting duct cells, which are GH dependent (21). The GH-IGF axis regulates various physiologic functions of the kidney and is involved in the development of renal hypertrophy and in the postischemic regeneration of the proximal renal tubule (21, 22). These functions of GH will require consideration when the therapeutic use of recombinant human growth hormone (rhGH) in children with growth retardation consequent to CRF is contemplated.

GROWTH HORMONE ADMINISTRATION TO GROWTH-RETARDED UREMIC RATS

In 1983, Mehls and Ritz (23) reported a significant increase in length and weight gain in rats made uremic by subtotal 5/6 nephrectomy after 1 and 2 weeks of supraphysiological doses of porcine GH administered intraperintoneally (i.p.). There was no concomitant increment in the IGF levels; however, the IGF carrier protein levels were increased after treatment. The discrepancy was attributable to methodological problems. No significant effect of physiologic doses of human GH were noted.

Mehls et al (24), in 1988, extended these studies to a larger group of animals who received rhGH i.p. for a 2 week period. The rhGH significantly improved, but did not normalize, the growth velocity and weight gain in uremic rats. Food consumption was not significantly affected by rhGH administration; however, food utilization was significantly increased, indicating an anabolic effect. The dry weight of skeletal muscle was increased in the group of rats receiving rhGH. No effect of rhGH on the serum creatinine level was noted; therefore, the increment in height was not attributable to an improvement in GFR by rhGH treatment. As in the previous study (23), the IGF levels remained unchanged after rhGH treatment whereas the IGF total protein binding capacity increased. The authors indicated that the latter observation required further elucidation.

Powell et al (25), in 1988, examined the effects of rhGH in the 5/6 nephrectomized rat model and essentially confirmed the findings in the previous reports from Mehls and colleagues (24, 25). Uremic rats given 4 weeks of rhGH manifested an increase in length without consuming additional food. There was no difference in the fasting glucose, or insulin levels, and the creatinine clearance remained unchanged, after rhGH administration. Those authors concluded that uremic rats treated with rhGH have an increase in length, use ingested calories more efficiently, and fail to develop insulin resistance. The normal IGF-I levels in the uremic rats suggested to the authors that perturbations in serum IGF-I levels are not a major cause for the growth failure in uremic rats.

Table 1. Effect of rhGH treatment on growth velocity (cm/yr) of growth-retarded children with chronic renal failure.

Reference	# Pt.	Growth Velocity		
		Prior 12 Mo (cm/yr)	rhGH 12 Mo (cm/yr)	Significance (p value)
Koch et al (J Ped '89)	5	4.9 ± 1.4	8.9 ± 1.2	0.006
Tonshoff et al (J Ped '90)	9*	4.4	8.0	<0.005
Rees et al (Arch Dis Child '90)	6	4.8	10.7	<0.01
Johansson et al (Acta Ped Scand '90)	22	4.8	10.0	<0.1

* Dialysis 8

Because dietary protein restriction may modulate the progressive decline of renal function, Nakano et al (26) investigated the effects of exogenous rat GH administered for 3 weeks to 75% nephrectomized rats receiving an 8% protein diet. Compared with the uremic control rats, those given rat GH had significantly improved growth, food efficiency, and serum albumin levels without any change in creatinine clearance despite the low-protein diet. In the previous studies (23-25), the rats were fed a 22% to 25% protein diet. These data of Nakano et al (26) suggested that children with CRF who were receiving a protein-restricted diet to delay the progression of renal failure would respond favorably to rhGH treatment with an increment in growth velocity.

Lastly, Kainer et al (27), using the same model as that described by Nakano et al (26), but with the addition of 1,25 dihydroxy vitamin D_3, noted a significant increase in the magnitude of hypercalciuria when GH and 1,25 dihydroxy vitamin D_3 were administered concomitantly. This finding raised the concern that the combined use of rhGH and 1,25 dihydroxy vitamin D_3 in growth-retarded children with CRF would result in sufficient hypercalciuria to produce nephrocalcinosis, thereby leading to further impairment of renal function. To date, no clinical phenomena in children treated with rhGH comparable to the observation in uremic rats have been reported. Interestingly, the combination of 1,25 dehydroxy vitamin D_3 and bovine GH in this model abolished the beneficial effect of GH.

rhGH ADMINISTRATION TO GROWTH-RETARDED CHILDREN WITH CHRONIC RENAL FAILURE

On the basis of the findings of Mehls and Ritz (23) an investigational new drug application was submitted by me to the Food and Drug Administration for the use of supraphysiologic doses of rhGH in growth retarded children with CRF. The initial 6-month data of five children with CRF treated with rhGH were reported at a symposium in 1987 (28). The annualized growth velocity increased from 4.94 ± 1.4 cm/yr for the year before treatment to 10.08 ± 1.97 cm/yr after treatment ($p<0.01$). A subsequent report published in 1989 (29) noted that the actual growth velocity after 1 yr of treatment in these five children was 8.9 ± 1.2 cm/yr ($p=0.006$) (Table 1). The long-term (3 year) outcome of nine patients with CRF treated with rhGH, which included the five children from the previous two reports (28, 29), indicated that the acceleration in growth velocity continues during the second and third year of rhGH treatment (30). The mean growth velocity of these nine patients increased from 5.0 ± 1.4 cm/yr to 8.5 ± 1.3 ($p=0.0001$), 8.2 ± 1.8 ($p<0.004$), and 8.1 ± 1.8 ($p<0.05$) cm/yr after 12, 24, and 36 months of rhGH treatment, respectively. The mean standard deviation score (SDS) improved from -3.19 ± 1.2 at the initiation of treatment to -1.29 ± 1.3 ($p<0.03$) after 36 months of treatment. Six of the seven patients who had been treated for >24 months had achieved sufficient acceleration in growth velocity to attain a SDS more positive than -2.00 and were above the 5th percentile for chronological age on the growth curve despite the fact that all were below the 5th centile at the initiation of treatment.

In addition to the increase in growth velocity, the patients exhibited an increment in weight and an increase in the mid-arm muscle circumference, indicating that rhGH produced an anabolic effect. The salutary effect of rhGH was achieved without any adverse impact on glucose tolerance or calculated creatinine clearance; however, two patients required initiation of dialysis at 18 and 30 months after initiation of rhGH treatment. Despite the acceleration in growth velocity, the bone age did not increase more than the increase in chronologic age, indicating that growth potential was preserved.

Rees et al (31) recently reported confirmatory results in six prepubertal children with preterminal CRF. The height SDS increased from -2.9 to -2.1 after 1 yr of daily rhGH treatment. Overnight GH profiles were normal before treatment; however, the IGF-I levels were below the normal range before treatment and increased to normal values after treatment. The mean calculated GFR was 18 ml/min/1.73 m^2 before treatment and remained unchanged. Although the parents reported that the children had an improvement in appetite, this impression was not confirmed by dietary assessment. The improvement in growth rate despite unchanged energy and protein intake suggested an increase in the efficiency of food utilization with rhGH. Those authors (31) concluded that the magnitude of improvement in growth rates after rhGH treatment obviated the need for subsequent controlled trials.

Similarly, Tonshoff et al (32, 33) reported their initial results on the use of rhGH in nine children with CRF, eight of whom were undergoing dialysis (seven continuous ambulatory peritoneal dialysis and one hemodialysis). Seven patients completed 1 year of treatment, two patients completed 9 months of treatment, and one patient completed 6 months of treatment. The height velocity increased from 4.4 cm/yr before treatment to 8.0 cm/yr (actual plus annualized) after treatment ($p<0.005$). No acceleration in bone age or increase in glucose intolerance was noted despite the increase in growth velocity. Somatomedin (Sm) bioactivity, IGF-I, IGF-II and IGF-binding protein levels increased after rhGH treatment; however, the increment in IGF-I levels was greater than the increment in the IGF-binding protein levels. Those authors (32, 33) hypothesized that the net increase in unbound IGF-I could explain the normalization in the Sm activity and that the acceleration in growth velocity could be attributed to the increased concentration of circulating IGF-I.

In a multicenter European study of 22 patients with CRF, Johansson et al (34) noted an increase in growth velocity from 4.8 cm/yr for the year prior to rhGH treatment to 10.0 cm/yr following one year of treatment ($p<0.01$).

An additional uncontrolled study on the use of rhGH in children with preterminal CRF are the data in the report of Wilson et al (35) of two severely growth-retarded children with cystinosis. During 1 year of rhGH treatment, the growth velocity was 9.0 and 9.3 cm/yr; however, data were not available regarding the growth velocity during the year before treatment and no information was presented detailing the precise degree of renal functional impairment. The patients were 10 and 11 4/12 years of age at the initiation of rhGH treatment, and those authors stated that the progression of renal failure was not altered by rhGH treatment.

The only controlled study reported to date was a placebo controlled, double-blind, cross-over trial of rhGH treatment in 20 prepubertal children with CRF reported recently by Hokken-Koelega et al (36). Placebo or rhGH were given for 6 months and then crossed over to the alternate therapy. Sixteen of the 20 patients completed the study: 9 conservative treatment and 7 dialysis therapy. There was a significant increase in growth velocity with rhGH treatment (5.2 ± 2.1 cm) compared to placebo (2.4 ± 0.4 cm) ($p<0.001$). The increase in growth velocity was similar in the dialysis treated and conservatively treated group.

In addition to the eight dialysis patients reported by Tonshoff et al (32, 33), Fine et al (37) reported the results of rhGH treatment in five growth-retarded children undergoing continuous cycling peritoneal dialysis (CCPD). Three of the five children manifested an acceleration in growth velocity after 6 to 12 months of thrice weekly rhGH treatment. The lack of a uniform effect in this small group of patients may be related to dosage schedule which was thrice weekly and not daily. Effective absorption of intraperitoneal (i.p.) rhGH (38) has led to preliminary studies with daily i.p. rhGH during the diurnal dwell in patients undergoing CCPD (39).

GROWTH FACTORS IN RENAL ALLOGRAFT RECIPIENTS

Pennisi et al (40), in 1979, evaluated Sm bioactivity and GH concentration in 10 growth-retarded, well-nourished pediatric allograft recipients. The Sm activity was clearly subnormal in 3 of 10 recipients, and there was a significant correlation between Sm activity and creatinine clearance. Serial determinations of Sm activity over a 24 hour period after administration of prednisone demonstrated that Sm activity decreased to subnormal values at 6 and 12 hours and returned to normal values by 24 hours. Insulin-induced hypoglycemia failed to produce a significant (>7 ng/ml) rise in the plasma GH concentration in four of eight recipients. The mean 24 hour GH concentrations tended to be lower in three of four poor responders. However, there was no correlation between the GH values and [1] growth velocity during the preceding year, [2] prednisone dosage, or [3] creatinine clearance. The authors concluded that growth failure in pediatric allograft recipients receiving daily prednisone may result from [1] partial GH deficiency, [2] reduced Sm activity resulting from diminished allograft function, and [3] decreased Sm levels after daily prednisone administration (40).

In 1988, Rees et al (41) performed overnight GH profiles in 17 adolescent renal allograft recipients with short stature and/or maturational delay receiving alternate day corticosteroid therapy. Decreased GH secretion was present in 8 of 17. However, there was no correlation between height velocity during the previous 6 months and [1] area of GH under the curve, [2] mean GH concentration, or [3] GH mean peak amplitude.

Similarly, there was no correlation between either the corticosteroid dose or GFR and growth velocity or any GH parameters. All concentrations of IGF-I were within normal limits for age and sex. Those authors (41) suggested that corticosteroid treatment was responsible for maturational and growth delay in pubertal renal allograft recipients and recommended either excluding corticosteroids from the immunosuppressive regimen or using rhGH in those recipients with stable renal function who were manifesting slow pubertal growth.

Tejani et al (42), in 1989, studied the L-DOPA stimulated GH response in 21 recipients who were either receiving daily prednisone or who had discontinued prednisone and were receiving cyclosporine monotherapy. In 4 of 21 recipients who were receiving >5 mg of prednisone daily, the peak-stimulated GH levels were <10 ng/dl.

Jabs et al (43), in 1990, evaluated plasma GH concentrations during sleep and after arginine and L-DOPA stimulation in eight poorly growing renal allograft recipients. Maximum GH concentration was inadequate both after pharmacologic stimulation and during sleep in four of eight recipients. In an additional two of eight, there were inadequate responses during sleep despite normal responses to pharmacologic stimulation. Plasma IGF-I levels were normal for age in all eight recipients. Those authors (43) concluded that abnormalities of GH secretion occur frequently in poorly growing recipients of successful renal transplants and that the usefulness of rhGH therapy should be investigated.

David-Neto et al (44) studied nocturnal spontaneous GH secretion and Sm levels (RIA) before and after converting 15 pediatric renal allograft recipients from an azathioprine/prednisone to an azathioprine/cyclosporine regimen. Insulin-induced hypoglycemia-stimulated GH response was normal before conversion and the discontinuation of prednisone. GH nocturnal spontaneous secretion was inversely correlated with the prednisone dosage. In 6 of 15, the GH nocturnal spontaneous secretion increased significantly after prednisone withdrawal. After conversion to azathioprine/cyclosporine and prednisone withdrawal, the growth rate increased significantly.

Lastly, Schaefer et al (45) studied pulsatile spontaneous GH secretion in 40 pubertal transplant recipients. GH peak amplitude was correlated with height velocity in the transplant recipients and a strong inverse relationship was observed between the GH peak amplitude and corticosteroid dosage in the transplant recipients. Those authors (45) concluded that pubertal growth failure despite successful transplantation appears to be due to corticosteroid-induced GH hyposecretion.

GLUCOCORTICOIDS AND GROWTH HORMONE

Studies by Kaufmann et al (46) implicated the hypothalamus as the site of glucocorticoid-induced inhibition of GH secretion. The serum GH response to GHRH was tested in seven normal individuals before and after 4 days of prednisone (20 mg, three times a day). After prednisone administration, the GH response to GHRH was markedly depressed. Those authors (46) concluded that the short-term administration of glucocorticoids decreases GHRH-induced GH secretion to a degree indistinguishable from basal secretion. Although the precise mechanism of the inhibition was not delineated, the authors proposed a local increase in somatostatin inhibitory activity.

The potential for exogenous GH to overcome the growth suppressive effects of glucocorticoids was demonstrated recently by Kovacs et al (47). Methylprednisolone (MP) caused a dose dependent reduction of length gain, weight gain and weight gain/food intake ratio in rats. With MP treatment endogenous GH secretion was inhibited, serum IGF-I concentration was decreased and the growth cartilage plate architecture was disturbed. Uremic rats manifested a reduction in growth which was further decreased following MP treatment. Concomitant exogenous rhGH in both uremic and control animals prevented the effects of MP on all the growth parameters evaluated.

These data supported the concept that the growth suppressive effect of glucocorticoids were mediated by perturbations in GH levels. Therefore, exogenous rhGH may be beneficial in both preventing and reversing the adverse consequences of glucocorticoids on growth.

rhGH ADMINISTRATION TO GROWTH-RETARDED RENAL ALLOGRAFT RECIPIENTS

Tejani et al (42), in 1989, reported the treatment of 4 patients who were receiving >5 mg prednisone daily and had peak stimulated GH levels of <10 ng/dl with thrice weekly rhGH for 3 to 6 months. Accelerated growth velocity was reported in 3 of the 4 recipients; however, precise growth data were not included in the report. Van Dop et al (48) in the same year, described the use of rhGH in one renal allograft recipient who had no evidence of GH deficiency but who had a growth rate of only 2 cm/yr while receiving 9 mg/m^2 of prednisone on alternate days. The recipient grew 8.7 cm during 12 months of rhGH treatment.

Rees et al (31), in 1990, reported the results of rhGH treatment of 6 prepubertal and 6 pubertal renal allograft recipients. Overnight GH profiles were depressed in 4/5 in the prepubertal group and 3/5 in the pubertal growth. The mean dose of alternate day prednisolone treatment was 14.9 mg/m^2 in the prepubertal group and 11.0 in the pubertal group. Daily rhGH resulted in an increase in growth velocity over the year prior to treatment from 2.3 to 6.1 cm/yr and 3.2 to 6.0 cm/yr in the prepubertal and pubertal groups respectively (Table 2).

Table 2. Effect of rhGH treatment on growth velocity (cm/yr) of growth-retarded renal allograft recipients.

Reference	# Pt.	Growth Velocity		
		Prior 12 Mo (cm/yr)	rhGH 12 Mo (cm/yr)	Significance (p value)
Rees et al (Arch Dis Child '90)	6* 6**	2.3 3.2	6.1 6.0	<0.005 <0.02
Johansson et al (Acta Ped Scand '90)	15* 13**	2.6 3.8	6.2 6.7	 <0.01
Fine et al (Pediatr Nephrol '91)	9	2.5 ± 2.1	5.7 ± 2.7	<0.0001
Van Dop et al	9	1.9 ± 1.1	7.2 ± 1.8	

* Prepubertal ** Pubertal

Our initial report in 1990 (49) noted an increment in growth velocity in 4 of 5 recipients. In the same year Johansson et al (34) reported the results of a multicenter center study in 15 prepubertal and 13 pubertal recipients. Following one year of daily rhGH treatment the mean growth velocity increased over the year prior to treatment from 2.6 to 6.2 cm/yr and 3.8 to 6.7 cm/yr in the prepubertal and pubertal groups respectively.

Our experience was updated in 1991 (50) to include 9 recipients who received either thrice weekly or daily rhGH for 6 to 30 months. The annualized growth velocity for the initial year of rhGH treatment was significantly greater than that of the preceding year (2.5 ± 2.1 vs 5.7 ± 2.7 cm/yr; $p<0.0001$).

In the report of Rees et al (31) and the reports of Fine et al (49, 50) there was no significant decline in GFR or increase in the number of episodes of graft dysfunction after rhGH treatment. Johansson et al (34) reported a decrease in graft function in 4/28 recipients. This was attributed to progression of chronic rejection in 2 recipients and non-compliance in 1 recipient. In one patient, the cause of the increase in the serum level was unknown.

Recently, Van Dop et al (51), sounded a cautionary note regarding the potential adverse impact of rhGH treatment on graft function. Six of 9 recipients who completed >12 months of either thrice weekly or 6 days per week rhGH treatment had an increase in growth velocity over the year prior to treatment from 2.1 ± 1.3 to 7.5 ± 2.0 cm/yr; however, 6 recipients had increases in the serum creatinine level within 8 weeks of commencing rhGH treatment and the creatinine clearance decreased in 5. Treatment was discontinued in 2 recipients who had biopsy proven chronic rejection prior to treatment. The serum creatinine levels returned to pretreatment values following discontinuation of treatment.

Although GH treatment may cause perturbations in lymphocyte subset levels in the peripheral blood and the response of lymphocytes to mitogenic stimulation (52-54), there are no data that GH produces any clinical immunologic effects. However, GH does produce an increase in GFR and RPF (55) and it is possible that hyperfiltration caused by GH may accelerate the decline in GFR in a chronically rejecting allograft. A controlled trial of the use of rhGH in prepubertal pediatric allograft recipients with optimal graft function which includes periodic measurements of the GFR is required to obtain definitive data on the impact of GH on allograft function.

GROWTH HORMONE AND RENAL FUNCTION

Acute GH infusion over a 2 hour period to either animals (56) or humans (57) failed to produce an increase in GFR/RPF; whereas, 1 week of GH twice daily to seven healthy men resulted in an increase in both GFR and RPF without any concomitant change in kidney size (58). The delay in response of GFR/RPF to GH was also noted by Hirschberg and Kopple (59) after the rhGH treatment of a GH-deficient patient. The delayed increase in GFR/RPF was correlated with the increase in plasma IGF-I levels and led the authors to hypothesize that it was IGF-I rather than GH that stimulated the increase in GFR/RPF. This hypothesis was advanced by the findings of Hirschberg et al (55). Those authors administered rhGH to seven normal adults and followed the GFR and RPF for the following 3 days. The rise in the GFR/RPF was delayed until day 2 when the GH levels had fallen and the IGF-I levels were elevated.

Acute infusion of IGF-I to rats by Hirschberg and Kopple (60) produced an increase in GFR/RPF concomitant with a decrease in renal vascular resistance. The response to IGF-I was blocked by indomethacin, but not somatostatin, indicating that the vasodilating effects of eicosinoids may mediate the effect of IGF-I on GFR/RPF and that the effect is unlikely to be mediated by either renin, insulin, glucagon, or GH - which are all affected by somatostatin. Similarly, the absence of a relationship between the renin-angiotensin-aldosterone system and GH/IGF-induced increase in GFR/RPF was noted by Haffner et al (61). Pretreatment of eight normal individuals with enalapril failed to abort the GH-induced increase in GFR/RPF.

It would appear, therefore, that GH/IGF induces the increase in GFR/RPF by stimulating the reserve renal function.

Haffner et al (62) administered rhGH for 3 days to seven healthy adults and seven patients with CRF. At 72 hours, the inulin clearance increased from 120 to 133 ml/min in the healthy adults but no increase was noted in the patients with CRF (21 to 22 ml/min). The absence of any renal reserve in the patients with CRF probably accounted for the lack of increase in GFR/RPF after GH administration.

Despite the absence of any adverse effect of rhGH on GFR in uremic rats and the lack of any adverse clinical consequences on renal function of children receiving rhGH, caution regarding this potential consequence is required.

Studies in transgenic mice noted an increase in glomerular size and progressive glomerulosclerosis in those mice expressing the GH and GHRH genes but only an increase in size in the mice transgenic for IGF-I (63). Renal failure was the primary factor contributing to the shortened life span in these animals (63, 64).

Studies by Doi et al (65) in mice transgenic for GH demonstrated that the accumulation of extracellular matrix components in the glomeruli of the transgenic mice were related to excessive production rather than reduction in turnover. These data provide a molecular basis for the GH-induced glomerulosclerosis in this animal model.

The potential importance of GH in the pathogenesis of glomerular scarring was emphasized by the studies of El Nahas et al (66). Wistar rats showed progressive proteinuria, hypertension, and renal failure as well as severe glomerular and tubulointerstitial scarring 120 days after subtotal nephrectomy, whereas GH-deficient Dwarf rats had only minimal proteinuria, mild functional renal impairment and moderate histological scarring. Therefore, the absence of GH appears to provide some form of protection against glomerular sclerosis and tubulointerstitial scarring in association with reduced renal mass.

Consequently, GH may be involved in the pathogenesis of glomerulosclerosis and accurate serial GFR measurements are required in patients receiving rhGH in order to assess the long term impact on renal function.

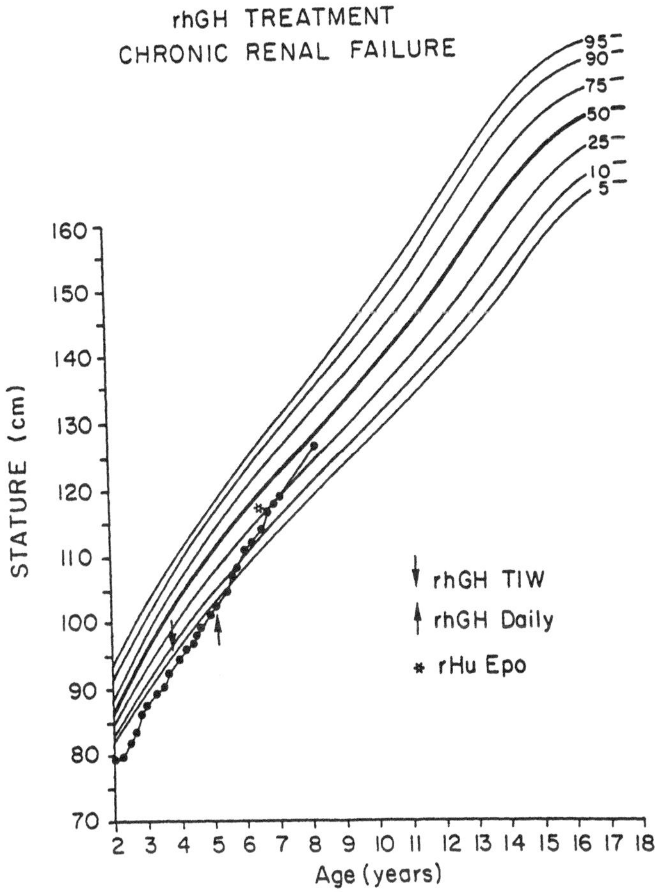

Figure 1. Growth chart of patient treated with rhGH, initially thrice weekly and subsequently daily. Accelerated growth continued following rHuEpo initiation despite a low GFR (* = rHuEpo treatment).

CONCLUSIONS

The potential short-term benefits of rhGH treatment are: [1] alleviation of the psychosocial consequences of marked impairment of linear growth and [2] delaying renal transplantation by eliminating growth retardation as an indication for "pre-emptive" engraftment, which currently accounts for almost one-quarter of all renal transplants performed in children in the United States (10). Although precise data regarding the indications for pre-emptive transplantation are not available, it seems likely that persistent growth retardation is among the common reasons for employing this intervention.

The availability of 1,25-dihydroxy vitamin D_3 for preventing the development of clinical renal osteodystrophy, rhGH to correct the growth retardation, and recombinant human erythropoietin (rHuEpo) to reverse the anemia of CRF have the combined potential to delay the clinical need for dialysis and transplantation and to prolong the duration of conservative treatment. The patient depicted in the Figure 1 illustrates this potential. He had had conservative treatment for more than 18 months following initiation of rHuEpo treatment despite having GFR comparable to that of patients receiving rhGH who required therapy for end-stage renal disease (dialysis). rHuEpo was not yet available when these patients required initiation of dialysis. During this 18-month period, continued rhGH treatment produced an increase in height. Perhaps in the future we will be able to significantly prolong the period of conservative management of CRF by reducing the clinical consequences of uremia in children - renal osteodystrophy, growth retardation, and anemia.

The long-term benefit of rhGH in children with CRF is that rhGH facilitates achievement of the genetic potential for height by improving the growth velocity to the extent that patients reach the 50th centile on the growth curve for mid-parental height. If this goal is achieved prior to the development of end-stage renal disease, then the possibility of these children obtaining normal adult heights following dialysis and/or transplantation will be enhanced. Long-term follow-up of the children currently receiving rhGH treatment is required to determine whether we can help these children reach that goal.

REFERENCES

1. Guthrie LG, Oxon MD: Chronic interstitial nephritis in childhood. Lancet, I: 585-588, 1897.
2. Riley CM: Thoughts about kidney hemotransplantation in children. J Pediatr, 65: 797-800, 1964.
3. Reinhart JB: The doctor's dilemma. J Pediatr, 77: 505-507, 1970.
4. Holliday MA, Chantler C, Potter DE (eds): Metabolism and growth in children with kidney insufficiency. Proc Int Conf, Carmel, California. Kidney Int, 14: 299-382, 1978.
5. Scharer K, Mehls O, Holliday M (eds): International Workshop on Chronic Renal Failure in Children, Heidelberg. Kidney Int, 24 (Suppl 15): 1-115, 1983.
6. Chesney R, Holliday M, Greifer I, Gruppe W, Gruskin A, McEnery P (eds): Third Int Workshop on Growth in Children with Renal Disease, Warenton, Virginia. Am J Kidney Dis, 7: 255-352, 1986.
7. Scharer K, Mehls O (eds): Proc Int Symp on Growth, Nutrition, and Endocrine changes in Children with Chronic Renal Failure, Heidelberg. Pediatr Nephrol, 5: 438-571, 1991.
8. Fine RN: Growth in children with renal insufficiency. In: "Clinical Dialysis" (2nd ed) (Ed AR Nissenson, RN Fine, DE Gentile), Appleton & Lange, East Norwalk, Connecticut, 1990, pp 667-675.
9. Kleinknecht C, Broyer M, Huot D, Marti-Henneberg C, Dartois A: Growth and development in nondialyzed children with chronic renal failure. Kidney Int, 24 (Suppl 15): S40, 1983.
10. North American Pediatric Renal Transplant Cooperative Study: Annual Report, 1991.

11. Czernichow P, Dauzet MC, Broyer M, Rappaport R: Abnormal TSH, PRL and GH response to TSH releasing factor in chronic renal failure. J Clin Endocrinol Metab, 43: 630-34, 1976.
12. Phillips LS, Pennisi AJ, Belosky DC, Uittenbogaart C, Ettenger RB, Malekzadeh MH, Fine RN: Somatomedin activity and inorganic sulfate in children undergoing hemodialysis. J Clin Endocrinol Metab, 46: 165-168, 1978.
13. Phillips LS, Kopple JD: Circulating somatomedin activity and sulfate levels in adults with normal and impaired kidney function. Metabolism, 30: 1091-1095, 1981.
14. Spencer EM, Uthne KO, Arnold WC: Growth impairment with elevated somatomedin levels in children with chronic renal insufficiency. Acta Endocrinol, 91: 36-48, 1979.
15. Phillips LS, Fusco AC, Unterman TG, Del Greco F: Somatomedin inhibitor in uremia. J Clin Endocrinol Metab, 59: 764-772, 1984.
16. Powell DR, Rosenfeld RG, Sperry JB, Baker BK, Hintz RL: Serum concentrations of insulin-like growth factor (IGF)-I, IGF-II and unsaturated somatomedin carrier proteins in children with chronic renal failure. Am J Kidney Dis, 10: 287-292, 1987.
17. Chawla RK, Parks JS, Rudman D: Structural variants of human growth hormone: Biochemical, genetic, and clinical aspects. Annu Rev Med, 34: 519-547, 1983.
18. Daughaday WH: Growth hormone: Normal synthesis, secretion, control, and mechanism of action. In: "Endocrinology" (Ed LJ De Groot), WB Saunders, Philadelphia, 1989, pp 318-329.
19. Flier JS, Moses AC: Diabetes in acromegaly and other endocrine disorders. In: "Endocrinology" (Ed LJ De Groot), WB Saunders, Philadelphia, 1989, pp 1389-1399.
20. D'Ercole AJ, Stiles AD, Underwood LE: Tissue concentrations of somatomedin C: Further evidence for multiple sites of synthesis and paracrine or autocrine mechanisms of action. Proc Natl Acad Sci USA, 81: 935-939, 1984.
21. Hammerman MR: Editorial review. The growth hormoneinsulinlike growth factor axis in kidney. Am J Physiol, 254: F503-F514, 1989.
22. Anderson G, Jennische E: IGF-I immunoreactivity is expressed by regenerating renal tubular cells after ischaemic injury in the rat. Acta Physiol Scand, 132: 453-457, 1988.
23. Mehls O, Ritz E: Skeletal growth in experimental uremia. Kidney Int, 21 (Suppl): S53-S62, 1983.
24. Mehls O, Ritz E, Hunziker EB, Eggli P, Heinrich U, Zapf J: Improvement of growth and food utilization by human recombinant growth hormone in uremia. Kidney Int, 33: 45-52, 1988.
25. Powell DR, Rosenfeld RG, Hintz RL: Effects of growth hormone therapy and malnutrition on the growth of rats with renal failure. Pediatr Nephrol, 2: 425-430, 1988.
26. Nakano M, Kainer G, Foreman JW, Ko D, Chan JCM: The effects of exogenous rat growth hormone therapy on growth of uremic rats fed an 8% protein diet. Pediatr Res, 26: 204-207, 1989.
27. Kainer G, Nakano M, Massi FS, Foreman JW and Chan JCM: Hypercalciuria due to combined growth hormone and calcitriol therapy in uremia: Effects of growth hormone on mineral homeostasis in 75% nephrectomized weanling rats. Pediatric Res, 30: 528-533, 1991.
28. Lippe B, Fine RN, Koch VH, Sherman BM: Accelerated growth following treatment of children with chronic renal failure with recombinant human growth hormone (Somatrem): A preliminary report. Acta Paediatr Scand, 343 (Suppl): 127-131, 1988.
29. Koch VH, Lippe BM, Nelson PA, Boechat MI, Sherman BM, Fine RN: Accelerated growth after recombinant human growth hormone treatment of children with chronic renal failure. J Pediatr, 115: 365-371, 1989.
30. Fine RN, Pyke-Grimm K, Nelson PA et al: Recombinant human growth hormone (rhGH) treatment of children with chronic renal failure (CRF): Long-term (one to three years outcome). Pediatr Nephrol, 5: 477-481, 1991.
31. Rees L, Rigden SPA, Ward G, Preece MA: Treatment of short stature in renal disease with recombinant human growth hormone. Arch Dis Child, 65: 856-860, 1990.
32. Tonshoff B, Mehls O, Schauer A, Heinrich U, Blum W, Ranke M: Improvement of uremic growth failure by recombinant human growth hormone. Kidney Int, 36 (Suppl): S201-S04, 1989.
33. Tonshoff B, Mehls O, Heinrich U, Blum W, Ranke MB, Schauerf A: Growth-stimulating effects of recombinant human growth hormone in children with end-stage renal disease. J Pediatr, 16: 561-566, 1990.
34. Johansson G, Sietnieke A, Janssens F, et al: Recombinant human growth treatment in short children with chronic renal disease, before transplantation or with functioning renal transplants: an interim report on five European studies. Acta Paediatr Scand (Suppl), 370: 36-42, 1990.

35. Wilson DP, Jelley D, Stratton R, Coldwell JG: Nephropathic cystinosis: Improved linear growth after treatment with recombinant human growth hormone. J Pediatr, 115: 758-761, 1989.
36. Hokken-Koelega ACS, Stijnen T, de Muinck Keizer-Schrama SMPF, Wit JM, Wolff ED, deJong MCJW, Donckerwolcke RA, Abbad NCB, Bot A, Blum WF, Drop SLS: Placebo-controlled, double-blind, cross-over trial of growth hormone treatment in prepubertal children with chronic renal failure. Lancet, 338: 585-590, 1991.
37. Fine RN, Koch VH, Boechat MI, et al: Recombinant human growth hormone (rhGH) treatment of children undergoing peritoneal dialysis. Perit Dial Int, 10: 209-214, 1990.
38. Fine RN, Fine SE, Sherman BM: Absorption of recombinant human growth hormone (rhGH) following intraperitoneal instillation. Perit Dial Int, 9: 91-93, 1989.
39. Kamil ES, Yadin O, Koch VH, et al: Intraperitoneal (IP) recombinant human growth hormone (met-hGH) treatment (Rx) of children undergoing peritoneal dialysis. XXXIInd Annual meeting, American Society of Nephrology, Washington, DC, December 3-6, 1989.
40. Pennisi AJ, Costin G, Phillips LS, et al: Somatomedin and growth hormone studies in pediatric renal allograft recipients who receive daily prednisone. Am J Dis Child, 133: 950-954, 1979.
41. Rees L, Greene SA, Adlard P, et al: Growth and endocrine function after renal transplantation. Arch Dis Child, 63: 1326-1332, 1988.
42. Tejani A, Butt KMH, Rajpoot D, et al: Strategies for optimizing growth in children with kidney transplants. Transplantation, 47: 229-233, 1989.
43. Jabs KL, Van Dop C, Harmon WE: Endocrinologic evaluation of children who grow poorly following renal transplantation. Transplantation, 49: 71-76, 1990.
44. David-Neto E, Vilares S, Lando V, et al: Conversion for azathioprine/prednisone to azathioprine/cyclosporin promotes catch-up growth in pediatric renal allograft recipients. Clin Transplant, 4: 229-234, 1990.
45. Schaefer F, Stanhope R, Preece MA, Scharer K: Pulsatile growth hormone secretion in peripubertal patients with chronic renal failure. J Pediatr, 119: 568-577, 1991.
46. Kaufmann S, Jones KL, Wehrenberg WB, Culler FL: Inhibition by prednisone of growth hormone (GH) response to GH-releasing hormone in normal men. J Clin Endocrinol Metab, 67: 1258-1261, 1988.
47. Kovacs G, Fine RN, Worgall S, Schaefer F, Hunziker EB, Skottner-Lindun A, Mehls O: Growth hormone prevents steroid-induced growth depression in health and uremia. Kidney Int, 40: 1032-1040, 1991.
48. Van Dop C, Donohoue PA, Bock GH, Ruley J: Enhanced growth with growth hormone therapy after renal transplantation. Pediatr Nephrol, 3: 468-469, 1989.
49. Fine RN, Koch VH, Nelson PA, et al: Recombinant human growth hormone (rhGH) treatment of children with renal insufficiency. Adv Nephrol, 19: 187-208, 1990.
50. Fine RN, Yadin O, Nelson, PA, Pyke-Grimm K, Boechat MI, Lippe BH, Sherman BM, Ettenger RB, Kamil E: Recombinant human growth hormone treatment of children following renal transplantation. Pediatric Nephrol, 5: 147-151, 1991.
51. Van Dop C, Jabs KL, Donohoue PA, Bock GH, Flvush BA, Harmon WE: Accelerated growth rates in children treated with growth hormone after renal transplantation. J Pediatr, 120: 244-250, 1992.
52. Rapaport R, Oleske J, Ahdieh H, Solomon S, Delfaus C, Denny T: Suppression of immune function in growth hormone-deficient children during treatment with human growth hormone. J Pediatr, 109: 343-439, 1986.
53. Ammann AJ, Sherman BM: Effect of growth hormone therapy on immune function. J Pediatr, 110: 663-664, 1987 (Letter).
54. Church JA, Costin G, Brooks J: Immune functions in children treated with biosynthetic growth hormone. J Pediatr, 115: 420-423, 1989.
55. Hirschberg R, Rabb, H, Bergano R, Kopple JD: The delayed effect of growth hormone on renal function in humans. Kidney Int, 35: 865-870, 1989.
56. Westby GR, Goldfarb S, Goldberg M, Agus ZS: Acute effects of bovine growth hormone on renal calcium and phosphate excretion. Metabolism, 26: 525-530, 1977.
57. Parving HH, Noer I, Mogensen CE, Svendsen PA: Kidney function in normal man during short-term growth hormone infusion. Acta Endocrinol, 89: 796-800, 1978.
58. Christiansen JS, Gammelgaard J, Orskov H, Andersen AR, Telmer S, Parving HH: Kidney function and size in normal subjects before and during growth hormone administration for one week. Eur J Clin Invest, 11: 487-490, 1981.

59. Hirschberg RR, Kopple JD: Increase in renal plasma flow and glomerular filtration rate during growth hormone treatment may be mediated by insulin-like growth factor I. Am J Nephrol, 8: 249-253, 1988.
60. Hirschberg R, Kopple JD: Evidence that insulin-like growth factor I increases renal plasma flow and glomerular filtration rate in fasted rats. J Clin Invest, 83: 326-330, 1989.
61. Haffner D, Ritz E, Mehls O, et al: Growth hormone induced rise in glomerular filtration rate is not obliterated by angiotensin-converting enzyme inhibitors. Nephron, 55: 63-68, 1990.
62. Haffner D, Zachariwicz S, Mehls O, Heinrich U, Ritz E: The acute effect of growth hormone on GFR is obliterated in chronic renal failure. Clin Nephrol, 32: 266-269, 1989.
63. Doi T, Striker LJ, Quaife C, et al: Progressive glomerulosclerosis develops in transgenic mice chronically expressing growth hormone and growth hormone releasing factor but not in those expressing insulin growth factor-I. Am J Pathol, 131: 398-403, 1988.
64. Wanke R, Hermanns W, Folger S, Wolf E, Brem G: Accelerated growth and visceral lesions in transgenic mice expressing foreign genes of the growth hormone family: An overview. Pediatr Nephrol, 5: 518-521, 1991.
65. Doi T, Striker LJ, Kimata K, Peten EP, Yamada Y, Striker GE: Glomerulosclerosis in mice transgenic for growth hormone. Increased mesangial extracellular matrix is correlated with kidney and mRNA levels. J Exp Med, 173: 1287-1290, 1991.
66. El Nahas AM, Basset AH, Cope GH, Le Carpenter JE: Role of growth hormone in the development of experimental renal scarring. Kidney Int, 40: 29-34, 1991.

GERIATRIC NEPHROLOGY

Chapter 10

THE AGEING KIDNEY: PRACTICAL CONSIDERATIONS IN THE MANAGEMENT OF THE ELDERLY PATIENT WITH RENAL DISEASE

RICHARD CHAN, MICHAEL F. MICHELIS

Division of Nephrology, Department of Medicine, Lenox Hill Hospital, New York, New York 10021, USA

FUNCTIONAL CHARACTERISTICS OF THE AGING KIDNEY

The changes in renal function that may accompany aging have been the subject of numerous studies over the past several decades (1, 2). These changes include decreases in glomerular filtration rate (3), and alterations in tubular function (4). The qualitative and quantitative aspects of these changes must be appreciated prior to developing strategies for treating elderly patients with renal disease. The alterations in renal function in elderly patients that affect therapeutic choices will be specifically referred to later in this chapter. The functional characteristics of the aging kidney will be summarized now, however, so that a proper orientation to the problem will be developed.

It is well recognized that glomerular filtration rate, as estimated by creatinine clearance (CrCl), decreases in many individuals as they age (1, 5). The decrease in CrCl may not be appreciated if serum creatinine (Cr) alone is monitored. This occurs because the decrease in muscle mass associated with aging results in decreased Cr production. If the decrease in Cr production parallels the decrease in CrCl, serum Cr may remain unchanged despite declining renal function.

Changes in renal tubular function also accompany aging. These include a decreased ability for renal sodium conservation during sodium depletion (6), limitation of urinary concentrating and diluting ability (7), and decreased distal tubular capacity for acid and potassium excretion (4, 8). In addition to the impaired renal sodium conservation that may result from structural alterations in the nephron, hormonal alterations which may accompany aging such as decreased renin and aldosterone secretion (9, 10), and increased activity of atrial natriuretic factor (11), can also affect renal sodium handling in elderly patients.

The decrease in urinary concentrating ability observed in elderly patients occurs, in part, as a result of renal structural changes which decrease medullary hypertonicity and limit maximal urinary concentration (7). Inability to adequately concentrate the urine may result in increased morbidity during extrarenal fluid loss from diarrheal states or febrile illnesses. On the other hand, dysfunction of the diluting segment of the nephron and alterations in the regulation of vasopressin secretion, may result in inappropriate water retention (12). Excess vasopressin secretion has been noted to occur spontaneously in older patients (13), and may also occur during stressful situations (14), in association with pulmonary disease (15), neoplastic disease (16), and with drugs that stimulate vasopressin secretion (17). Hypoosmolar syndromes can become particularly severe when older patients are given obligatory free water during intravenous therapy with dilute fluids (18).

Distal renal tubular dysfunction may cause an impairment in hydrogen ion and potassium secretion. Acidosis secondary to renal hydrogen ion retention has been well described in instances of chronic renal interstitial disease (4, 19). Potassium retention can develop either in association with renal tubular diseases or secondary to the decreased secretion of renin and aldosterone which may accompany aging (8, 20, 21). Some data suggest that hyporeninemic hypoaldosteronism may result from gradual fluid accumulation (22). Recent studies by our group are consistent with this hypothesis in that patients with this disorder, who received chronic diuretic therapy, demonstrated increases in plasma renin activity, during a captopril stimulation test (23), associated with a decrease in atrial natriuretic factor (Figure 1). The above alterations in renal function must be considered when developing specific diagnostic or therapeutic plans in elderly patients with renal disease.

SPECIAL CLINICAL SITUATIONS

Five important clinical situations will now be reviewed in regard to the special problems presented by elderly renal patients with these disorders: [1] systolic and diastolic hypertension, [2] radiocontrast nephrotoxicity, [3] conditions requiring the use of nonsteroidal antiinflammatory drugs, [4] factors predisposing to interstitial nephritis, and [5] dialysis therapy in the aged.

Systolic and diastolic hypertension

Elevations of systolic and diastolic blood pressure in the elderly are often observed in association with increased peripheral vascular resistance and decreased cardiac output

(24). Data from many recent long-term studies strongly confirm the impression that antihypertensive therapy decreases cardiovascular morbidity and mortality in elderly patients (25-27). Drug therapy can employ beta-adrenergic blocking agents, as well as vasodilatory agents which currently include alpha$_1$-adrenergic blocking agents, calcium channel blocking agents, and converting enzyme inhibitors (CEI). Centrally acting agents may also be quite useful in the management of elderly hypertensives, but are often used cautiously since sedation or confusion may occur. Diuretics can also play a significant role in the management of hypertension in the elderly. Recent results from the systolic hypertension in the elderly program (SHEP) demonstrated diuretics to be effective, low-cost antihypertensive agents, and not associated with significant adverse effects on lipid profiles (27). Other long-term trials have also reported little change or even a lowering of serum cholesterol levels following antihypertensive therapy with diuretics (28).

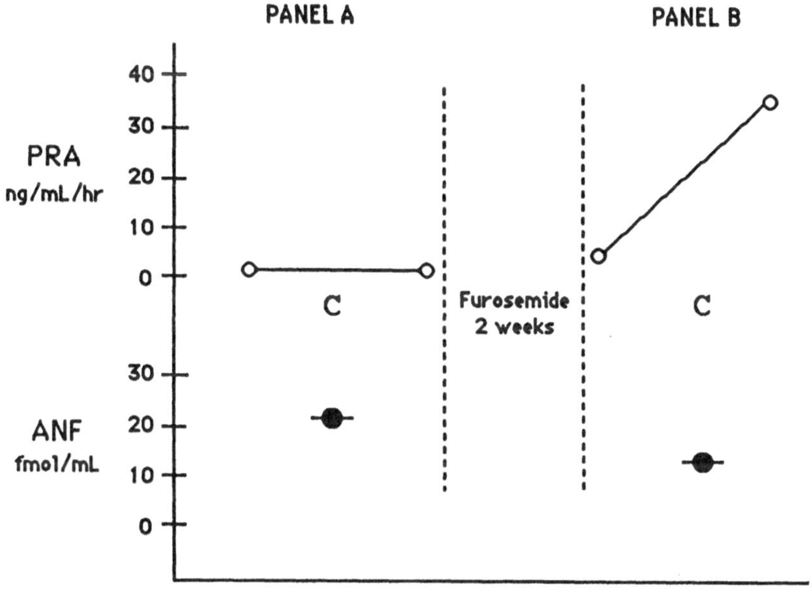

Figure 1. Panel A illustrates initial lack of response of plasma renin activity (PRA) to captopril and plasma level of atrial natriuretic factor (ANF). Panel B shows responsiveness of PRA to captopril and ANF level post-chronic diuresis with furosemide. C=captopril test (25 mg of oral captopril with measurements at 0 time and 60 minutes).

Negative aspects of diuretic therapy in elderly renal patients include excessive volume depletion and hypokalemia (29). Intravascular volume deficits may be associated with orthostatic hypotension which may result in confusion, dizziness, and even serious trauma secondary to falls (30). Such changes may be avoided by the use of lower doses of either thiazide diuretics or loop diuretics, depending on the degree of renal dysfunction. Hypokalemia may cause concern since serious cardiac arrhythmias can occur in association with this disorder (31). In patients with adequate renal function, routine potassium supplementation may avoid this complication. Further, recent studies have shown that low dose diuretic therapy can effectively lower blood pressure while avoiding troublesome side-effects such as hypokalemia (32).

Postsynaptic $alpha_1$-adrenergic blocking agents such as prazosin, and the longer-acting agents terazosin and doxazosin, may be useful for lowering blood pressure and also for afterload reduction in patients with congestive heart failure. The use of these drugs has been associated with orthostatic hypotension and syncope, but this can be avoided by initiation of therapy at low doses and very gradual dose alterations. Initiation of therapy with bedtime dosing as drug tolerance is being developed, may avoid falls during more active parts of the day. Recent reports have indicated a beneficial effect on the lipid profile of patients during doxazosin therapy (33). $Alpha_1$-adrenergic blocking agents have also been successfully employed in the management of benign urinary bladder outlet obstruction and impotence (34). Older agents, such as hydralazine, may also be useful in regard to control of hypertension in elderly patients, and may have less side effects, particularly at lower doses. Tachycardia, which can occur with hydralazine usage, is actually less common in older patients.

Beta-adrenergic blocking agents such as propranolol, nadolol, and atenolol, have been widely used in the treatment of hypertension. A variety of negative effects have been associated with the use of these agents. These include decreases in peripheral circulation, adverse changes in lipid profiles, difficulties in the management of diabetic patients, and precipitation of episodes of bronchospasm. These problems may be avoided by careful patient selection and meticulous patient follow-up. Furthermore, important beneficial effects have been associated with the use of drugs in this group such as those described in studies which suggest that metoprolol may result in improvement in morbidity and mortality in postmyocardial infarction patients (35). This may occur because of the antiarrhythmic and oxygen-sparing effects of these drugs (36). Agents with significant renal excretion, such as atenolol and pindolol, should be used with care and in reduced dosage in elderly renal failure patients (37).

Calcium channel blocking agents have also gained widespread use in the management of elderly patients with hypertensive or cardiovascular disorders. It has also been suggested that these agents may have beneficial effects in patients with progressive diabetic nephropathy (38). More commonly used agents include verapamil, nifedipine, diltiazem, and nicardipine (Table 1).

Table 1. Calcium-channel blockers for hypertension*

Drug	Initial Dosage
Diltiazem - Cardizem SR (Marion Merrell Dow)	60-120 mg bid
Isradipine - DynaCirc (Sandoz)	2.5 mg bid
Nicardipine - Cardene (Syntex)	20 mg tid
Nifedipine - Procardia XL (Pfizer)	30 mg qd
Verapamil -	80 mg tid
Calan (Searle)	
Isoptin (Knoll)	
sustained release:	
Calan SR (Searle)	180 mg qd
Isoptin SR (Knoll)	
Verelan (Lederle)	240 mg qd

* modified from The Medical Letter® 33: 51, 1991 and reprinted by special permission of the publisher.

Sublingual nifedipine has also been used to treat accelerated hypertension, while diltiazem has been employed in the management of angina. These agents may be useful in treating hypertension in elderly patients with varying levels of renal dysfunction, including patients on chronic dialysis therapy. Side effects such as the development of edema and constipation (a problem of particular importance to the elderly), may complicate the use of these drugs. Also, these agents may produce cardiac conduction disorders, especially when used in conjunction with beta-adrenergic blocking agents (39). Newer calcium channel blocking agents, such as isradipine and felodipine, have been reported to be free of adverse effects on cardiac conduction (40).

Converting enzyme inhibitors are a newer group of antihypertensive agents which have been thought to be particularly useful in elderly hypertensive patients (41, 42). With increasing use of CEIs, however, decreases in renal function during the use of these agents have been noted (43, 44). The pathophysiology of the alterations in renal function observed, may result from removal of the vasoconstrictor effects of angiotensin II on the postglomerular arteriole, the constriction being a protective effect which may maintain glomerular filtration in the presence of decreased renal perfusion. Such decreases in renal function have been described with the use of CEIs in patients with bilateral renal artery stenosis or unilateral renal artery stenosis in a patient with a solitary kidney. Because atherosclerosis is common in the elderly, renal artery disease may predispose patients of advanced age to CEI-induced renal insufficiency (44). This risk may be heightened with concomitant use of diuretics or when elderly patients are dehydrated from other causes. Indeed, it has recently been suggested that reversible decreases in renal function in elderly patients who are receiving CEI-type drugs occur more commonly in association with intrarenal perfusion deficits than in association with renal artery stenosis (45). We, therefore, recommend the monitoring of serum Cr after initiation, or dose adjustment, of CEI therapy, when concomitant diuretics are prescribed, or if clinical circumstances associated with the possibility of dehydration occur. An example of reversible azotemia when diuretics and CEI-type drugs are used simultaneously is illustrated in (Figure 2) (43). Renal function improved as diuretic dosage was decreased while use of the CEI was continued. Hyperkalemia may also occur in association with CEI therapy (8, 46).

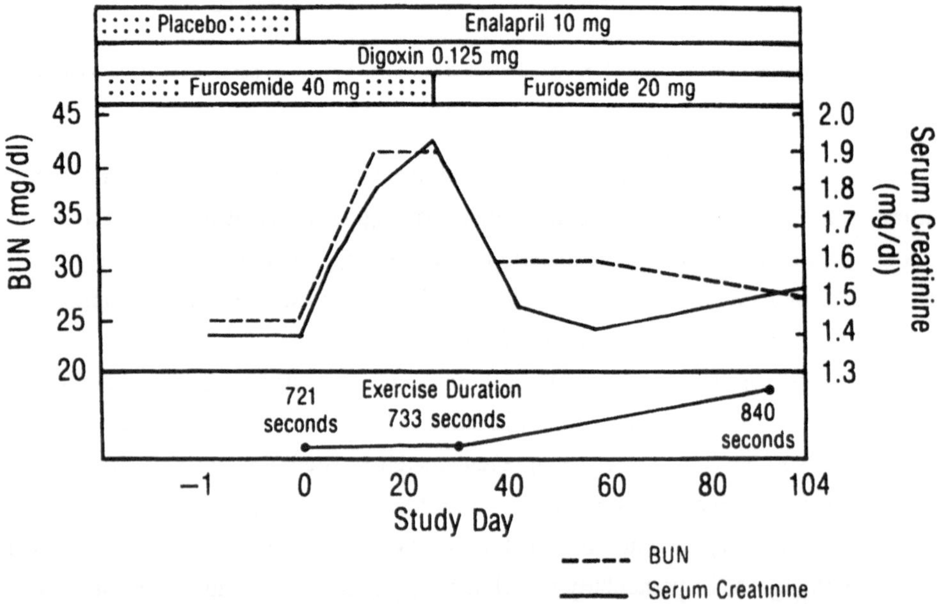

Figure 2. Reversal of azotemia by decrease of diuretic dosage in a patient on CEI therapy (reprinted by special permission, Warner NJ, Rush JE, Keegan ME. Tolerability of enalapril in congestive heart failure. Am J Cardiol, 63: 35D,1989).

Commonly used CEIs include captopril, enalapril, and lisinopril, as well as newer agents such as benazepril, fosinopril, and ramipril (Table 2). The newer CEIs seem to be characterized by a longer duration of action and varying degrees of hepatic versus renal excretion (47). Drugs with greater hepatic excretion may require less dose adjustment in elderly patients with renal insufficiency (48). However, it should not be assumed that these same elderly patients are free of subclinical decreases in hepatic function. Unusual side-effects with the use of CEIs in the elderly, such as captopril-associated mania, have also been reported (49).

Table 2. Converting enzyme inhibitors for hypertension*

Drug	Daily Dosage	Dosage for Renal Impairment
Benazepril - Lotensin (Ciba)	Initial: 10 mg Usual: 20-40 mg qd or bid Maximum: 80 mg	Serum creatinine >3 mg/dl: 5-40 mg
Captopril - Capoten (Squibb)	Initial: 25 mg bid or tid Usual: 25-150 mg bid or tid Maximum: 450 mg	Decreased
Enalapril - Vasotec (Merck)	Initial: 5 mg Usual: 10-40 mg qd or divided Maximum: 40 mg	Serum creatinine >3 mg/dl: 2.5-40 mg
Fosinopril - Monopril (Mead Johnson)	Initial: 10 mg Usual: 20-40 qd or bid Maximum: 80 mg	No change
Lisinopril - Prinivil (Merck) Zestril (Stuart)	Initial: 10 mg Usual: 20-40 mg qd Maximum: 80 mg	Serum creatinine >3 mg/dl: 5-40 mg
Ramipril - Altace (Hoechst)	Initial: 2.5 mg Usual: 5-10 mg qd or bid Maximum: 20 mg	Serum creatinine >2.5 mg/dl: 1.25-5 mg

* modified from The Medical Letter® 33:84, 1991 and reprinted by special permission of the publisher.

Radiocontrast-induced nephrotoxicity in the elderly

Atherosclerotic vascular disease occurs commonly in the elderly. Older patients may require complex diagnostic studies (e.g. coronary angiography, renovascular studies, etc.) and renal failure due to radiocontrast-induced nephrotoxicity can occur (50). Recent studies suggest that this type of renal failure is uncommon (51), but certain patients may be at greater risk than others. These high-risk individuals include patients with congestive heart failure, diabetes mellitus, advanced arteriosclerosis, decreased renal function, dehydration, or patients with a history of prior radiocontrast-induced renal dysfunction (52). In such patients, the use of previously described protective regimens (e.g. mannitol & furosemide) should be considered (50, 51). In patients in whom dehydration is evident, adequate hydration should be provided prior to the initiation of such prophylactic measures. Although it has been suggested that newer nonionic contrast agents may be associated with a lower incidence of radiocontrast-induced nephrotoxicity, a recent study has not supported this conclusion (53). Current data suggesting that radiocontrast-induced intrarenal vasoconstriction may be mediated by endothelin and counteracted by atrial natriuretic factor deserve further scrutiny (54).

The following two protocols may be employed in patients where the possibility of radiocontrast-induced renal failure is a matter of concern. In older patients, serum creatinine levels of 2.0 mg/dL, or greater, may be associated with significant renal dysfunction, and therefore warrant the use of these regimens. The protocols differ in the inclusion or exclusion of mannitol, which may be deleted in those patients where an increase in intravascular volume may precipitate acute pulmonary edema. In both protocols, the aim is to produce a high urine flow rate, and thereby protect the kidney. These protocols may be especially useful in those individuals who are expected to receive large doses of radiocontrast material, or who must undergo repeated procedures.

- *FUROSEMIDE AND MANNITOL* (used in patients with minimal, to no risk of congestive heart failure): furosemide 100 mg per mg/dL creatinine (maximum 300 mg furosemide) in 500 ml 20% mannitol infused at 20 ml/hr, to begin one hour pre-procedure, and continued 3-4 hours post-procedure.
- *FUROSEMIDE IN D5%/W* (used in patients with significant risk of congestive heart failure): furosemide 100 mg per mg/dL creatinine (maximum 300 mg furosemide) in 500 ml D5%/W infused at 20 ml/hr, to begin one hour pre-procedure, and continued 3-4 hours post-procedure.

A drainage catheter should be inserted into the bladder during the infusion period to facilitate voiding and accurate measurement of intake and output. During and following the infusion, sufficient replacement fluid should be administered hourly to avoid significant negative fluid balance, which in itself may have adverse renal effects.

Non-steroidal anti-inflammatory agents in the elderly

Non-steroidal anti-inflammatory drugs (NSAIDs) have gained wide popularity as analgesic agents over the last decade. A variety of untoward effects have been noted including gastrointestinal bleeding and cutaneous eruptions (55). Concern about the renal effects of these drugs in the elderly followed several reports of renal dysfunction occurring during their use (56-58). These drugs are known to interfere with prostaglandin (PG) synthesis and may decrease urine volume resulting in fluid retention and worsening hypertension in situations where PG effect on glomerular hemodynamics is maintaining urine flow in a compensatory manner (56, 59, 60). These clinical situations include dehydration, congestive heart failure, and decreased renal perfusion due to large vessel disease.

Other reported complications of NSAID therapy include minimal change nephropathy, heavy proteinuria, and interstitial disease which can be associated with papillary necrosis. A recent report by Sandler, et al indicated that the risk of renal insufficiency associated with daily use of NSAIDs was particularly apparent in males over 65 years of age (61). An editorial by Wagner points out, however, that these data were barely statistically significant, that there was no dose-response effect, and that the finding may represent a special situation where NSAIDs were used as part of the therapy of complicated medical problems which had chronic renal disease as part of their clinical picture (62). NSAID therapy can also be associated with the occurrence of hyperkalemia (8, 21).

A variety of NSAIDs are now available for clinical use. Differences in their pharmacologic activity and metabolism may be important in regard to avoidance of renal toxicity secondary to these agents (56). For example, the unusual metabolism of sulindac may result in a decreased potential for renal toxicity (63, 64). Since the nephrotoxic events related to the use of these drugs are still not completely understood however, caution should be used with all agents in this group. Further, careful use of low doses of these agents and frequent determination of body weight, blood pressure, and renal function tests are indicated.

Acute interstitial nephritis in the elderly

The renal interstitium of elderly patients comprises a greater proportion of total renal mass than that of younger individuals (65). This results from processes leading to nephron loss secondary either to renal injury incurred during life, or from senescent changes associated with aging (66). The function of renal tubular structures which lie within the interstitium may already be impaired in elderly patients, as evidenced by decreased capacity for urinary concentration and acid excretion. Because drug-induced acute interstitial nephritis is frequently reversible when the offending agent is withdrawn, heightened awareness of this disorder may prevent further decreases of renal tubular function, as well as acute renal failure, in elderly patients.

Acute interstitial nephritis (AIN) in the elderly renal patient is characterized by an abrupt decrease in renal function. This can occur either following institution of therapy with a new drug, or during chronic use of therapeutic agents with the potential to adversely affect the kidney.

The clinical manifestations of AIN may mimic an allergic reaction. The development of fever, rash, and eosinophilia, in conjunction with azotemia, may signal the presence of this disorder. It should be noted that eosinophilia can also be observed in patients with cholesterol emboli (67).

Urinary findings of AIN include gross or microscopic hematuria, and proteinuria. Even nephrotic-range proteinuria in conjunction with AIN can be seen in association with the use of NSAIDs (56). The presence of eosinophils in the urine as detected by Wright's stain or Hansel's stain, is strongly suggestive of AIN (68). Because elderly patients may frequently not exhibit these signs of AIN, a high index of suspicion should be maintained. In some cases, gallium-67 renal scanning may be a useful diagnostic measure. The diagnosis of AIN is definitively made by renal biopsy. Histopathologic findings typically include an acute inflammatory response, with migration of lymphocytes and plasma cells into the renal interstitium, and sparing of glomeruli and tubules (69).

Drugs are now a frequently identifiable cause of AIN in the elderly (70). Classically, the penicillins have been implicated in causing AIN. However, the underlying pathophysiology of AIN is immune-mediated, and the list of drugs associated with AIN includes not only all classes of antibiotics, but many NSAIDs, and even antihypertensives such as diuretics, and the sulfhydryl-containing CEIs (Table 3).

Table 3. A partial listing of agents which could cause interstitial nephritis in the elderly.

Antibiotics	Diuretics
penicillin & derivatives	furosemide
cephalosporins	thiazides
ciprofloxacin	triamterene
sulfonamides	
others	Miscellaneous
	allopurinol
Nonsteroidal Antiinflammatory Drugs	captopril
ibuprofen	arbamazepine
indomethacin	cimetidine
naproxen	
others	

Because elderly patients frequently use multiple medications from the above categories, attention to proper drug dosing following assessment of creatinine clearance and hepatic function is mandatory. When considering a diagnosis of AIN in elderly patients, a review of their current medications should be performed with attention to recent additions to their medical regimen or chronically used drugs known to be associated with AIN. A trial of withdrawal of a suspected agent is then warranted. In severe cases of renal dysfunction, the use of corticosteroids has been associated with improvement in renal function (71).

Dialysis therapy in the elderly

HEMODIALYSIS-ASSOCIATED PROBLEMS

Hemodialysis has become a standard means of successful renal replacement therapy for older chronic renal failure patients (72, 73). A recent study suggests that older patients may be as tolerant of hemodialysis therapy as their younger counterparts (74). Special problems which may relate to the usefulness of hemodialysis in the elderly are outlined in Table 4.

Table 4. Problems which may limit the usefulness of hemodialysis therapy in the elderly

Cardiovascular disease
Anemia
Hypertension
CNS syndromes

Patients placed on hemodialysis who have advanced cardiovascular disease may have more difficulty tolerating dialysis because of hypotension which invariably occurs during therapy (75). This may be especially problematic in patients with borderline perfusion of cerebral vessels, coronary vessels, or vessels in the extremities. On the other hand, the current popularity of bicarbonate-containing solutions has resulted in a decrease in the incidence of intradialytic hypotension (76). Perfusion problems during hemodialysis were formerly compounded by the coincident anemia of chronic renal failure, which may also produce adverse effects in older patients with poor circulation. The use of erythropoietin has mitigated this problem, but difficulties still remain. Some concern exists in regard to the possibility of an excessive increase in red blood cell levels with erythropoietin therapy which, because of changes in viscosity, may predispose to thrombosis of essential vessels, including those involved with the dialysis access (77).

The hypertensive elderly renal failure patient may require antihypertensive agents for interdialytic blood pressure control, which may then excessively decrease blood pressure during the hemodialysis treatment. Further, the use of commonly used antihypertensive agents may cause problems with orthostatic hypotension in older patients and result in thrombosis of both vascular access or other essential vessels. Central nervous system dysfunction, including those dementias associated with aging, may also interfere with both the acceptance of, and rehabilitation from, hemodialysis therapy. Further, patients given to unpredictable movements or emotional outbursts may endanger themselves during the hemodialysis procedure by their unexpected behavior.

The decision to employ chronic hemodialysis therapy will require special consideration in regard to the timing of the creation of a vascular access in older patients. In the elderly with advanced renal insufficiency, serum creatinine may not rise to the levels seen in younger patients. Therefore, thought should be given to vascular access surgery at lower serum creatinine values. Measurement of 24 hour creatinine clearance to assess renal functional status would seem to be essential in this age group. In addition, the sclerotic vascular changes attendant to aging may require more prolonged periods for dialysis fistulas to mature, as well as causing more technical difficulties when surgical placement of dialysis grafts are attempted. Further, proportionately more grafts will be required for hemodialysis access in older patients. Lastly, on a positive note, the limited time devoted to hemodialysis and the decreased patient involvement required for the performance of staff-assisted in-center dialysis may appeal to some elderly patients.

CONTINUOUS AMBULATORY PERITONEAL DIALYSIS-ASSOCIATED PROBLEMS

Although chronic peritoneal dialysis as a treatment modality for end-stage renal failure has been increasingly used in elderly patients (78), the institution of this form of renal replacement therapy should be carefully considered in each patient. Because continuous ambulatory peritoneal dialysis (CAPD) requires active patient participation, elderly patients with impaired cognitive function may be unsuitable for self-dialysis; however, a spouse can often be effectively trained to assist in the CAPD process.

Problems associated with the use of CAPD therapy in the elderly can be varied (79). Inability to manipulate CAPD equipment properly may predispose elderly patients to an increased frequency of peritonitis. Constipation, which is not infrequent in elderly patients, may impede drainage of dialysate from the abdomen. The more frequent occurrence of diverticulitis in older patients may cause difficulty in the evaluation of peritoneal signs in CAPD patients. In addition, age-associated decreases in the tone of the abdominal musculature may predispose the elderly patient on CAPD to intestinal herniation as a result of repeated instillation of dialysate into the peritoneal cavity. Furthermore, CAPD-associated protein losses may pose special problems for the elderly whose protein intake may already be limited by a variety of factors, including economic ones (80).

Nevertheless, the use of CAPD in elderly patients with end-stage renal failure has been quite successful. Nissenson (79) recently reviewed the international experience with this therapeutic modality in over 8,000 elderly CAPD patients. Overall complication rates of CAPD in elderly patients were similar when compared to that in younger patients; however, hospitalizations were more common in the elderly, and hospital stays were longer in these patients.

Recent data has suggested that survival of older patients on CAPD may actually be better than that on hemodialysis (81). Beneficial features of CAPD over hemodialysis may be influenced by several factors. To begin, placement of abdominal catheters for CAPD by a variety of techniques (82) may be less problematic in elderly patients whose vascular disease limits the creation of a suitable access for hemodialysis. Because CAPD is associated with continuous fluid and solute removal, it may have advantages in elderly patients who typically have atherosclerotic changes of medium and large arteries. The more abrupt changes in intravascular fluid volume and electrolytes that occur in hemodialysis may predispose elderly patients to hypotensive episodes and their complications, such as angina, cardiac arrhythmias, and cerebrovascular insufficiency. Such complications may be avoided by the use of CAPD. CAPD also obviates the use of heparin, and may also be associated with less rigorous approaches to diet and fluid restriction, which may be problematic in older patients. More liberal fluid intake may also avoid constipation, which, as noted above, is a frequent complaint of the elderly.

CAPD patients may also tend to demonstrate higher red blood cell counts, which may reflect, in part, the absence of the blood loss which occurs with hemodialysis. This decreased tendency toward anemia may cause symptomatic improvement in the elderly, but this benefit of peritoneal dialysis has been lessened by the use of erythropoietin in hemodialysis patients. Further, blood pressure control may be more consistent with CAPD, because of continuous fluid removal, thereby limiting the use of antihypertensive agents and avoiding their troublesome side-effects. Recent reports suggest that beta-2 microglobulin is cleared by CAPD (83). However, beta-2 microglobulin may now also be removed by newer hemodialysis devices (84). This capability may be less important to older patients whose course on dialysis may be somewhat shortened by their advanced age.

REFERENCES

1. Rowe JW, Andres R, Tobin JD, Norris AH, Shock NW: The effect of age on creatinine clearance in men: A cross-sectional and longitudinal study. J Gerontol, 31: 155-163, 1976.
2. Epstein M: Effects of aging on the kidney. Fed Proc, 38: 168-171, 1979.
3. Lindeman RD, Tobin JD, Shock NW: Longitudinal studies on the rate of decline in renal function with age. J Am Geriatr Soc, 33: 278-285, 1985.
4. Adler S, Lindeman RD, Yiengst MJ, Beard E, Shock NW: Effect of acute acid loading on urinary acid excretion by the aging human kidney. J Lab Clin Med, 72: 278-289, 1968.
5. Lindeman RD, Tobin JD, Shock NW: Association between blood pressure and the rate of decline in renal function with age. Kidney Int, 26: 861-868, 1984.
6. Epstein M, Hollenberg NK: Age as a determinant of renal sodium conservation in normal men. J Lab Clin Med, 87: 411-417, 1976.
7. Rowe JW, Shock NW, DeFronzo RA: The influence of age on the renal response to water deprivation in man. Nephron, 17: 270-278, 1976.
8. Michelis MF: Hyperkalemia in the elderly. Am J Kid Dis, 16: 296-299, 1990.
9. Noth RH, Lassman MN, Tan SY: Age and the renin-aldosterone system. Arch Intern Med, 137: 1414-1417, 1977.
10. Tsunoda K, Abe K, Goto T, Yasujima M, Sato M, Omata K, Seino M, Yoshinaga K: Effect of age on the renin-angiotensin-aldosterone system in normal subjects: Simultaneous measurement of active and inactive renin, renin substrate, and aldosterone in plasma. J Clin Endocrinol Metab, 62: 384-389, 1986.
11. Ohashi M, Fujio N, Nawata H, Kato KI, Ibayashi H, Kangawa K, Matsuo H: High plasma concentrations of human atrial natriuretic polypeptide in aged men. J Clin End Met, 64: 81-85, 1987.
12. Lindeman RD, Lee TD, Jr., Yiengst, MJ, Shock NW: Influence of age, renal disease, hypertension, diuretics, and calcium on the antidiuretic responses to suboptimal infusions of vasopressin. J Lab Clin Med, 68: 206-223, 1966.
13. Goldstein CS, Braunstein S, Goldfarb S: Idiopathic syndrome of inappropriate antidiuretic hormone secretion possibly related to advanced age. Ann Int Med, 99: 185-188, 1983.
14. Kennedy PGE, Mitchell DM, Hoffbrand BI: Severe hyponatremia in hospital inpatients. Br Med J, 2: 1251-1253, 1978.
15. Sladen A, Laver MB, Pontoppidan H: Pulmonary complications and water retention in prolonged mechanical ventilation. N Engl J Med, 279: 448-453, 1968.
16. Bartter FC, Schwartz WB: The syndrome of inappropriate secretion of antidiuretic hormone. Am J Med, 42: 790-806, 1967.
17. Gardenswartz MH, Berl T: Drug induced changes in water excretion. The Kidney, 14: 19-23, 1981.
18. DeVita MV, Gardenswartz MH, Konecky A, Zabetakis PM: Incidence and etiology of hyponatremia in an intensive care unit. Clin Nephrol, 34: 163-166, 1990.
19. Lathem W: Hyperchloremic acidosis in chronic pyelonephritis. N Engl J Med, 258: 1031-1036, 1958.
20. Nadler JL, Lee FO, Hsueh W, Horton R: Evidence of prostacyclin deficiency in the syndrome of hyporeninemic hypoaldosteronism. N Engl J Med, 314: 1015-1020, 1986.
21. Tan SY, Burton M: Hyporeninemic hypoaldosteronism. Arch Int Med, 141: 30-33, 1981.
22. Oh MS, Carroll HJ, Clemmons JE, Vagnucci AH, Levison SP, Whang ESM: A mechanism for hyporeninemic hypoaldosteronism in chronic renal disease. Metabolism, 23: 1157-1166, 1974.
23. Muller FB, Sealey JE, Case DB, Atlas SA, Pickering TG, Pecker MS, Preibisz JJ, Laragh JH: The captopril test for identifying renovascular disease in hypertensive patients. Am J Med, 80: 633-644, 1986.

24. Messerli FH, Sundgaard-Riise K, Ventura HO, Dunn FG, Glade LB, Frohlich ED: Essential hypertension in the elderly: Haemodynamics, intravascular volume, plasma renin activity, and circulating catecholamine levels. Lancet, II: 983-985, 1983.
25. Amery A, Birkenhager W, Brixko P, Bulpitt C, Clement D, Deruyttere M, De Schaepdryver A, Dollery C, Fagard R, Forette F: Mortality and morbidity results from the European Working Party on High Blood Pressure in the Elderly trial. Lancet, I: 1349-1354, 1985.
26. Dahlof B, Lindholm LH, Hansson L, Schersten B, Ekbom T, Wester PO: Morbidity and mortality in the Swedish Trial in Old Patients with Hypertension (STOP-Hypertension). Lancet, 338: 1281-1285, 1991.
27. SHEP Cooperative Research Group: Prevention of stroke by antihypertensive drug treatment in older persons with isolated systolic hypertension. Final results of the systolic hypertension in the elderly program. JAMA, 265: 3255-3264, 1991.
28. Moser M: Hypertension treatment results in minority patients. Am J Med, 88 (suppl 3B): 24S - 31S, 1990.
29. Pascual J, Lrofino L, Liano F, Marcen R, Naya MT, Orte L, Ortuno J: Incidence and prognosis of acute renal failure in older patients. J Am Geriatr Soc, 38: 25-30, 1990.
30. Tinetti ME, Speechley M: Prevention of falls among the elderly. N Engl J Med, 320: 1055-1059, 1989.
31. Hollifield JW, Slaton PE: Thiazide diuretics, hypokalemia and cardiac arrhythmias. Acta Med Scand, suppl 647: 67-73, 1981.
32. Kaplan NM: The case for low dose diuretic therapy. AJH, 4: 970-971, 1991.
33. Pool JL: Effects of doxazosin on serum lipids: A review of the clinical data and molecular basis for altered lipid metabolism. Am Heart J, 121(pt 2): 251-260, 1991.
34. Le Duc A, Cariou G, Baron C, Cukier J, Quentel P, Faure G, Rambeaud JJ, Navratil H, Costa P, Richaud JJ: A multicenter, double-blind, placebo-controlled trial of the efficacy of prazosin in the treatment of dysuria associated with benign prostatic hypertrophy. Urol Int, 45 suppl 1: 56-62, 1990.
35. Ryden L, Ariniego R, Arnman K, Herlitz J, Hjalmarson A, Holmberg S, Reyes C, Smedgard P, Svedberg K, Vedin A, Waagstein F, Waldenstrom A, Wilhelmsson C, Wedel H, Yamamoto M: A double-blind trial of metoprolol in acute myocardial infarction. Effects on ventricular arrhythmias. N Engl J Med, 308: 614-618, 1983.
36. Green KG: British MRC trial of treatment for mild hypertension—a more favorable interpretation. AJH, 4: 723-724, 1991.
37. Frishman WH: Beta-adrenergic receptor blockers. Adverse effects and drug interactions. Hypertension, 11(Supp II): II-21-II-29, 1988.
38. Bakris GL: Effects of diltiazem or lisinopril on massive proteinuria associated with diabetes mellitus. Ann Int Med, 112: 707-710, 1990.
39. Tjoa HI, Kaplan NM: Treatment of hypertension in the elderly. JAMA, 264: 1015-1018, 1990.
40. Kuhlkamp V, Maier F, Seipel L. Electrophysiologic effects of the calcium antagonist isradipine, a double-blind placebo-controlled study. Int J Cardiol, 30(2): 215-220, 1991.
41. Niarchos AP, Laragh JH: Renin dependency of blood pressure in isolated systolic hypertension. Am J Med, 77: 407-414, 1984.
42. Jenkins AC, Knill JR, Dreslinski GR: Captopril in the treatment of the elderly hypertensive patient. Arch Intern Med, 145: 2029-2031, 1985.
43. Warner NJ, Rush JE, Keegan ME: Tolerability of enalapril in congestive heart failure. Am J Cardiol, 63: 33D-37D, 1989.
44. Hricik DE, Browning PJ, Kopelman R: Captopril-induced functional renal insufficiency in patients with bilateral renal-artery stenoses or renal artery stenosis in a solitary kidney. N Engl J Med, 308: 373-376, 1983.
45. Toto RD, Mitchell HC, Lee HC, Milam C, Pettinger WA: Reversible renal insufficiency due to angiotensin converting enzyme inhibitors in hypertensive nephrosclerosis. Ann Int Med, 115: 513-519, 1991.
46. DeVita MV, Han H, Chan R, Zabetakis PM, Gleim GW, Michelis MF: Drug use and the elderly in relation to changing etiologies of hyperkalemia. Ger Nephrol Urol, 1: 41-45, 1991.
47. Sica DA, Cutler RE, Parmer RJ, Ford NF: Comparison of the steady-state pharmacokinetics of fosinopril, lisinopril and enalapril in patients with chronic renal insufficiency. Clin Pharmacokinet, 20(5): 420-427, 1991.

48. Hui KK, Duchin KL, Kripalani KJ, Chan D, Kramer P, Yanagawa N: Pharmacokinetics of fosinopril in patients with various degrees of renal function. Clin Pharm Therap, 49: 457-467. 1991.
49. Patten S, Brager N, Sanders S: Manic symptoms associated with the use of captopril. Can J Psych, 36: 314-315, 1991 (Letter).
50. Berkseth RO, Kjellstrand CM: Radiologic contrast-induced nephropathy. Med Clin N Am, 68: 351-371, 1984.
51. Rich MW, Crecelius CA: Incidence, risk factors, and clinical course of acute renal insufficiency after cardiac catheterization in patients 70 years of age or older. Arch Intern Med, 150: 1237-1242, 1990.
52. Byrd L, Sherman RL: Radiocontrast-induced acute renal failure: a clinical and pathophysiologic review. Medicine, 58: 270-279, 1979.
53. Nora N, Berns A: Renal failure following cardiac angiography: a prospective study of diatrizoate and iopamidol. Kidney Int, 35: 414, 1989.
54. Margulies KB, Hildebrand FL, Heublein DM, Burnett Jr JC: Radiocontrast increases plasma and urinary endothelin. J Am Soc Nephrol, 2: 1041-1045, 1991.
55. Griffin MR, Ray WA, Schaffner W: Nonsteroidal anti-inflammatory drug use and death from peptic ulcer in elderly persons. Ann Intern Med, 109: 359-363, 1988.
56. Clive DM, Stoff JS: Renal syndromes associated with nonsteroidal antiinflammatory drugs. N Engl J Med, 310: 563-572, 1984.
57. Blackshear JL, Napier JS, Davidman M, Stillman MT: Renal complications of nonsteroidal antiinflammatory drugs: identification and monitoring of those at risk. Semin Arthritis Rheum, 4: 163-175, 1985.
58. Gurwitz JH, Avorn J, Ross-Degnan D, Lipsitz LA: Nonsteroidal anti-inflammatory drug-associated azotemia in the very old. JAMA, 264: 471-475, 1990.
59. Garella S, Matarese RA: Renal effects of prostaglandins and clinical adverse effects of nonsteroidal anti-inflammatory agents. Medicine, 63: 165-81, 1984.
60. Badr KF, Ichikawa I: Prerenal failure: a deleterious shift from renal compensation to decompensation. N Engl J Med, 319: 623-629, 1988.
61. Sandler DP, Burr FR, Weinberg CR: Nonsteroidal anti-inflammatory drugs and the risk for chronic renal disease. Ann Int Med, 115: 165-172, 1991.
62. Wagner EH: Nonsteroidal anti-inflammatory drugs and renal disease—still unsettled. Ann Int Med, 115; 227-228, 1991.
63. Whelton A, Stout RL, Spilman PS, Klassen DK: Renal effects of ibuprofen, piroxicam, and sulindac in patients with asymptomatic renal failure. A prospective, randomized, crossover comparison. Ann Int Med, 112: 568-576, 1990.
64. Ciabattoni G, Cinotti GA, Pierucci A, Simonetti BM, Manzi M, Pugliese F, Barsotti P, Pecci G, Taggi F, Patrono C: Effects of sulindac and ibuprofen in patients with chronic glomerular disease. Evidence for the dependence of renal function on prostacyclin. N Engl J Med, 310: 279-283, 1984.
65. McLachlan MSF, Guthrie JC, Anerson CK, Fulker MJ: Vascular and glomerular changes in the ageing kidney. J Pathol, 121: 65-78, 1977.
66. Takazakura E, Sawabu N, Handa A, Takada A, Shinoda A, Takeuchi J: Intrarenal vascular changes with age and disease. Kidney Int, 2: 224-230, 1972.
67. Kassirer JP: Atheroembolic renal disease. N Engl J Med, 280: 812-818, 1969.
68. Nolan CH, Angel M, Kelleher A: Eosinophiluria: a new method of detection and definition of the clinical spectrum. N Engl J Med, 315: 1516-1519, 1986.
69. Heptinstall RH, Kissane JM, McCluskey RT, Porter KA: Interstitial nephritis. In: "Pathology of the Kidney" (Ed RH Heptinstall), Little Brown & Company, Boston,1974, pp 821-836.
70. Linton AL, Clark WF, Driedger AA, Turnbull DI, Lindsay RM: Acute interstitial nephritis due to drugs. Review of the literature with a report of nine cases. Ann Int Med, 93: 735-741, 1980.
71. Galpin JE, Shinaberger JH, Stanley TM, Blumenkrantz MJ, Bayer AS, Friedman GS, Montgomerie JZ, Guze LB, Coburn JW, Glassock RJ: Acute interstitial nephritis due to methicillin. Am J Med, 65: 756-765, 1978.
72. Chester AC, Rakowski TA, Argy WP Jr., Giacalone A, Schreiner GE: Hemodialysis in the eighth and ninth decades of life. Arch Intern Med, 139: 1001-1005. 1979.
73. Eggers PW: Mortality rates among dialysis patients in Medicare's end-stage renal disease program. Am J Kidney Dis, 15: 414-421, 1990.

74. Capuano A, Sepe V, Cianfrone T, Castellano T, Andreucci VE: Cardiovascular impairment, dialysis strategy and tolerance in elderly and young patients on maintenance hemodialysis. Nephrol Dial Transplant, 5: 1023-1030, 1990.
75. Daugirdas JT: Dialysis hypotension: A hemodynamic analysis. Kidney Int, 39: 233-246, 1991.
76. Veech RL: The untoward effects of the anions of dialysis fluids. Kidney Int, 34: 587-597, 1988.
77. Shinaberger JH, Miller JH, Gardner PW: Disadvantages and risks of normal hematocrit (Hct) hemodialysis (HD). Kidney Int, 25: 264, 1989 (Abstract).
78. Panarello G, De Baz E, Cecchin F, Tesio F: Dialysis for the elderly: Survival and risk factors. Adv Perit Dial, 5: 49-51, 1989.
79. Nissenson AR: Chronic peritoneal dialysis in the elderly. Ger Nephrol and Urol, 1: 3-12, 1991.
80. Schilling H, Wu G, Pettit J, Harrison J, McNeill K, Siccion Z, Oreopoulos DG: Nutritional status of patients on long-term CAPD. Perit Dial Bull, 5: 12-18, 1985.
81. Maiorca R, Vonesh E, Cancarini GC, Cantaluppi A, Manili L, Brunori G, Camerini C, Feller P, Strada A: A six year comparison of patient and technique survivals in CAPD and HD. Kidney Int, 34: 518-524, 1988.
82. Handt AE, Ash SR: Longevity of Tenckhoff catheters placed by the VITEC peritoneoscopic technique. Perspect Perit Dial, 2: 30-33, 1984.
83. Gagnon RF, Somerville P, Kaye M: ß-microglobulin serum levels in patients on long term dialysis. Perit Dial Bull, 7: 29-31, 1987.
84. Floege J, Bartsch A, Schulze M, Shaldon S, Koch KM, Smeby LC: Clearance and synthesis rates of $ß_2$-microglobulin in patients undergoing hemodialysis and in normal subjects. J Lab Clin Med, 118: 153-165, 1991.

ACUTE RENAL FAILURE

Chapter 11

THE PATHOGENESIS OF TYPICAL, DIARRHEA-ASSOCIATED, HEMOLYTIC UREMIC SYNDROME

MARY B. LEONARD, EDUARDO RUCHELLI, AND
BERNARD S. KAPLAN

Division of Nephrology, Department of Pediatrics, and Department of Pathology, The Children's Hospital of Philadelphia, University of Pennsylvania, Philadelphia, Pennsylvania, 19104, USA

Hemolytic uremic syndrome (HUS) is an important cause of renal failure, morbidity and mortality and is classified broadly into typical (epidemic, diarrhea-associated or D+) and atypical (sporadic or D-) forms (1, 2). Atypical forms more closely resemble thrombocytopenic thrombotic purpura (TTP) than do typical forms. There is a distinctive form of HUS (typical, D+, Shiga-like toxin-associated HUS) (1-3) which occurs mainly in childhood and is characterized by the rapid onset of acute hemolysis, thrombocytopenia, and acute renal injury. These are preceded by a prodromal illness of acute gastroenteritis, usually with bloody diarrhea. Renal failure predominates over brain involvement. Typical HUS is uncommon in blacks. Typical HUS is associated with infection by organisms that produce Shiga-like toxins (SLT), especially Escherichia coli 0157:H7 (3). Most cases have a neutrophilia. The endothelial injury and thrombotic microangiopathy predominantly involve glomeruli (4). The immediate prognosis is excellent and recurrences are rare (1, 2, 5, 6).

Typical, D+ HUS is distinguished from the typical form of TTP less by the clinical features that are common to each (fever, thrombocytopenia, hemolysis, neurologic involvement, and renal manifestations), than by its gestalt. Features of the TTP pentad occur in asynchronous combinations and the onset is usually gradual. Antecedent bloody diarrhea is uncommon and brain involvement predominates. Blacks are frequently affected. TTP occurs mainly in adults. The prognosis of TTP was poor before the use of plasmapheresis (7).

Atypical HUS (sporadic, variant or D- HUS) is a catch-all category of several variants of HUS (1, 6). These include recurrent forms, inherited HUS, HUS associated with pregnancy, oral contraceptives, antitumor drugs, malignancy, cyclosporin, lupus erythematosus, or AIDS (Table 1). The onset is insidious, there is no seasonal variation, and the prodromes are nonspecific (8). The thrombotic microangiopathy is predominantly arteriolar and hypertension is often severe and difficult to treat (1-3). Recurrences occur and the prognosis is poor (1, 2, 5).

An etiological classification of HUS is shown in Table 1. The clinical aspects of HUS are the subject of many reviews and will be discussed briefly.

Table 1. Etiologic classification of HUS.

IDIOPATHIC		
SECONDARY		
Infections		
	Good evidence:	Escherichia coli 0157:H7 (SLT-1,2)
		Shigella dysenteriae type 1
		Shigella pneumoniae
	Circumstantial:	Salmonella typhi; Campylobacter jejuni; Yersinia pseudotuberculosis; Pseudomonas; Bacteroides; A.hydrophilia
		portillo, coxsackie, echo, influenza, Ebstein Barr, and rotoviruses; HIV; microtatabiote
Inherited		
	Autosomal recessive *	
	Autosomal dominant *	
Drug-associated		
	cyclosporin; mitomycin; oral contraceptives; quinine	
Pregnancy-associated		
Transplant-associated *		
Malignancy-associated		

* Recurrent episodes may occur in patients with D- HUS, in autosomal recessive or dominant inheritance of HUS, and in some cases post-transplantation. (Reproduced from Kaplan BS, Cleary TG, Obrig TG: Recent advances in understanding the pathogenesis of the hemolytic uremic syndromes. Pediatr Nephrol, 4: 276-283, 1990, with permission).

EXTRARENAL MANIFESTATIONS OF HUS

The acute colitis is usually transient. Surgical complications are uncommon and include rectal prolapse, toxic megacolon, bowel wall necrosis, intussusception, perforation and stricture (8-10). Colonic gangrene is often fatal. HUS patients have abdominal pain and it can be difficult to distinguish HUS from appendicitis, inflammatory bowel disease, or intussusception (8). However, several patients owe their survival to removal of a segment of gangrenous colon. Specimens of colon show a spectrum of edema, submucosal hemorrhage, ulcerated mucosa, pseudomembrane formation, thrombosis of submucosal and intramural vessels and transmural infarction (8-11). Radiographic features include filling defects, thumb printing, pseudotumors and marginal serrations (12). Hepatic involvement is difficult to evaluate. The serum albumin may be low secondary to intestinal and urinary losses, and hemolysis may cause indirect hyperbilirubinemia. Transaminases are often mildly and transiently elevated, secondary to hypoxia, hemolysis or peritonitis (8, 10, 13). Cholestatic jaundice is uncommon (13). Fibrin microthrombi have been observed in liver specimens (11). Microthrombi and necrosis may involve pancreatic exocrine and endocrine glands (10, 11, 14). Insulin dependent diabetes mellitus and/or pancreatitis occur in some cases (10, 15, 16). Cardiac involvement occurs as complications of hypertension, fluid overload, electrolyte disturbances, myocarditis, or microthrombi (11).

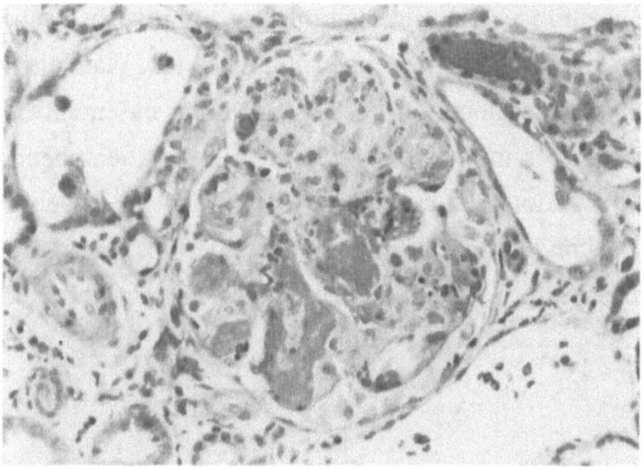

Figure 1. The characteristic glomerular lesion consists of endothelial cell swelling, a widened subendothelial space, narrowed capillary lumens, and variable numbers of thrombi.

Mucocutaneous manifestations include ulcers of the buccal mucosa and gums, dry cracked lips, and erythematous necrotic lesions of skin, penis, and perianal area (17). Many patients have mild central nervous system symptoms that include irritability, lethargy, behavioral changes, ataxia and dizziness (18-20). Major neurologic symptoms of stupor, coma, generalized or local seizures, hemiplegia, decerebrate posturing, dystonic posturing, cortical blindness and hallucinations occur in 14% to 50% of patients (10-20). Hypertension (21), and metabolic and fluid derangements (20), contribute to CNS involvement. In one half to two thirds of patients with CNS symptoms, hyponatremia, hypocalcemia, and acidemia have been implicated (19, 20). CT scan abnormalities include diffuse edema, large vessel infarction, multiple small infarctions and parenchymal hemorrhage (18). Large cerebral vessel thromboses and fibrin microthrombi are rarely found at autopsy (11, 18, 20). CNS involvement is associated with an increased morbidity and mortality (18-20).

HISTOPATHOLOGY

Three patterns of renal histopathologic changes have been identified and these can be correlated with the clinical picture and prognosis (4).

Thrombotic microangiopathy (TMA) with glomerular involvement is the most common pattern (Figure 1). Glomerular capillary lumina may be occluded by thrombi and there may be areas of necrosis in the tufts. Mesangiolysis may occur and the mesangium may have a foamy appearance (21). Electron microscopy reveals a subendothelial space with pale, fluffy substances, fibrin-like material and lipids. Platelets may approximate capillary walls and basement membranes. The glomerular basement membrane is intact (21, 22). Arteriolar changes include discrete widening of the subendothelial space to marked swelling of the endothelial cell with narrowing of the lumen. Patchy or diffuse cortical necrosis is a second variant (Figure 2). The interlobar arteries are spared but the inter-lobular and arcuate arteries are often occluded by fibrous endarteritis and fibrinoid necrosis.

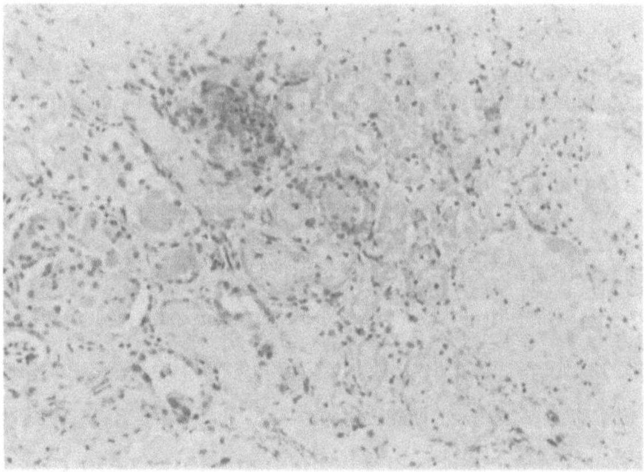

Figure 2. The glomeruli are almost unrecognizable in this area of cortical necrosis. This patient was anuric for several months but gradually recovered renal function and now has serum creatinine of 1.5 mg/dl.

In the third pattern, arterial TMA, there is severe involvement of arterioles and interlobular arteries with ischemic changes in glomeruli (Figure 3). Early arteriolar changes are intimal edema, proliferation, thrombosis and necrosis. Later changes include fibrous endarteritis in medium-sized arteries and onion skin laminar changes in arterioles. The ischemic glomeruli have split capillary walls, diffusely wrinkled glomerular basement membranes and widened subendothelial spaces. The mesangial matrix and cells are unremarkable. Some glomeruli have no fibrin; others have scattered deposits in capillary loops or in the subendothelial spaces of arterioles and arteries.

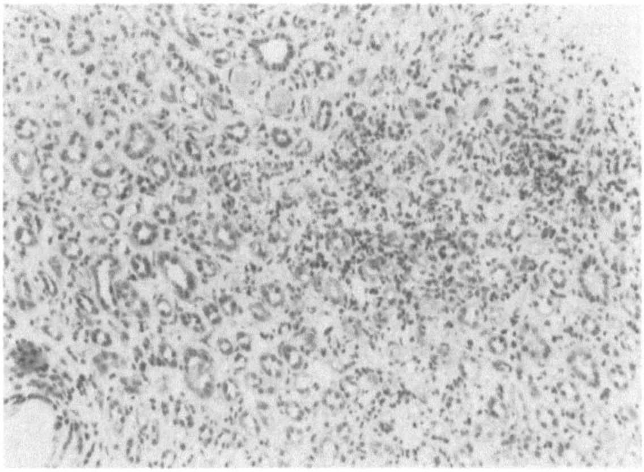

Figure 3. Arterial thrombotic microangiopathy (TMA). Note severe injury to the arteriole with intimal edema, proliferation, thrombosis and necrosis. This patient had a recurrent, atypical form of hemolytic uremic syndrome (HUS). She died post-renal transplantation from a massive intracerebral thrombosis.

Occasional patients have severe tubulo-interstitial disease with foci of inflammation and tubular damage (Figure 4).

The clinical characteristics of age, presentation, hypertension and outcome correlate with the morphologic variants (4). Typical HUS is associated with patchy cortical necrosis or predominantly glomerular involvement (23). Atypical HUS correlates both with arterial TMA, and with glomerular TMA complicated by marked arterial involvement.

PATHOGENESIS

The denominator in all forms of HUS is vascular endothelial cell injury and dysfunction (24). The normal endothelial cell monolayer forms a selective permeability barrier and a nonthrombogenic surface that isolates blood components from the highly thrombogenic subendothelial space and has dynamic regulatory functions (25). These dynamic cells synthesize and secrete substances that regulate immune responses and modulate vascular tone and reactivity (25). Endothelial injury can increase thrombogenicity, facilitate leukocyte adhesion, produce mediators, and induce new functions. Many of the integral proteins are on the endothelial cell surface and have short half-lives, thereby localizing regulation. Antithrombotic substances include prostacyclin (PGI_2), thrombomodulin, tissue plasminogen activator (TPA), and heparin-like molecules which activate antithrombin III. Prothrombotic substances, many of which are altered in HUS, include tissue factor, platelet activating factor, tissue plasminogen activator-inhibitor (TPA-I), and von Willebrand factor (2, 26-36). Vascular injury in HUS starts with endothelial injury and progresses to platelet activation and local intravascular thrombosis.

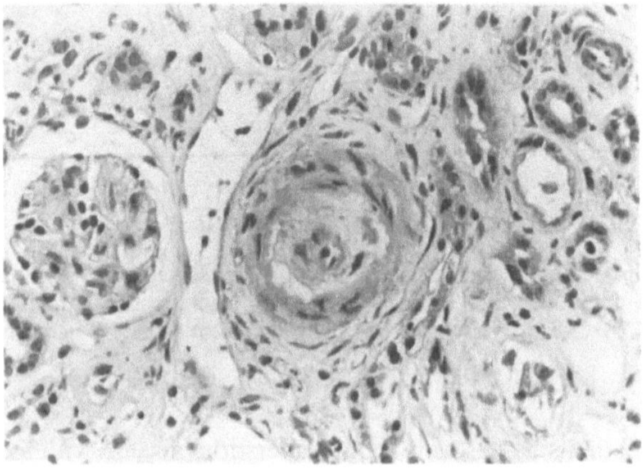

Figure 4. Note tubulo-interstitial disease with a focus of inflammation and tubular damage in a biopsy specimen from a patient with typical (D+) hemolytic uremic syndrome (HUS).

Shiga-like toxin-induced endothelial cell injury in typical HUS

A strain of Escherichia coli produces a cytotoxin that is active on Vero cells, and is distinct from the enterotoxins of Escherichia coli (37). The enterohemorrhagic Escherichia coli that produce large amounts of these cytotoxins are called verotoxin-producing Escherichia coli (VTEC). Karmali et al (3) found that 75% of patients with D+ HUS had evidence of infection with VTEC compared with none of controls. Escherichia coli 0157:H7, the most common serotype associated with HUS, produces large amounts of cytotoxin and is implicated in many outbreaks of hemorrhagic colitis and HUS (38, 39).

Verotoxins are related to Shiga toxin (ST), the exotoxin produced by Shigella dysenteriae type 1, are often called Shiga-like toxins (6, 40), and have been extensively characterized (40). Human VTEC strains produce one or both of two different verotoxins, VT1 (SLT-1) and VT2 (SLT-2). Shiga toxin and SLT-1 are almost identical. SLT-2 is structurally and functionally related, but is immunologically distinct. Anti-Shiga toxin antibodies neutralize SLT-1 but not SLT-2. All three toxins bind to the glycolipid receptor, glycosphingolipid globotriosyl ceramide (Gb3). The toxins consist of an A subunit and five B subunits. The B subunits bind to the Gb3 receptor. The A unit is internalized by receptor-mediated endocytosis, is processed, and then directly inhibits protein synthesis and causes cell death, by inactivating the 60S ribosomal subunit. The receptor is in human kidneys (41) but not in all mammalian kidneys (41).

Many patients who have VTEC-associated enterocolitis do not progress to full-blown HUS. The propensity to develop HUS has been studied in relation to the presence or absence of the P1 blood group antigen which contains the same galactose ceramide linkage as the Gb3 receptor. An excess of patients with HUS have weak or absent expression of blood group P1 (42). It has been suggested that in individuals with strong expression of the P1 antigen, larger amounts of the absorbed SLT may be bound by red blood cells thereby decreasing the potential injury to endothelial cells. Furthermore, because mature erythrocytes do not synthesize protein, they may be resistant to the cytotoxic effects of SLTs.

Studies in animal models and in endothelial cell cultures have delineated the effects of SLTs on endothelial cells. Continuous peritoneal infusion of SLT-2 in rabbits produced diarrhea with colonic edema, hemorrhage, necrosis and ulceration which resemble the intestinal lesions seen in humans with hemorrhagic colitis (43). Scattered foci of hemorrhage, consistent with endothelial damage, are seen in the CNS, but glomeruli are unaffected. Gb3 receptors are present in rabbit gut mucosa but not in their kidneys. The ultrastructural changes in the capillaries, in rabbits given parenteral SLT-1, were similar to the characteristic swelling of endothelial cells and widened subendothelial spaces found in HUS (44). Gb3 is a major component of glycolipids in human kidneys, and is found in greater density in the cortex than in the medulla in a distribution that correlates with the lesions in HUS (41).

Purified Shiga toxin is directly cytotoxic to human umbilical vessel endothelial cells (HUVEC) with a time and dose-dependent reduction in the number of viable, attached cultured cells (45). Nonconfluent, actively dividing endothelial cells bind twice as much toxin, and are more sensitive than confluent, quiescent cells. Protein synthesis is terminated in nonconfluent cells in 2 hours while confluent cells continue to synthesize protein at a steady, but partially reduced rate for three or more days. Inhibition of protein synthesis and cell death results in cell detachment with exposure, *in vivo*, of thrombogenic factors. This cytotoxic response is neutralized by anti-Shiga toxin antibody or heat denaturation of the toxin. SLT-1 also inhibits protein synthesis in human renal microvascular endothelial cells *in vitro* (46). The endothelial cell perturbations caused by ST and SLT may cause alterations in the synthesis and regulation of cell wall components necessary to maintain a normal nonthrombogenic state. It has been suggested that the holotoxin A-subunit may operate through signal transduction mechanisms in quiescent cells (6). Vascular endothelial cells are quiescent (45) and therefore, the toxic effects *in vivo* may be a result of dysfunction and/or destruction of quiescent cells and/or detachment of dividing cells.

Much evidence supports the notion that SLTs are a necessary component for the pathogenesis of typical HUS; however, SLT may not be a sufficient requirement. It is possible that SLT permits initiation, or potentiates other mechanisms of cell injury, such as thrombogenesis, endotoxins (lipopolysaccharide = LPS), cytokines, or neutrophil-mediated injury.

Platelet activation

Because thrombocytopenia, renal microvascular thrombi, and fibrin deposits are constant findings in HUS, generalized intravascular coagulation was implicated as an important pathogenetic event.

However, coagulation studies usually reveal normal prothrombin and partial thromboplastin times, normal or elevated factors V and VIII (1), normal fibrinogen turnover and elevated fibrin split products (1, 47).

Intravascular activation of platelets occurs in typical and atypical forms of HUS (2, 48). Platelet survival is shortened and platelets circulate in an exhausted, degranulated state (49). Platelet activation may persist for weeks after the platelet count has returned to normal. In cases with recurrent episodes there is evidence of recurring platelet activation (48). Despite the disparate clinical pictures in typical and atypical forms of HUS, both subgroups have evidence of intravascular platelet activation and impaired platelet aggregation.

Potential mechanisms that may account for platelet activation include deficient prostacyclin (PGI_2) activity (2, 29, 32), abnormal VIII: von Willebrand factor patterns (26), endothelial cell damage with exposure of the thrombogenic subendothelium (6), SLT- or neuraminidase-induced platelet aggregation (27), circulating platelet aggregating factor/s (28), and cytokine-mediated thrombogenesis (50, 51). These complex, overlapping, cellular processes are tightly regulated and closely integrated.

Prostanoids

Prostacyclin, synthesized by endothelial cells from arachidonic acid, is a potent vasodilator and a powerful inhibitor of platelet aggregation and adhesion. Prostacyclin is produced locally after endothelial injury, and limits platelet activation and localizes thrombus formation (25). Many mechanisms of PGI_2 dysregulation have been implicated in HUS (2). Possibilities include an inhibitor of PGI_2 deficiency of a plasma factor required for PGI_2 production, or excessively rapid degradation of PGI_2. Many of these observations are anecdotal and often pertain to atypical cases of HUS and to TTP. Although *in vitro* studies show that plasma from HUS patients cannot support PGI_2 synthesis (29, 48), this has not been confirmed *in vivo* (30). The antiaggregatory effects of increased PGI_2 may be opposed by relatively increased platelet release of thromboxane (TxA_2) (30, 48). Abnormalities of PGI_2 are found in a few kindreds of HUS but there is no clear pattern (31, 32).

Factor VIII: von Willebrand factor (VWF) multimers

Endothelial cells and megakaryocytes synthesize VWF, an adhesive protein required for platelet-platelet interactions at sites of vessel injury and for platelet attachment to subendothelium.

The VIII-VWF levels are markedly increased in typical and atypical HUS presumably because of endothelial injury (26). The patterns normalizes with clinical improvement but persist in patients with recurrent or progressive disease (33). The largest multimers are usually decreased either because of binding to platelets or enhanced proteolytic degradation (34). Unusually large multimers are also detected in HUS and TTP perhaps because of leakage from damaged endothelial cells. These unusually large multimers can induce aggregation of platelets in situations with raised fluid shear stress such as intravascular coagulation (52). Elastase, released by activated neutrophils, cleaves VWF *in vitro* (53) and it is of interest that patients with typical HUS have elevated neutrophil counts and markedly increased serum elastase levels (52). Increased turnover of platelets with platelet activation and release of VWF-containing alpha granules, may also contribute to elevated VWF levels.

The significance of these alterations in multimers is not clear. It is suggested that patients with typical HUS may have enhanced proteolysis with relatively fewer ultra-large multimers, and may be at decreased risk for major thrombotic events. In contrast, the presence of ultra-large multimers may predict thrombotic episodes, especially in some patients with atypical forms of HUS (54).

Platelet aggregating factors

Platelet aggregating factors (PAF) are found in some patients with HUS and more convincingly in TTP (28, 48). Plasma from 6 of 11 typical HUS patients caused platelet aggregation which was inhibited by normal adult IgG (28). Incubation of normal plasma with SLT caused platelet aggregation. This required IIA and IIIB platelet surface glycoproteins and was inhibited by prostacyclin (27). Although platelet aggregating activity is demonstrated in typical and atypical HUS patients, the effect is weak, and because it does not correlate with disease activity, the role of PAF in pathogenesis may be minimal (48).

Defective fibrinolysis

Tissue plasminogen activator (t-PA) is produced by endothelial cells; tissue plasminogen activator inhibitor (t-PAI) is produced by endothelial cells and platelets. Platelet activation, therefore, may cause decreased local fibrinolysis. An inhibitor of glomerular fibrinolysis, tPAI-1, which can be removed by peritoneal dialysis, is detected in sera of patients with HUS (33, 36).

Endothelium-derived vasoactive substances

Endothelial cells synthesize endothelium-derived relaxation factor (EDRF), and endothelin, a potent vasoconstrictor, which have important functions in microcirculatory hemodynamics (55, 56). These are closely integrated with the prostanoid and coagulation cascades. EDRF and prostacyclin have similar characteristics; both act locally, are very labile, and inhibit platelet aggregation. Unlike prostacyclin, EDRF impedes platelet adhesion to endothelial surfaces. Free hemoglobin binds and inactivates EDRF, and therefore hemoglobinemia possibly inactivates EDRF and exacerbates platelet aggregation. Ischemia also reduces EDRF production. Inactivation and decreased production of EDRF in HUS may therefore further decrease renal blood flow and glomerular filtration rate in HUS.

Release of endothelin may be enhanced at sites of endothelial injury, platelet aggregation, and clot formation. This results in further increases in renal vascular resistance. Lipopolysaccharide (LPS) stimulates endothelin release (57). Kidney biopsy specimens from HUS patients often have insufficient structural damage to account for the oliguric renal failure and hypertension and therefore vasoactive substances may play a role (58). Urine endothelin levels are elevated in patients with HUS and the highest concentrations are in those with hypertension, anuria or oliguria. The endothelin levels decrease to normal with recovery (58).

Lipid peroxidation

Lipid peroxides may affect many steps in the pathogenetic cascade that culminates in HUS. They injure vascular endothelium (59), have a procoagulant effect through thrombin generation (60), inhibit antithrombin III (61), and may inhibit PGI_2 synthesis (62). Reduced arachidonic acid and increased diene conjugates in found erythrocyte membranes in HUS is consistent with free radical-induced injury (63, 64). Activated neutrophils may be the source of the free radicals.

Cyclosporin

The possible mechanisms whereby cyclosporin may induce HUS (56) include endothelial cell vacuolization, necrosis and thrombosis, increased TxA_2 production, decreased PGI_2 production, endothelin production, and impaired effect of EDRF. Cyclosporin also enhances platelet aggregation and thromboxane release from platelets. Therefore, it would seem that cyclosporine has a role in the pathogenesis of post-transplantation HUS, but HUS can occur post-transplantation, whether or not the patient has been treated with cyclosporin.

Endotoxin and cytokines

Lipopolysaccharide (LPS) may be involved in the integration of many of the microthrombotic and inflammatory mechanisms in HUS. LPS-induced renal vascular injury occurs in the generalized Schwartzman reaction in which there is disseminated intravascular coagulation and bilateral cortical necrosis (65). Fibrin deposits seen in kidneys and histopathologic similarities with HUS suggest that LPS derived from bacteria in a damaged gastrointestinal tract produce a similar reaction in patients with bloody diarrhea and HUS. Circulating LPS was found in patients with Shigella-associated HUS

(66). These patients had a high mortality, extreme leukemoid reaction, disseminated coagulopathy and cortical necrosis (67).

Recognition of the procoagulant, antifibrinolytic, and synergistic proinflammatory effects of LPS and cytokines, which are enhanced by SLT, has reestablished a possible role for LPS in the pathogenesis of typical HUS. Significantly elevated titres of agglutinins and IgM antibodies against Escherichia coli 0157-derived LPS were found in 91% of the patients with SLT-associated HUS (68).

LPS stimulates mononuclear cells to produce tumor necrosis factor (TNF) and interleukin-1 (IL-1). LPS and TNF also induce IL-1 expression in endothelial cells which further concentrate IL-1 locally (69). LPS, TNF and IL-1 induce endothelial cell damage through three proposed mechanisms: [1] direct toxicity (70), [2] neutrophil activation, chemotaxis, and adherence to endothelial cells (71, 72) and [3] establishment of a local procoagulant and antifibrinolytic state (73).

LPS produces time- and dose-dependent bovine endothelial cell injury *in vitro* with cell detachment and lysis (74). LPS mediated injury is enhanced by protein synthesis inhibition with cyclohexamide. Although it was proposed that Shiga toxin may be the direct cause of protein inhibition (45), SLT and LPS from Shigella dysenteriae type 1 is not directly cytotoxic to HUVEC, and LPS does not augment SLT-mediated cytotoxicity (74). Neither IL-1 nor TNF are directly cytotoxic to HUVEC but cytotoxic effects can be achieved by the addition of cyclohexamide (75). These results are substantiated by observations that addition of TNF increased the cytotoxicity of SLT *in vitro* (74). IL-1 and TNF disrupt endothelial cell morphology and cytoskeletal structures (73).

An integral role for neutrophils is illustrated by the prevention of the vascular injury in the Schwartzman reaction by prior induction of neutropenia (76) and in a modified Schwartzman reaction induced by slow infusion of endotoxin (77).

LPS, TNF and IL-1 have major effects on neutrophils. IL-1 and TNF stimulate increased surface adhesiveness for neutrophils by induction and synthesis of a transient endothelial leukocyte adhesion molecule (ELAM-1) (73). *In vitro* activation of neutrophils adherent to HUVEC results in endothelial cell detachment (71). Neutrophil-derived proteases, rather than O_2 radicals, digest endothelial cell surface proteins, including fibronectin, and permit circulating blood components access to the thrombogenic subendothelium (71). Neutrophil-mediated injury is markedly enhanced by preincubation with LPS (72). LPS directly stimulates neutrophil adherence to endothelial cells and primes neutrophils for an enhanced response to chemotactic factors. Neutrophil-mediated injury may not occur unless the endothelial cell has been subtly altered or harmed (78).

Endothelial injury caused by SLT may account for early endothelial changes, followed by endotoxin, cytokine and neutrophil mediated injury.

In vitro studies in the modified generalized Schwartzman reaction show evidence of neutrophil activation and exhaustion with enzyme release, lipid peroxidation, impaired chemotaxis, poor aggregation and increased procoagulant content (79). Studies of neutrophils from patients with HUS support a role for neutrophil adhesion and neutrophil-mediated endothelial injury (80) by activated neutrophils which can cause fibronectin degradation (71). Serum levels of neutrophil elastase are increased and there are degranulated circulating neutrophils (53, 81). A leukocytosis correlates with poor outcome in D+ HUS (82). There is therefore clear evidence for an important role for neutrophils in the pathogenesis of typical HUS.

SLT, LPS, IL-1 and TNF all increase expression of procoagulant tissue factor on the surface of endothelial cells (83-86). IL-1, TNF and LPS also decrease thrombomodulin and increase t-PAI (69). LPS and IL-1 increase PAFs (87). This tips the balance markedly toward fibrin deposition, local intravascular coagulation and defective fibrinolysis. IL-1 Infusions result in fibrin deposition on intact endothelial cells (88) and TNF infusions cause intraglomerular leukocyte and platelet aggregation and infiltration with endothelial damage and increasing concentrations of serum creatinine (89).

Many of the abnormalities seen in HUS such as neutrophilia, lipid peroxidation, increased VWF proteolysis, impaired fibrinolysis, microthrombosis and endothelial cell damage, can be explained by the effects of LPS, TNF and IL-1. However, not all patients with endotoxemia develop HUS. Therefore, because the SLTs can uniquely inhibit protein synthesis, they may enhance the cytopathic effects of LPS, IL-1 and TNF. It is also possible that they may perturb the endothelial cell enough to initiate LPS-enhanced neutrophil activation. In this context, a single sublethal dose of LPS given to rats 3 days after intravenous SLT resulted in increased lethal effects (90).

TREATMENT

Supportive therapy is responsible for the decline in the acute mortality rate of patients with D+ HUS from 40% in the 1960's to present rates of between 4 and 12 percent. The mortality rate for patients with autosomal recessive HUS has not changed over the past 15 years and remains at about 65%. More than 90% of patients with dominantly inherited HUS either die or develop chronic renal failure (91).

There is no specific treatment for the colitis, and anti-peristaltic agents and antibiotics are not recommended. Fluids and electrolytes must be managed carefully according to the general principles established for acute renal failure. Dehydration from diarrhea and vomiting must be carefully treated and overhydration and hyponatremia must be avoided. The value of early dialysis has never been evaluated prospectively. Hyperkalemia, hyperphosphatemia, and metabolic acidosis can be managed medically, but if this fails, dialysis or hemofiltration is indicated. Five to ten ml/kg body weight of packed red blood cells can be transfused slowly if the hemoglobin level decreases below 6 g/dl. Thrombocytopenia does not usually rarely require treatment with platelet transfusions unless the patient is actively bleeding, or has profound thrombocytopenia, or is about to undergo an operation. Hypertension may respond to fluid removal or vasodilators may be required. Administration of carbohydrates and essential amino acids is recommended and inanition may be an indication for early onset of dialysis in a catabolic, oliguric patient. Commercial immune globulin preparations have not been proven to be effective in eliminating organisms from the bowel and do not contain anti-SLT II antibodies. Surgery is indicated if ischemic bowel lesions are suspected. Hyperglycemia, ketonemia and acidosis must be treated with insulin.

Neither anti-thrombotic, fibrinolytic and anti-platelet measures, nor the use of fresh frozen plasma, have proven to reduce the acute mortality rate or the long-term morbidity. Fresh frozen plasma is contraindicated in patients with Shigella pneumoniae-associated HUS (92). Plasmapheresis is recommended for the treatment of TTP (7), is not indicated for treatment of typical HUS, but may be beneficial in atypical forms of HUS.

RENAL TRANSPLANTATION

Recurrences post-transplant are rare in patients who have had the typical, D+ HUS, whether living related or cadaver donor kidneys are used, or whether or not cyclosporin is given (93). These conclusions may not apply to patients with atypical or inherited forms of HUS, or in those who have had a pretransplant recurrence of HUS (94).

REFERENCES

1. Kaplan BS, Proesmans W: The hemolytic uremic syndrome of childhood and its variants. Semin Hematol, 24: 148-160, 1987.
2. Barratt TM, Dillon MJ, Hardisty RM, Levin M, Nokes TJC, Smith C, Stroobant P, Walters MDS: The role of platelet-derived growth factors in the pathogenesis of the haemolytic-uraemic syndrome. In: "Recent Advances in Pediatric Nephrology" (Eds K Murakami, T Kitagawa, K Yabuta, T Sakai), Excerpta Medica, Amsterdam, 1987, pp 577-580.

3. Karmali MA, Petric M, Lim C, Fleming PC, Arbus GS, Lior H: The association between idiopathic hemolytic uremic syndrome and infection by Verotoxin-producing Escherichia coli. J Infect Dis, 151: 775-782, 1985.
4. Habib R, Levy M, Gagnadoux MF, Broyer M: Prognosis of the hemolytic uremic syndrome in children. Adv Nephrol, 11: 99-128, 1982.
5. Kaplan BS: Hemolytic uremic syndrome with recurrent episodes: an important subset. Clin Nephrol, 8: 495-498, 1977.
6. Kaplan BS, Cleary TG, Obrig TG: Recent advances in understanding the pathogenesis of the hemolytic uremic syndromes. Pediatr Nephrol, 4: 276-283, 1990.
7. Rock GA, Shumak KH, Buskard NA, Blanchette VS, Kelton JG, Nair RC, Spasoff RA: Comparison of plasma exchange with plasma infusion in the treatment of thrombotic thrombocytopenic purpura. N Engl J Med, 325: 393-397, 1991.
8. Whitington PF, Friedman AL, Chesney RW: Gastrointestinal disease in the hemolytic-uremic syndrome. Gastroenterology, 76: 728-733, 1979.
9. Brandt ML, O Regan S, Rousseau E, Yazbeck S: Surgical complications of the hemolytic-uremic syndrome. J Pediatr Surg, 25: 1109-1112, 1990.
10. Grodinsky S, Telmesani A, Robson WLM, Fick G, Scott RB: Gastrointestinal manifestations of hemolytic uremic syndrome: recognition of pancreatitis. J Pediatr Gastroenterol Nutr, 11: 518-524, 1990.
11. Upadhyaya K, Barwick K, Fishaut M, Kashgarian M, Siegel NJ: The importance of nonrenal involvement in hemolytic-uremic syndrome. Pediatrics, 65: 115-120, 1980.
12. Peterson RB, Meseroll WP, Shrago GG, Gooding CA: Radiographic features of colitis associated with the hemolytic-uremic syndrome. Radiology, 118: 667-671, 1976.
13. Jeffrey G, Kibbler CC, Baillod R, Farrington K, Morgan MY: Cholestatic jaundice in the haemolytic-uraemic syndrome: a case report. Gut, 26: 315-319, 1985.
14. Primhak RA, Taitz LS, Variend S, Webb DHK, Cser A: Necrosis of the pancreas in the haemolytic uraemic syndrome. J Clin Pathol, 37: 655-658, 1984.
15. Andreoli SP, Bergstein JM: Development of insulin-dependent diabetes mellitus during the hemolytic-uremic syndrome. J Pediatr, 100: 541-545, 1982.
16. Burns JC, Berman ER, Fagre JL, Shikes RH, Lum GM. Pancreatic islet cell necrosis: association with hemolytic-uremic syndrome. J Pediatr, 100: 582-584, 1982.
17. Ehlayel MS, Akl KF: Mucocutaneous manifestations of the hemolytic-uremic syndrome. Clin Pediatr, 30: 208-210, 1991.
18. Hahn JS, Havens PL, Higgins JJ, O Rourke PP, Estroff JA, Strand R: Neurological complications of hemolytic-uremic syndrome. J Child Neurol, 4: 108-113, 1989.
19. Bale JF Jr, Brasher C, Siegler RL: CNS manifestations of the hemolytic-uremic syndrome. Relationship to metabolic alterations and prognosis. Am J Dis Child, 134: 869-872, 1980.
20. Sheth KJ, Swick HM, Haworth N: Neurological involvement in hemolytic-uremic syndrome. Ann Neurol, 19: 90-93, 1986.
21. Shigematsu H, Dikman SH, Churg J, Grishman E, Duffy JL: Mesangial involvement in hemolytic-uremic syndrome. A light and electron microscopic study. Am J Pathol, 85: 349-362, 1976.
22. Courtecuisse V, Habib R, Monnier C: Nonlethal hemolytic and uremic syndromes in children: an electron-microscope study of renal biopsies from six cases. Exp Mol Pathol, 7: 327-347, 1967.
23. Richardson SE, Karmali MA, Becker LE, Smith CR: The histopathology of the hemolytic uremic syndrome associated with verocytotoxin-producing Escherichia coli infections. Hum Pathol, 19: 1102-1108, 1988.
24. de Chadarevian JP, Kaplan BS: The hemolytic uremic syndrome of childhood. In: "Perspectives in Pediatric Pathology" (Eds H Rosenberg, R Bolande), Yearbook Medical Publishing, Chicago, 1978, pp. 565-502.
25. Cotran RS: Endothelial cells. In: "Textbook of Rheumatology" (Eds WN Kelley, ED Harris Jr, S Ruddy, CB Sledge), WB Saunders Publishing Company, Philadelphia, 1989, pp 389-415.
26. Moake JL, Byrnes JJ, Troll JH, Rudy CK, Weinstein MJ, Colannino NM, Hong SL: Abnormal VIII: von Willebrand factor patterns in the plasma of patients with the hemolytic-uremic syndrome. Blood, 64: 592-598, 1984.
27. Rose PE, Armour JA, Williams CE, Hill FGH: Verotoxin and neuraminidase induced platelet aggregating activity in plasma: their possible role in the pathogenesis of the haemolytic uraemic syndrome. J Clin Pathol, 38: 438-441, 1985.

28. Monnens L, van de Meer W, Langenhuysen C, van Munster P, van Oostrom C: Platelet aggregating factor in the epidemic form of hemolytic-uremic syndrome in childhood. Clin Nephrol, 24: 135-137, 1985.
29. Levin M, Elkon KB, Nokes TJC, Buckle AM, Dillon MJ, Hardisty RM, Barratt TM: Inhibitor of prostacyclin production in sporadic haemolytic uraemic syndrome. Arch Dis Child, 58: 703-708, 1983.
30. Tonshoff B, Momper R, Kuhl PG, Schweer H, Scharer K, Seyberth HW: Increased thromboxane biosynthesis in childhood hemolytic uremic syndrome. Kidney Int, 37: 1134-1141, 1990.
31. Jorgensen KA, Pedersen RS: Familial deficiency of prostacyclin production stimulating factor in the hemolytic uremic syndrome of childhood. Thromb Res, 21: 311-315, 1981.
32. Remuzzi G, Marchesi D, Misiani R, Misiani R, Mecca G, de Gaetano, Donati MB. Familial deficiency of a plasma factor stimulating vascular prostacyclin activity. Thromb Res, 16: 517-525, 1979.
33. Rose PE, Enayat SM, Sunderland R, Short PE, Williams CE, Hill FGH: Abnormalities of factor VIII related protein multimers in the haemolytic uraemic syndrome. Arch Dis Child, 59: 1135-1140, 1984.
34. Mannucci PM, Lombardi R, Lattuada A, Ruggenenti P, Vigano GL, Barbui T, Remuzzi G: Enhanced proteolysis of plasma von Willebrand factor in thrombotic thrombocytopenic purpura and the hemolytic syndrome. Blood, 74: 978-983, 1989.
35. Bergstein JM, Kuederli U, Bang NU: Plasma inhibitor of glomerular fibrinolysis in the hemolytic-uremic syndrome. Am J Med, 73: 322-327, 1982.
36. Bergstein JM, Bang NU: Plasminogen activator inhibitor-1 (PAI-1) is the circulating inhibitor of fibrinolysis (PAI-HUS) in the hemolytic uremic syndrome (HUS). Kidney Int, 37: 254, 1989 (Abstract).
37. Konowalchuk J, Speirs JI, Stavric S: Vero response to a cytotoxin of Escherichia coli. Infect Immun, 18: 775-779, 1977.
38. Riley LW, Remis RS, Helgerson SD, McGee HB, Wells JG, Davis BR, Hebert RJ, Olcott ES, Johnson LM, Hargrett NT, Blake PA, Cohen ML: Hemorrhagic colitis associated with a rare Escherichia coli serotype. N Engl J Med, 308: 681-685, 1983.
39. Neill MA, Tarr PI, Clausen CR, Christie DL, Hickman RO: Escherichia coli 0157:H7 as the predominant pathogen associated with the hemolytic uremic syndrome: a prospective study in the Pacific Northwest. Pediatrics, 80: 37-40, 1987.
40. Cleary TG, Lopez EL: The Shiga-like toxin-producing Escherichia coli and hemolytic uremic syndrome. Pediatr Infect Dis J, 8: 720-724, 1989.
41. Boyd B, Lingwood C: Verotoxin receptor glycolipid in human renal tissue. Nephron, 51: 207-210, 1989.
42. Taylor CM, Milford DV, Rose PE, Roy TCF, Rowe B: The expression of blood group P1 in post-enteropathic haemolytic uraemic syndrome. Pediatr Nephrol, 4: 59-61, 1990.
43. Barrett TJ, Potter ME, Wachsmuth IK: Continuous peritoneal infusion of Shiga-like toxin II (SLT II) as a model for SLT II-induced diseases. J Infect Dis, 159: 774-777, 1989.
44. Richardson SE, Jagadha VB, Smith CR, Becker LE, Petric M, Karmali MA: Comparative pathology of the hemolytic uremic syndrome associated with Verotoxin-producing Escherichia coli infection and experimental disease in rabbits produced by parenteral VT challenge. Presented at an International Symposium and Workshop on Verocytotoxin-producing Escherichia coli infections, Toronto, July 12-15, 1987 (Abstract AMV-5).
45. Obrig TG, Del Vecchio PJ, Brown JE, Moran TP, Rowland BM, Judge TK, Rothman SW: Direct cytotoxic action of Shiga toxin on human vascular endothelial cells. Infect Immun, 56: 2373-2378, 1988.
46. Barley-Maloney L, Obrig T, Daniel T: Human renal microvascular endothelial cells (HRMEC) are targets for hemolytic uremic syndrome (HUS)-associated verotoxin (VT). Am J Soc Nephrol, 1: 515, 1990 (Abstract).
47. Katz J, Krawitz S, Sacks PV, Levin SE, Thomson P, Levin J, Metz J: Platelet, erythrocyte and fibrinogen kinetics in the hemolytic-uremic syndrome of infancy. J Pediatr, 83; 739-748, 1973.
48. Walters MDS, Levin M, Smith C, Nokes TJC, Hardisty RM, Dillon MJ, Barratt TM: Intravascular platelet activation in the hemolytic uremic syndrome. Kidney Int, 33: 107-115, 1988.
49. Fong JSC, Kaplan BS: Impairment of platelet aggregation in hemolytic uremic syndrome: evidence for platelet exhaustion. Blood, 60: 564-570, 1982.

50. Cotran RS, Pober JS: Effects of cytokines on vascular endothelium: their role in vascular and immune injury. Kidney Int, 35: 969-975, 1989.
51. Bussolino F, Camussi G, Baglioni C: Synthesis and release of platelet-activating factor by human vascular endothelial cells treated with tissue necrosis factor or interleukin 1 alpha. J Biol Chem, 263: 11856-11861, 1988.
52. Moake JL, Turner NA, Stathopoulos NA, Nolasco LH, Hellums JD: Involvement of large plasma von Willebrand factor (vWF) multimers and unusually large vWF forms derived from endothelial cells in shear stress-induced platelet aggregation. J Clin Invest, 78: 1456-1461, 1986.
53. Kaplan BS, Mills M: Elevated serum elastase and alpha-1-antitrypsin levels in hemolytic uremic syndrome. Clin Nephrol, 30: 193-196, 1988.
54. Helmsworth M, Ragin CS, Sherbotie J, Kaplan BS: Abnormal factor VIII: von Willebrand (VIII:vWF) multimers in patients with hemolytic uremic syndrome (HUS) or thrombocytopenic thrombotic purpura (TTP) may predict thrombotic episodes. VIII Congress International Pediatric Association, Toronto, Canada, August 27. Pediatr Nephrol, 3: c182, 1989 (Abstract 10-006).
55. Brenner BM, Troy JL, Ballermann BJ: Endothelium-dependent vascular responses. J Clin Invest, 84: 1373-1378, 1989.
56. Luscher TF, Bock HA, Yang Z, Diederich D: Endothelium-derived relaxing and contracting factors: perspectives in nephrology. Kidney Int, 39: 575-590, 1991.
57. Sugiura M, Inagami T, Kon V: Endotoxin stimulates endothelin-release *in vivo* and *in vitro* as determined by radio immunoassay. Biochem Biophys Res Commun, 161: 1220-1227, 1989.
58. Siegler RL, Edwin SS, Christofferson RD, Mitchel MD: Endothelin in the urine of children with the hemolytic uremic syndrome. Pediatrics, 88: 1063-1065, 1991.
59. Yagi K, Ohkawa H, Ohishi N, Yamashita M, Nakashima T: Lesions of aortic intima caused by intravenous administration of linoleic acid hydroperoxide. J Appl Biochem, 3: 58-65, 1981.
60. Barrowcliffe TW, Gray E, Kerry PJ, Gutteridge JMC: Triglyceride-rich lipoproteins are responsible for thrombin generation induced by lipid peroxides. Thromb Haemost, 52: 7-10, 1984.
61. Gray E, Barrowcliffe TW: Inhibition of antithrombin III by lipid peroxides. Thromb Res, 37: 241-250, 1985.
62. Moncada S, Vane JR: Pharmacology and endogenous roles of prostaglandin endoperoxides, thromboxane A_2, and prostacyclin. Pharmacol Rev, 30: 293-331, 1978.
63. Powell HR, Groves V, McCredie DA, Yong A, Pitt J: Low red cell arachidonic acid in hemolytic uremic syndrome. Clin Nephrol, 27: 8-10, 1987.
64. Situnayake RD, Crump BJ, Thurnham DI, Taylor CM: Further evidence of lipid peroxidation in post-enteropathic haemolytic-uraemic syndrome. Pediatr Nephrol, 5: 387-392, 1991.
65. Thomas L, Good RA: Studies on the generalized Schwartzman reaction. I. General observations concerning the phenomenon. J Exp Med, 96: 605-613, 1952.
66. Koster F, Levin J, Walker L, Tung KS, Gilman RH, Rahaman MM, Majid MA, Islam S, Williams JC Jr: Hemolytic uremic syndrome after shigellosis. Relation to endotoxemia and circulating immune complexes. N Engl J Med, 298: 927-933, 1978.
67. Koster FT, Boonpucknavig V, Sujaho S, Gilman RH, Rahaman MM: Renal histopathology in the hemolytic-uremic syndrome following shigellosis. Clin Nephrol, 21: 126-133, 1984.
68. Bitzan M, Moebius E, Ludwig K, Muller-Wiefel D, Heesemann J, Karch H: High incidence of serum antibodies to Escherichia coli 0157 lipopolysaccharide in children with hemolytic-uremic syndrome. J Pediatr, 119: 380-385, 1991.
69. Libby P, Ordovas JM, Auger KR, Robbins AH, Birinyi LK, Dinarello CA: Endotoxin and tumor necrosis factor induce interleukin-1 gene expression in adult human vascular endothelial cells. Am J Pathol, 124: 179-185, 1986.
70. Harlan JM, Harker LA, Reidy MA, Gajdusek CM, Schwartz SM, Striker GE: Lipopolysaccharide-mediated bovine endothelial cell injury *in vitro*. Lab Invest, 48: 269-274, 1983.
71. Harlan, JM, Killen PD, Harker LA, Striker GE, Wright DG: Neutrophil-mediated endothelial injury *in vitro*. Mechanisms of cell detachment. J Clin Invest, 68: 1394-1403, 1981.
72. Smedly LA, Tonnesen MG, Sandhaus RA, Haslett C, Guthrie LA, Johnson RB Jr, Henson PM, Worthen GS: Neutrophil-mediated injury to endothelial cells. Enhancement by endotoxin and essential role of neutrophil elastase. J Clin Invest, 77: 1233-1243, 1986.
73. Cotran RS, Pober JS: Effects of cytokines on vascular endothelium: their role in vascular and immune injury. Kidney Int, 35: 969-975, 1989.

74. Tesh VL, Samuel JE, Perera LP, Sharefkin JB, O Brien AD: Evaluation of the role of Shiga and Shiga-like toxins in mediating direct damage to human vascular endothelial cells. J Infect Dis, 164: 344-352, 1991.
75. Pohlman TH, Harlan JM: Human endothelial cell response to lipopolysaccharide, interleukin-1, and tumor necrosis factor is regulated by protein synthesis. Cell Immunol, 119: 41-52, 1989.
76. Stetson CA Jr: Studies on the mechanism of the Schwartzman phenomenon. Certain factors involved in the production of the local hemorrhagic necrosis. J Exp Med, 93: 489-504, 1951.
77. Bertani T, Abbate M, Zoja C, Corna D, Remuzzi G: Sequence of glomerular changes in experimental endotoxemia: a possible model of hemolytic uremic syndrome. Nephron, 53: 330-337, 1989.
78. Brigham KL, Meyrick B: Granulocyte-dependent injury of pulmonary endothelium: a case of miscommunication? Tissue Cell, 16: 137-155, 1984.
79. Vedanarayanan VV, Kaplan BS, Fong JSC: Neutrophil function in an experimental model of hemolytic uremic syndrome. Pediatr Res, 21: 252-256, 1987.
80. Forsyth KD, Simpson AC, Fitzpatrick MM, Barratt TM, Levinsky RL: Neutrophil-mediated endothelial injury in haemolytic uraemic syndrome. Lancet, II: 411-414, 1989.
81. Milford D, Taylor CM, Rafaat F, Halloran E, Dawes J: Neutrophil elastases and haemolytic uraemic syndrome. Lancet, II: 1153, 1989.
82. Walters MDS, Matthei IU, Kay R, Dillon MJ, Barratt TM: The polymorphonuclear leukocyte count in childhood hemolytic uraemic syndrome. Pediatr Nephrol, 3: 130-134, 1989.
83. Colucci M, Balconi G, Lorenzet R, Pietra A, Locati D, Donati MB, Semeraro N: Cultured human endothelial cells generate tissue factor in response to endotoxin. J Clin Invest, 71: 1893-1896, 1983.
84. Bevilacqua MP, Pober JS, Majeau GR, Cotran RS, Gimbrone MA Jr: Interleukin 1 (IL-1) induces biosynthesis and cell surface expression of procoagulant activity in human vascular endothelial cells. J Exp Med, 160: 618-623, 1984.
85. Moore KL, Andreoli SP, Esmon NL, Esmon CT, Bang NU: Endotoxin enhances tissue factor and suppresses thrombomodulin expression of human vascular endothelium *in vitro*. J Clin Invest, 79: 124-130, 1987.
86. Conway EM, Bach R, Rosenberg RD, Konigsberg WH: Tumor necrosis factor enhances expression of tissue factor mRNA in endothelial cells. Thromb Res, 53: 231-241, 1989.
87. Morrison DC, Ryan JL: Endotoxins and disease mechanisms. Ann Rev Med, 38: 417-432, 1987.
88. Naworth PP, Handley DA, Esmon CT, Stern DM: Interleukin 1 induces endothelial cell procoagulant activity while suppressing cell surface anticoagulant activity. Acad Sci (USA), 83: 3460-3467, 1986.
89. Bertani T, Abbate M, Zoja C, Ghezzi P, Remuzzi G: Tumor necrosis factor as a new mediator of glomerular injury. Kidney Int, 33: 311, 1988 (Abstract).
90. Barrett TJ, Potter ME, Wachsmuth IK: Bacterial endotoxin both enhances and inhibits the toxicity of Shiga-like toxin II in rabbits and mice. Infect Immun, 57: 3434-3437, 1989.
91. Kaplan BS, and Kaplan P: Hereditary hemolytic-uremic syndrome. In: "Birth Defects Encyclopedia" (Ed ML Buyse), Alan R Liss, New York, 1990, pp 858-859.
92. Taylor CM, Milford DV, Rose PE, Roy TCF, Rowe B: The expression of blood group P1 in post-enteropathic haemolytic uraemic syndrome. Pediatr Nephrol, 4: 59-61, 1990.
93. Bassani CE, Ferraris J, Gianantonio CA, Ruiz S, Ramierey J: Renal transplantation in patients with classical haemolytic-uraemic syndrome. Pediatr Nephrol, 5: 607-611, 1991.
94. Hebert D, Kim E-M. Sibley RK, Mauer MS: Post-transplantation outcome of patients with hemolytic-uremic syndrome: update. Pediatr Nephrol, 5: 162-167, 1991.

Chapter 12

INCIDENCE, RISK FACTORS, PREVENTION AND TREATMENT OF RADIOCONTRAST-INDUCED NEPHROPATHY

BRIAN LEAKER

Department of Medicine, University College, Middlesex School of Medicine, The Rayne Institute, London WC1 6JJ, England

Radiocontrast-induced renal failure has been reported as the third leading cause of hospital acquired renal failure (1). It may be defined as an acute impairment of renal function followed by exposure to radiocontrast materials in the absence of other causes of renal impairment. It should be recognised that renal failure may arise from other causes in high risk patients despite radiocontrast studies (2). Where carefully controlled studies have been performed (3) renal dysfunction has been reported following radiologic procedures both with and without infusion of contrast agents. Thus many studies, especially when uncontrolled or retrospective, may overestimate the true incidence and risks of contrast nephropathy.

INCIDENCE

The true incidence of contrast nephropathy is difficult to estimate. It varies between 0 to 0.5% in normal patients to 15 to 100% in patients with pre-existing renal disease (4-6). The incidence is thought to be increasing perhaps because of increasing use of radiocontrast agents in imaging and because of increasing awareness with routine testing of renal function post procedures. The estimates of incidence vary with the type of study, type of procedure and presence of underlying risk factors. Of six prospective studies reviewed by Parfrey et al (7), only three had control groups. Many studies have defined the presence of renal dysfunction as a doubling of serum creatinine (7).

However, if smaller rises of serum creatinine are used in this definition (for example a rise of >44 μmols/l), then clearly more cases will be diagnosed and included. The type of imaging procedure may be an important factor with reported increase in risk with angiography but little or no difference between intravenous pyelography and CT scanning (6).

The incidence of contrast nephropathy appears to be directly related to the presence of underlying risk factors and is proportional to the degree of renal insufficiency. In a recent controlled prospective study (7), contrast nephropathy was found in 5% of patients with mild renal insufficiency (serum creatinine >150 μmol/l) and 8% in diabetics with renal insufficiency (serum creatinine 150-400 μmols/l). However, all these patients were carefully hydrated prior to the procedure and the degree of renal failure observed was mild.

Other uncontrolled studies have reported an incidence of approximately 20% in patients with renal insufficiency (4, 8, 9). In addition, in a study (10) of patients with severe renal dysfunction (mean serum creatinine 500 μmol/l) undergoing coronary angiography, the incidence was approximately 50% and in a further study of diabetic patients with renal insufficiency undergoing intravenous pyelography the incidence was found to be between 90 to 100% (11).

RISK FACTORS

Pre-existing renal disease, diabetes, hypovolaemia (2, 7, 12), multiple myeloma (13-15), volume (7, 16, 17) and type of contrast agents (17) and cardiac failure (16, 18-20) have all been reported as risk factors for the development of contrast nephropathy. The risk of developing contrast nephropathy is minimal in the absence of any of these risk factors. However, there are few controlled prospective studies and analysis of both independent and relative risks of each factor is therefore incomplete. In a large retrospective study of 8,000 patients (17) the following independent risk factors were identified by regression analysis: age; proteinuria; abnormal serum creatinine prior to the study; pre-existing renal disease; use of the contrast agent Renografin-76 (meglumine diatrizoate). Of these pre-existing renal disease was associated with a 6.6 times increased risk of developing contrast nephropathy. A similar retrospective study employing regression analysis (16) in high risk patients with abnormal renal function (serum creatinine >2 mg/dl) identified independent risk factors as Grade IV heart failure, multiple contrast studies within 72 hours of each other, dose of radiocontrast agents and diabetes.

A prospective study in 183 elderly patients (>70 years) identified contrast volume, diabetes and abnormal serum creatinine as independent risk factors (21).

All of these studies were uncontrolled and the retrospective studies involved reviews of case records over a ten year period. The limitation of such studies is clear and in addition there was no information supplied as to the extracellular fluid volume-status of patients prior to radiologic procedures. The study by Rich and Crecelius (21) suffered from employing a small sample size and also the exclusion of 10% of patients in the study because of a lack of follow up data.

Several studies have shown that risk factors are additive (17, 18, 22). Cochrane et al (22) reported that the incidence of contrast nephropathy increased from 5% with 1 or 2 risk factors to 50% with 5 risk factors.

Pre-existing renal disease

This remains the principal pre-disposing risk factor with over 90% of cases occurring in this group. Both the incidence and severity of contrast nephropathy are related to the degree of pre-existing renal damage (23). However, the true risk of developing contrast nephropathy is difficult to estimate because of the widely varying figures quoted in different studies. Van Zee et al (24) have reported a stepwise increase in incidents with degree of renal insufficiency; serum creatinine <1.5 mg/dl, incidence 0.6%, serum creatinine 1.5-4.5 mg/dl, incidence 3%, serum creatinine >4.5 mg/dl, incidence 31%.

The relatively low risk quoted by Parfrey et al (7) in a randomised controlled study may be attributable to the few patients included with severe renal insufficiency, i.e. serum creatinine >400 μmol/l; also their method of excluding a number of patients (with other predisposing conditions for renal failure) from analysis may deliberately under-estimate the incidence of contrast nephropathy in these high risk patients. Nevertheless the risk of acute renal insufficiency was reported as approximately 5 times increased in patients receiving contrast agents compared with controlled patients who did not receive contrast agents.

Other studies albeit retrospective have reported a greater incidence and severity of contrast nephropathy including a proportion of patients who required acute dialysis (16, 18, 25). Further, in two large prospective studies (19, 20) there was an exponential increase in the risk of contrast nephropathy with the degree of renal dysfunction. In both of these studies the baseline serum creatinine was the only independent risk factor for contrast nephropathy although it should be emphasised that the numbers of patients with abnormal renal function was small.

Diabetes

Diabetes has been reported as an independent risk factor in retrospective studies (11, 26). However there are only two recent prospective controlled studies of diabetics with and without renal disease. In the absence of renal insufficiency recent carefully controlled studies have reported no increase in incidence of contrast nephropathy (7). These authors have also reported a rather lower incidence of contrast nephropathy in diabetic and non diabetic nephropathy. However the number of patients studied with proven diabetic nephropathy was small and of these only one patient had severe renal insufficiency (serum creatinine >400 μmol/l). In a prospective controlled study of contrast nephropathy in diabetics with severe renal impairment Manske et al (10) reported that at least 50% of patients developed contrast nephropathy defined as a rise in serum creatinine at 48 hours at least 25% over the baseline serum creatinine. Although the authors reported that renal failure was reversible in most cases, 9 out of 59 patients required acute dialysis following radiocontrast exposure with 10 out of 59 patients remaining on dialysis at follow up.

To date there are no studies comparing the relative risks of contrast nephropathy in patients with pre-existing non-diabetic renal disease and in patients with diabetic renal impairment.

It would appear that from retrospective data (24) and recent controlled prospective studies (7, 10) that diabetics at any given level of renal impairment are at increased risk of contrast nephropathy. In diabetics with severe renal impairment contrast nephropathy may precipitate the need for dialysis (10).

Contrast Volume

Radiologic studies may use repeated doses of increased quantities of radiocontrast dye where special views for therapeutic manoeuvres, such as angioplasty, are performed. The volume of contrast media used has been reported as directly related to contrast nephropathy in some studies (10, 16, 18) but not others (9, 11, 27, 28).

Taliercio et al (16) showed that contrast volume was an independent risk factor for contrast nephropathy and further that in patients receiving >125 mls of contrast agent the incidence was 19% compared with only 2% in those patients receiving <125 mls of contrast agent. In a recent prospective study contrast volume was identified as an independent risk factor in elderly patients >70 years (21). Further a reduction of the volume of contrast agent used in high risk patients has been associated with a lower incidence of contrast nephropathy (29).

Myeloma

Myeloma has been reported as a risk factor for contrast nephropathy. However most large series report a low incidence of contrast nephropathy (13-15). Patients with myeloma may have other underlying risk factors such as hypovolaemia and abnormal renal function. The relative risk of myeloma itself producing contrast nephropathy is therefore slight in the absence of abnormal renal function.

NON-IONIC VERSUS IONIC CONTRAST MEDIA

There is little doubt that the incidence and severity of minor adverse reactions is reduced by the use of non-ionic agents (for reviews see 27, 28, 30). In addition there is a significant reduction in cardiac complications such as hypotension, dysrhythmias and pulmonary oedema with the use of non-ionic agents (19, 31, 32).

Early studies have suggested that non-ionic contrast agents are associated with a lower incidence of contrast-induced nephrotoxicity. However, nephrotoxicity has been reported with the use of these agents (20, 33-37). Several recent prospective randomised studies have addressed this question. In three recent randomised prospective studies of patients undergoing cardiac catheterisation no difference in nephrotoxicity was noted between patients randomised to receive ionic and non-ionic contrast media. In the first study (19), all patients were adequately hydrated with intravenous fluids prior to the procedure. However, although patients were randomised and stratified to high and low risk groups equally, the number of patients at high risk (elevated serum creatinine) was low (14% had serum creatinine >133 μmol/l). This finding was echoed in two recent studies which again failed to find any significant difference between ionic and non-ionic agents (31, 32). Again in these studies (31, 32) only a small percentage of patients were studied with renal dysfunction (12% and 15% respectively). Patients at high risk (serum creatinine >350 μmols/l) were excluded from the study by Barrett et al (31).

In conclusion, there is no definite evidence that use of non-ionic contrast media are less nephrotoxic in patients at high risk of developing contrast nephropathy. The greatly increased cost of these agents (38) cannot be justified in terms of reduced renal side effects.

CLINICAL COURSE

Contrast nephropathy should be suspected following a documented change in serum creatinine after administration of contrast agents. In most cases, contrast nephropathy is mild, reversible, non oliguric and of short duration. Serum creatinine usually rises within 24 hours of the procedure and peaks at 48 to 96 hours before falling to baseline within 7 to 10 days. This presentation of non oliguric renal dysfunction is perhaps the commonest form of contrast nephropathy seen today and probably reflects a milder renal injury resulting from better methods of hydration and preventative measures prior to contrast use (for reviews, 23, 39).

Studies including patients with advanced renal impairment have reported a high incidence of oliguric renal failure following contrast use. It would appear that urinary volumes simply reflect the degree of renal injury and are not related to contrast nephropathy *per se*. Irreversible renal failure is unusual even in patients who require short term dialysis and thus should prompt a search for other underlying causes.

Nevertheless permanent renal dysfunction following contract nephropathy has been reported in up to 1/3rd of patients in one study (40) with irreversible renal failure in several patients (9, 10, 18, 26, 40).

Serial measurements of serum creatinine are the most cost effective means of diagnosing and detecting contrast nephropathy and such changes are often apparent within 24 hours. Changes in urinary sediment are not diagnostic and are an insensitive test. In addition persistent nephrograms 24 hours after administration of contrast are often seen in contrast nephropathy (41) but are non specific (6).

The diagnosis of contrast nephropathy is one of exclusion and thus other potential causes of acute renal failure need to be addressed (2, 3, 7). Hypovolaemia, congestive heart failure, renal obstruction were all quoted by Parfrey et al (7) as causes of acute renal failure in a control group of patients who underwent radiological procedures without contrast agents.

Cholesterol emboli causing progressive renal failure should be considered in the differential diagnosis of contrast nephropathy (37). In this condition progressive renal failure usually occurring 1-4 weeks after angiography may result from cholesterol micro-emboli released following catheter related trauma. Clinical signs such as fluctuating or accelerated hypertension may develop and *livedo reticularis* of the lower limbs is pathognomic when present. Renal failure is usually irreversible and renal biopsy findings of cholesterol micro-emboli are diagnostic.

PREVENTION OF CONTRAST NEPHROPATHY

Although many suggestions for prevention of contrast nephropathy have been made in the literature (for review see 23, 39, 42), there have been few controlled studies performed to support these claims. These measures include specific therapy such as adequate hydration prior to the procedure, saline diuresis during and post procedure, concomitant therapy with either loop diuretics or mannitol infusion and reduction of dosage of contrast media in patients at high risk. Non-specific measures include avoiding other potential nephrotoxic agents (especially prostaglandin inhibitors) and minimising other risk factors that may exacerbate renal hypoperfusion such as hypotension and cardiac failure.

The most important preventative measure is to avoid unnecessary radiographic procedures involving contrast agents in patients at high risk. Dehydration or extracellular fluid volume depletion prior to the procedure should be avoided and, where necessary, hypovolaemia should be corrected. Repetitive procedures involving contrast agents should not be performed until serum creatinine levels return to normal levels. In the retrospective study reported by Cochrane et al (22) repetitive studies were associated with a twofold increased risk of contrast nephropathy. This may be particularly important in coronary angiography where balloon angioplasty is often performed subsequent to the original procedure. Further, other drugs which interfere with renal blood flow, especially non steroidal anti-inflammatory agents, should be stopped at an appropriate time before the procedure.

Experimental evidence of the value of these preventative measures has been reported in animal models of contrast nephropathy. In these studies (43-45) a combination of volume depletion, prostaglandin inhibitors (indomethacin) and contrast agents invariably produced renal failure. However, contrast agents or indomethacin treatment alone did not produce renal failure in a volume depleted animal.

Saline infusion prior to and during the procedure has been shown in animals (44) and man (12) to reduce the incidence of contrast nephropathy. In the study by Eisenberg et al (12) the incidence of contrast nephropathy was reduced to zero by the infusion of saline (500 mls/hr). However the study was uncontrolled thus limiting the viability of their conclusions. The lower incidence of contrast nephropathy reported in recent prospective controlled studies (7, 19) may in part be due to volume correction prior to the procedure and to modest volume expansion during the procedure. Gomes et al (18) did not find that saline infusion prevented contrast nephropathy although all their patients received intravenous volume replacement therapy and there was no control group to make a comparison with. There has been no randomised controlled study to confirm the presumed beneficial effect of volume replacement therapy. However in reported studies where there was no volume replacement therapy the incidence of contrast nephropathy was much higher (17). In addition the concomitant use of loop diuretics such as furosemide (44) has been shown to have a protective effect in an animal model although other experimental studies have not shown any benefit from acute saline infusions with or without concomitant mannitol infusions (43).

Similar studies combining saline infusion with either mannitol or furosemide have been attempted in man. In studies claiming a reduction in incidence of contrast nephropathy with mannitol infusion (46, 47) no control group was studied and the incidence of contrast nephropathy in both diabetics and non diabetics was extremely high. A small, retrospective and non randomised study (6 pts in each group) claimed benefit with mannitol infusion (48) whilst a similar regimen employed in a larger controlled study failed to reduce the incidence of contrast nephropathy (49). The relative benefits of using furosemide are also hard to assess as there are no controlled studies reported.

Other therapeutic measures, such as infusion of atrial natriuretic peptide (ANP) (50) and combined infusions of dopamine and atrial natriuretic peptide (51), have been used to attenuate acute renal failure in animal studies.

In a recent randomised study (52) the effects of either atrial natriuretic peptide or mannitol infusion were compared in a small group of patients (n = 21) with renal dysfunction who underwent cardiac angiography. There was no control group included unfortunately and no difference in contrast-induced renal failure was noted between each treatment group. Only patients with diabetes developed contrast nephropathy. Both ANP and mannitol prevented the renal vasconstrictive effect of contrast agent and yet did not seem to prevent the development of contrast nephropathy. Only diabetic patients showed a vasodilator response to ANP or mannitol. Thus further clinical studies are required to adequately evaluate the value of these newer agents in the prevention of contrast nephropathy. As previously discussed, the volume of contrast agents used has been identified as an independent risk factor in contrast nephropathy. In a large prospective controlled trial Cigarroa et al (29) reported a dose dependent reduction in the incidence of contrast nephropathy from 2% (where the volume of the contrast agent was carefully limited) to 21% where excess contrast agent was used. In this study the maximum dosage of contrast agents allowed during cardiac catheterization was calculated according to an empirical formula including body weight and serum creatinine. All patients who developed contrast nephropathy in this study were diabetics with abnormal renal function.

SUMMARY

There is a paucity of convincing data obtained from properly designed clinical trials to support many of the therapeutic manoeuvres that have claimed to reduce the incidence of contrast nephropathy. Recommendations made by authors in recent reviews and editorials (23, 37, 39, 42) have merely reiterated similar advice which is based in most cases on personal opinion. Nevertheless these recommendations have *ipso facto* become established in current clinical practice (39).

Clearly efforts should be directed at patients identified as being at high risk, namely those with abnormal renal function, in particular diabetics with abnormal renal function, and patients with severe heart failure. It would be sensible to avoid the concomitant use of other nephrotoxic agents, particularly drugs that interfere with renal blood flow such as prostaglandin inhibitors. Correction of hypovolaemia prior to the procedure and mild volume expansion with a saline infusion during the procedure is simple, safe and probably offers the best protection against contrast nephropathy. There is little evidence to support the concomitant use of furosemide, mannitol infusions or other renal vasodilator therapy. Contrast dose should be adjusted according to simple published guidelines and care should be taken not to exceed the maximum safe dose (29). Finally spacing of radiographic procedures and allowing renal function to return to baseline before further exposure to contrast media may also be of benefit.

REFERENCES

1. Hou SH, Bushinsky HA, Wish JB, Cohen JJ, Harrington JT: Hospital acquired renal insufficiency. Am J Med, 74: 243-248, 1983.
2. Knapp MS: Renal failure after contrast radiography. Br Med J, 287: 3-4, 1983.
3. Cramer BC, Parfrey PS, Hutchinson TA, et al: Renal function following infusion of radiologic contrast material. Arch Intern Med, 145: 87-89, 1985.
4. Eisenberg RL, Band WD, Hedgecock MW: Renal failure after major angiography. Am J Med, 68: 43-46, 1980.
5. Kumar S, Hull JD, Lathi S et al: Low incidence of renal failure after angiography. Arch Intern Med, 141: 1268-1270, 1981.
6. Byrd L, Sherman RL: Radiocontrast-induced renal failure. A clinical pathophysiologic review. Medicine (Balt), 58: 270-279, 1979.

7. Parfrey PS, Griffiths SW, Barrett BJ et al: Contrast material-induced renal failure in patients with diabetes mellitus, renal insufficiency or both. N Eng J Med, 320: 143-149, 1989.
8. Teruel JL, Marcan R, Onaindia JM, Serrano A, Quereda C, Orturo J: Renal function impairment caused by intravenous urography: a prospective study. Arch Intern Med, 141: 1271-1274, 1981.
9. D'Elia JA, Gleann RE, Alday M et al: Nephrotoxicity from angiograph contrast material: a prospective study. Am J Med, 72: 719-725, 1982.
10. Manske CL, Sprafka JM, Strong JT, Wong Y: Contrast nephropathy in azotemic diabetic patients undergoing coronary angiography. Am J Med, 89: 615-620, 1990.
11. Harkonen S, Kjellstrand CM: Exacerbation of diabetic renal failure following intravenous pyelography. Am J Med, 63: 939-946, 1977.
12. Eisenberg RL, Bank WO, Hedgock MW: Renal failure after major angiography can be avoided with hydration. Am J Roentgenol, 136: 859-861, 1981.
13. DeFronzo RA, Humphrey RL, Wright JR, Cooke CR: Acute renal failure in multiple myeloma. Medicine, 54: 209, 1975.
14. Myers GH, Witter DM: Acute renal failure after excretory urography in multiple myeloma. Am J Roentgenol, 113: 583, 1971.
15. Vix VA: Intravenous pyelography in multiple myeloma. Review of 52 studies in 40 patients. Radiology, 87: 896, 1966.
16. Taliercio CP, Vliestra RE, Fisher LO, Burnett JC: Risks for dysfunction with cardiac angiography. Ann Intern Med, 104: 501-504, 1986.
17. Swartz RD, Rubin JE, Leeming EW, Silva P: Renal failure following major angiography. Am J Med, 65: 31-37, 1978.
18. Gomes AS, Baker JD, Martin Paredoo V et al: Acute renal dysfunction after arteriography. Am J Roentgenol, 145: 1249-1253, 1985.
19. Schwab SJ, Heatley MA, Pieper KS et al: Contrast nephrotoxicity: a randomized controlled trial of a non-ionic and an ionic radiographic contrast agent. N Eng J Med, 320: 149-153, 1989.
20. Davidson CT, Hlatky M, Morris KG et al: Cardiovascular and renal toxicity of a nonionic radiographic contrast agent after cardiac catheterization. Ann Intern Med, 110: 119-124, 1989.
21. Rich MW, Crecelius CA: Incidence, risk factors, and clinical course of acute renal insufficiency after cardiac catheterization in patients 70 years of age or older. A prospective study. Arch Intern Med, 150 (6): 1237-1242, 1990.
22. Cochrane ST, Wong WS, Roe DJ: Predicting angiography-induced acute renal function impairment: clinical risk model.Am J Roentgenol, 141: 1027-1033, 1983.
23. Berkseth RO, Kjellstrand CM: Radiologic contrast-induced nephropathy. Med Clin North Am, 68: 351-370, 1984.
24. Van Zee BE, Hoy WE, Talley TE, Jaenike JR: Renal failure associated with intravenous pyelography in non-diabetic and diabetic patients. Ann. Intern Med, 89: 51-54, 1978.
25. Kove BC, Watson AJ, Gimeneney LF, Kadir S: Acute renal failure following percutaneous transhepatic cholangiography; a retrospective study. Arch Intern Med, 146: 1405-1407, 1986.
26. Weinrauch LA, Healy RW, Leland RW et al: Coronary angiography and acute renal failure in diabetic azotemic nephropathy. Arch Intern Med, 86: 56-59, 1977.
27. Bush WH, Swanson DP: Acute reactions to intravascular contrast media: types, risk factors, recognition, and specific treatment. Am J Roentgenol, 157: 1153-1161, 1991.
28. McLennan BL, Stolberg HO: Intravascular contrast media. Ionic versus non-ionic: current status. Contemporary Radiology, The Radiologic Clinics of North America, 29: 437-454, 1991.
29. Cigarroa RG, Lange RA, Williams RH, Hillis LD: Dosing of contrast material to prevent contrast nephropathy in patients with renal disease. Am J Med, 86: 649-652, 1989.
30. McClennan BL: Ionic and non-ionic iodinated contrast media: evolution and strategies for use. Am J Roentgenol, 155: 225-233, 1990.
31. Barrett BJ, Pargrey PS, Vavasour HM, O'Dea F, Kent G, Stone E: A comparison of non ionic, low osmolality radio contrast agents with ionic high osmolality agents during cardiac catheterization. N Eng J Med, 326: 431-436, 1992.
32. Steinberg EP, Moore RD, Powe NR, Gopalan R et al: Safety and cost effectiveness of high osmolality as compared with low osmolality contrast material in patients undergoing cardiac angiography. N Eng J Med, 326: 425-430, 1992.
33. Kinnison ML, Powe NR, Steinberg EP: Results of randomized controlled trials of low- vs high-osmolality contrast media. Radiology, 170: 381-389, 1989.

34. Foster CJ, Griffen JF: A comparison of the incidence of cardiac arrhythmias produced by two intravenous contrast media in coronary artery disease. Clin Radiol, 38: 399-401, 1987.
35. Denys BG, Reddy PS, Uretsky BF: Nephrotoxicity of a nonionic (iopamidol) versus an ionic (diatrizoate) contrast agent in the patient after cardiac transplant with moderate cyclosporine-induced renal insufficiency. Am J Cardiol, 64: 404-406, 1989.
36. McCullough M, Davies P, Richardson R: A large trial of intravenous Conray 325 and niopam 300 to assess immediate and delayed reactions. Br J Radiol, 62: 260-265, 1989.
37. Cronin RE: Southwestern Internal Medicine Conference: Renal failure following radiologic procedures. Am J Med Sci, 298: 342-366, 1989.
38. Hirschfield JW (Ed): Low osmolality contrast agents - Who needs them? N Eng J Med, 326: 482-484, 1992.
39. Berns AS: Nephrotoxicity of contrast media. Kidney Int, 36: 730-740, 1989.
40. Kleinknecht D, Landais P, Goldfarb B: Pathophysiology and clinical aspects of drug-induced tubular necrosis in man. Contr Nephrol, 55: 145, 1987.
41. Older RA, Korobkin M, Cleeve DM, Schaaf R, Thompson W: Contrast-induced acute renal failure: persistent nephrogram as clue to early detection. Am J Roentgenol, 134: 339-342, 1980.
42. Brezis M, Epstein FH: A closer look at radiocontrast-induced nephropathy. N Eng J Med, 320 (3): 179-181, 1989.
43. Vari RC, Natarajan LA, Whitescarver SA, Jackson BA, Ott CE: Induction, prevention and mechanisms of contrast media-induced acute renal failure. Kidney Int, 33: 699-707, 1988.
44. Heyman SN, Brezis M, Greenfeld Z, Rosen S: Protective role of furosemide and saline in radicontrast-induced acute renal failure in the rat. Am J Kidney Dis, 14 (No 5): 377-385, 1989.
45. Heyman SN, Brezis M, Reubinoff CA, Greenfeld Z, Lechene C, Epstein FH, Rosen S: Acute renal failure with selective medullary injury in the rat. J Clin Invest, 82: 401-412, 1988.
46. Anto HR, Chou SY, Porush JG, Shapiro WB: Infusion intravenous pyelography and renal function: effects of hypertonic mannitol in patients with chronic renal insufficiency. Arch Intern Med, 141: 1652-1656, 1981.
47. Shafti T, Chon S, Porush JG et al: Infusion intravenous pyelography and renal function. Arch Intern Med, 138: 1218-1221, 1978.
48. Old CW, Lehrner LM: Prevention of radiocontrast-induced acute renal failure with mannitol. Lancet, I: 885, 1980 (Letter).
49. Vosnides G, Kalogeropoulous V, Spanos H. et al: Radiocontrast-induced deterioration of renal function in patients with chronic renal failure. Eighth International Congress of Nephrology, Athens, University Studio Publishing Co, 1981, p.306 (Abstract).
50. Margulies KB, McKinley LJ, Cavero PG & Burnett JC Jr: Induction and prevention of radiocontrast-induced nephropathy in dogs with heart failure. Kidney Int, 38: 1101-1108, 1990.
51. Conger JD, Falk SA, Yuan BH, Schrier RW: Atrial natriuretic peptide and dopamine in a rat model of ischaemic acute renal failure. Kidney Int, 35: 1126-1132, 1989.
52. Kurnik BR, Weisberg LS, Cuttler IM, Kurnik PB: Effects of atrial natriuretic peptide versus mannitol on renal blood flow during radiocontrast infusion in chronic renal failure. J Lab Clin Med, 116: 27-36, 1990.

CHRONIC RENAL FAILURE

Chapter 13

USE OF RECOMBINANT HUMAN ERYTHROPOIETIN IN THE ANEMIA OF PROGRESSIVE RENAL FAILURE

JOSEPH W. ESCHBACH AND JOHN W. ADAMSON

University of Washington School of Medicine, Seattle, WA, New York Blood Center, New York, NY, USA

INTRODUCTION

The anemia of progressive renal failure (A/PRF) is now correctable through therapy with recombinant human erythropoietin (rHuEpo). While the prevalence of this anemia is not as great as in end-stage renal disease, its significance is greater than previously appreciated, since failure to correct this anemia can lead to disability that may not be corrected by dialysis and to unnecessary red cell transfusions. The purpose of this chapter will be to review the clinical manifestations of this anemia, its diagnosis, pathophysiology, therapy, and the beneficial and adverse consequences of rHuEpo therapy.

CLINICAL MANIFESTATIONS

Anemia almost always develops during the course of renal insufficiency, regardless of the diagnosis, although patients with polycystic kidney disease and nephrosclerosis, in general, have a less severe anemia. Chronic rejection of a renal transplant is becoming a more recognized cause of the A/PRF. Most patients are not symptomatic of anemia until the hematocrit or hemoglobin decreases to less than 30% and 10 gm%, respectively. Fatigue, coldness, and anorexia are the main symptoms, while angina and shortness of breath may develop depending on the degree of exertion and age of the patient. Despite the statement that this anemia rarely is symptomatic, can usually be managed by other hematinics and therefore does not require therapy with rHuEpo (1), in our experience these symptoms often develop gradually, and patients, especially younger ones, may adjust to or compensate for these symptoms, particularly if the anemia progresses slowly.

Once the anemia is corrected with rHuEpo, all patients, in retrospect, recognize how symptomatic they had been.

Prior to rHuEpo therapy, these symptoms were thought to be secondary to uremia. These symptoms are eliminated with correction of the anemia (hematocrit 35-40) and can allow the patient with progressive renal failure (PRF) to continue their usual activities, including full time physical work. However, when renal dysfunction progresses to an endogenous creatinine clearance of 4-6 ml/min, anorexia returns indicating the need for dialysis therapy (2).

DIAGNOSIS AND PATHOPHYSIOLOGY

The A/PRF is frequently not diagnosed until other causes of anemia have been excluded (3). It should be considered in the workup of all patients with anemia, regardless of whether other causes of anemia coexist, such as iron deficiency, which may occur in up to 25% of patients with the A/PRF (4). The serum creatinine is always greater than 2 mg/dl; the anemia is hypoplastic, i.e., it is characterized by a normochromic, normocytic peripheral blood smear that may contain irregular shaped red cells, or schistocytes (5); the reticulocyte count is rarely more than twice normal when corrected for the severity of the anemia; the bone marrow may disclose a decrease in erythroid cells relative to the granulocytic series; and serum erythropoietin levels are rarely more than twice "normal", yet inappropriately low for the degree of anemia. Anemia usually develops after the loss of more than one-half of kidney function. This hypoplastic anemia must be differentiated from that of the hemolytic uremic syndrome. In the latter syndrome, the serum creatinine is also elevated, but the reticulocyte count is increased 3-4 fold, serum erythropoietin levels are usually elevated greater than 2 fold, and red cell survival, if measured, is 1/4 of normal or less. Bone marrow morphology discloses moderate-marked erythroid hyperplasia.

The anemia is primarily due to erythropoietin deficiency, presumably due to disease-induced damage to the erythropoietin producing renal cortical, peritubular, capillary endothelial cells (6, 7). Mild hemolysis may also exist, as shown by isotopic red cell labelling studies (8, 9). In advanced uremia, blood loss can also contribute to the anemia by way of platelet dysfunction (10), which allows for more gastrointestinal and cutaneous blood loss. Uremic inhibition of red cell production has been suggested, since *in vitro* studies of erythropoiesis have demonstrated impaired heme synthesis or growth of erythroid colonies [from Colony-Forming Units-Erythroid (CFU-E)] in the presence of uremic serum. Fisher et al observed an increased inhibition of CFU-E associated with a decline in the hematocrit and a rise in serum creatinine levels in PRF (11). However, *in vitro* inhibition of murine or canine CFU-E by human uremic serum is probably non-specific, since granulopoiesis and megakaryopoiesis are also inhibited *in vitro* by uremic serum (12). When either sheep or human marrow cells are cultured with erythropoietin in the presence of autologous uremic serum, there is no inhibition of erythropoiesis when compared to normal controls (13, 14). Furthermore, this anemia is easily corrected by erythropoietin (2, 15-23), and one patient with the A/PRF, later studied when she had normal renal transplant function and was no longer anemic, had a similar erythropoietic response - as quantitated by changes in ferrokinetics, reticulocyte count and plasma levels of transferrin receptor protein - to the same amount of rHuEpo (24). Therefore, if uremic inhibition of erythropoiesis does occur, it probably plays little role in the A/PRF.

The platelet defect improves when the anemia improves, either by red cell transfusions or rHuEpo therapy (25, 26). Red cell survival, as measured by ^{51}Chromium labelling, will also improve following near correction of the anemia (21, 23, 27). Routine transplant immunosuppression with prednisone, azathioprine and cyclosporin does not contribute to the anemia in chronic transplant rejection (24). Therefore, erythropoietin deficiency appears to be the primary cause of this anemia.

ERYTHROPOIETIN THERAPY

A. Erythropoietic response

RHuEpo was first used in clinical trials in patients with A/PRF in the United States in early 1987 (15). As of early 1992, there have been twelve published studies reporting the intravenous or subcutaneous use of rHuEpo in a total of 126 patients with the A/PRF (2, 16-23, 28, 29), including four patients with anemia related to chronic transplant rejection (30). Eighty-six patients with the A/PRF were treated as part of a United States multicenter trial which included many of those reported in individual studies (15). The authors have also had experience with treating this anemia in an additional 20 patients with the A/PRF.

The hematocrit at baseline, when rHuEpo therapy was initiated, varied between 21% to 31% for 123 patients, with a mean (±SD) of 26.7±2.4%. Following 3-5 months of rHuEpo therapy, with 50, 100, or 150 U/Kg, given intravenously (i.v.) or subcutaneously (s.c.), thrice weekly, the mean hematocrit was 36.8±3.6%. The red cell mass increases without an increase in total blood volume (16, 17).

B. Dosing

Doses of rHuEpo required to induce an erythropoietic response have varied from 50 to 150 units (U)/Kg, thrice weekly, i.v., although a fixed dose (1500 U) was also reported (28).

There is a relationship between the rHuEpo dose and the rate of rise in hematocrit. In general, 50, 100 and 150 U/Kg, i.v., three times a week results in a daily hematocrit rise of 0.13%, 0.20% and 0.26%, respectively (15). Once the target hematocrit was obtained (33-40) the dose usually was reduced. Treatment duration has varied between 4 weeks (28) to over one year, and, theoretically, lasts until dialysis is required.

Some patients have been on rHuEpo for greater than 3 years and have yet to require dialysis. No secondary failures to rHuEpo have been reported and antibody formation to rHuEpo has not been reported. The same dose of rHuEpo should be continued when dialysis is needed, since the dose requirements do not change regardless of whether the patient requires peritoneal or hemodialysis (27).

Ferrokinetic studies also indicate that the erythropoietic response, as determined by the reticulocyte count and erythron transferrin uptake, following 150 U/Kg, i.v., is similar in patients with the A/PRF and hemodialysis patients (18). Most patients respond and increase their hematocrit to the target range within 12 weeks. The response to rHuEpo may be blunted if infection is present (27).

C. Route of injection

Most of the studies reported initially used rHuEpo i.v., three times a week, but investigators and sponsors soon realized that s.c. injections preserved the forearm veins for the arteriovenous fistulae eventually needed for hemodialysis, and that s.c. injections allowed for self-administration at home.

The route of administration should be s.c. for several reasons. Besides the ability to self-administer, evidence also suggests that s.c. dosing is more efficacious than i.v. administration.

One study indicated that the rate of rise in hematocrit was identical between 4 patients receiving 150 U/Kg i.v. and 4 patients receiving 100 U/Kg s.c. (18). Pharmacokinetic studies indicate that s.c. injection, although achieving lower peak levels of rHuEpo than i.v. injection, results in a more prolonged therapeutic blood level. For instance, the T1/2 after the first i.v. injection of rHuEpo is 7.69±1.11 hrs, and this shortens to 4.6 hrs after 24 doses (17), whereas s.c. injection of 50 U/kg will maintain Epo levels above baseline for more than 3 days (31).

D. Frequency of dosing

The frequency of administration reported varies: thrice weekly, twice weekly, and weekly. Our approach is to teach patients to self administer rHuEpo and to begin therapy at 4000 U (approximately 57 U/Kg for a 70 Kg person) thrice weekly. Patients are then monitored every 2 weeks for hematocrit and blood pressure, and the frequency reduced to twice weekly when the hematocrit rises to 32-35. If the hematocrit continues to rise above 35-38, the frequency is then reduced to weekly. The frequency and dose can then be titrated to maintain the target hematocrit between 35-40. Occasionally the frequency can be every other week.

CONSEQUENCES OF THERAPY

A. Hypertension

The consequences of therapy and correction of the anemia have been extensively studied. The two major concerns have been whether hypertension would be accentuated [as was shown in the rHuEpo trials in hemodialysis patients (32, 33)], or more difficult to manage, and whether renal function would decline at an accelerated rate due to hemodynamic changes as suggested in an animal model (34). Of the initial 11 reported studies of rHuEpo use in the A/PRF, blood pressure either increased and/or patients required more antihypertensive medication in 8 studies. Two studies showed no difference in the incidence of aggravation in hypertension between placebo and rHuEpo treated patients (2, 23) and one study did not detail blood pressure responses (21). Of these 123 treated patients, 43 were defined as becoming more hypertensive and/or requiring more antihypertensive medication, an incidence of 35% during the induction phase of rHuEpo therapy. This is similar to that reported in the hemodialysis population. On the other hand, the multicenter US study of i.v. rHuEpo therapy, which included 6 of the studies reported separately did not show a significant incidence of hypertension in the rHuEpo treated patients compared to those treated with placebo (15). Hemodynamic studies in 7 patients with the A/PRF disclosed that while the mean arterial pressure increased from 106 to 117 mm Hg following correction of the anemia with rHuEpo, total peripheral vascular resistance increased and there was no change in left ventricular end diastolic diameter (35).

B. Effect on renal function

Almost all studies have documented the course of renal function during rHuEpo therapy. There have been no patients who have had an acceleration in their expected rate of decline in renal function, as determined by serial measurements of serum creatinine, 1/serum creatinine or creatinine clearance. Many studies used retrospective serum creatinine values to compare the slope of 1/cr before rHuEpo therapy to the slope after therapy, and no significant differences in the rate of decline were observed. Lim et al (36) noted that the rate of decline in rHuEpo treated patients was similar to that of patients with the A/PRF not treated with rHuEpo, and to non-anemic patients with PRF. Frenken et al (29) noted that correction of A/PRF resulted in renal vasodilation of the efferent arterioles. These authors observed that 25 mg of captopril given orally when anemic before rHuEpo therapy resulted in an increase in effective renal plasma flow (PAH clearance) and reduced blood pressure without change in GFR (inulin clearance). Following correction of the anemia, there was no change in GFR but 25 mg of captopril now failed to increase effective renal plasma flow, yet still retained its systemic hypotensive effect (29).

C. Iron deficiency

Iron deficiency can develop easily unless supplemental iron is ingested. Absolute or functional iron deficiency was noted in the majority of patients in several studies, particularly during the induction phase of rHuEpo therapy. Oral iron can maintain iron stores during the maintenance phase of rHuEpo therapy (19), unless superimposed acute blood loss occurs.

D. Other possible adverse effects

There have been no consistent adverse consequences with rHuEpo in A/PRF except for the occasional increase in blood pressure, which can be managed with new or additional antihypertensive medication. Whole blood viscosity increases, but increases as a function of the rise in hematocrit and has not resulted in symptoms or signs of decreased tissue perfusion, even in patients with known peripheral vascular disease, such as patients with diabetes mellitus (22). Platelet levels have usually been unchanged following rHuEpo therapy, although a transient rise was noted in one study (19). There have been no reports of vascular clotting following correction of the anemia, and no reports that arteriovenous fistulae, created for initiation of hemodialysis, clot due to the normal hematocrit.

OTHER BENEFITS OF THERAPY

A. Quality of life

Quality of life, as determined by subjective questionnaires, has increased in most patients whose anemia is corrected with rHuEpo. In our experience, patients are able to continue working (if previously employed) despite the development of severe renal failure (BUN levels as high as 160 mg/dl) and better adjust to the initiation of dialysis. It is important to adjust dialysis schedules to minimize the impact on the patient's work schedule. The ideal form of overall treatment is for the patient to receive a kidney transplant just prior to the time dialysis is needed (Figure 1).

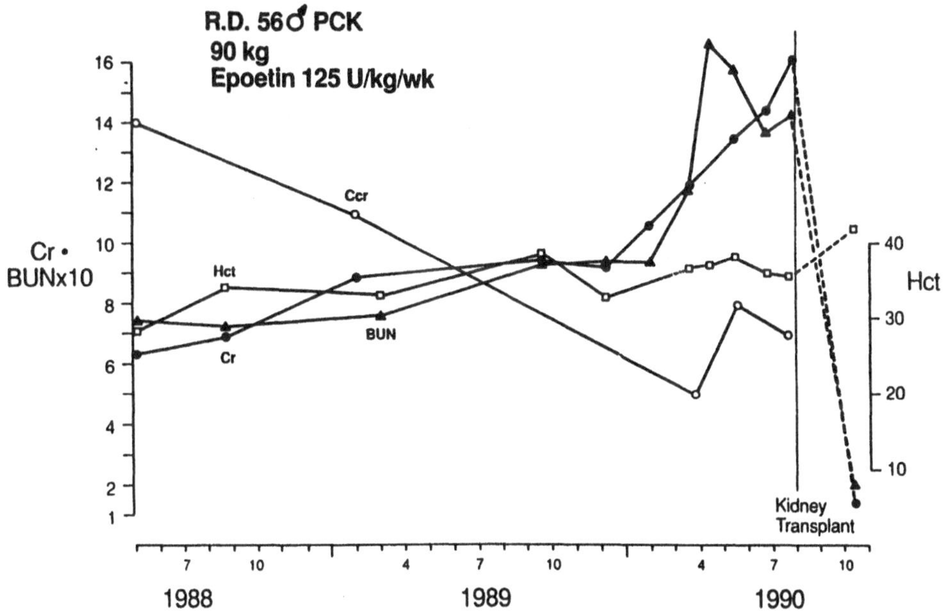

Figure 1. Recombinant human erythropoietin therapy (125 U/Kg/week, subcutaneously) in a patient with the anemia of progressive renal failure (polycystic renal disease). Despite marked azotemia, he was able to work full time until he received a cadaveric kidney transplant. Dialysis was never required.

By preventing the disabling effects of anemia in the presence of PRF by treating with rHuEpo, patients should be able to continue working. There may be enough time to obtain a suitable HLA matched kidney for transplantation. Dialysis can therefore be avoided and minimal time is lost from work for health problems.

B. Red cell survival

Red cell survival has been quantitated by ^{51}Chromium labelling of patients' red cells before and after correction of anemia (21, 23, 27).

In 28 patients with a mean baseline hematocrit of 26.6%, the T1/2 was 22.5 days. After three to eight months of rHuEpo therapy, the mean hematocrit was 37.9% with a ^{51}Chromium T1/2 of 26.8 days (normal range 28-32 days). Renal function, as determined by creatinine clearance or 1/serum creatinine X 100, expressed as ml/min, varied between 13.4 to 20 at baseline and 10.3 to 17 3-8 months after beginning rHuEpo therapy. Therefore, despite increasing renal failure, rHuEpo improved red cell survival almost to normal. Lim et al (27) calculated that the improvement in red cell survival accounted for 1/3 of the increase in hematocrit achieved by rHuEpo therapy and resulted in a lower rHuEpo requirement to maintain the target hematocrit than if red cell survival had not improved.

C. Exercise capacity

Exercise tolerance has been quantitated in 17 patients (17, 23). At a baseline hematocrit of 28.0% and 25.2%, oxygen utilization (VO_2 max.) was 16.0 and 13.5 ml/Kg/min, respectively, for a duration of 6.3 minutes in the latter study (23). After the hematocrit had increased to 38% and 36.1%, VO_2 max increased to 17.5 and 18.0 ml/Kg/min respectively, with the duration of exercise now increased to 9.8 minutes. Although this was a significant improvement in exercise tolerance, it was far from optimal, since the predicted VO_2 max only increased from 61.6 to 66.9% of normal (23).

D. Cardiovascular function

Treadmill ergometry in 10 patients with the A/PRF disclosed that the duration of exertion was 6.7±4.0 minutes at a baseline hematocrit of 25.2±3.5%; this increased to 8.9±4.6 minutes at a hematocrit of 36.1±2.7% following rHuEpo therapy (23). When anemic, 7 patients could not continue on the treadmill because of angina, claudication or dyspnea, whereas following the improved hematocrit, fatigue was the major reason for stopping the test.

SUMMARY

The A/PRF is primarily an erythropoietin deficiency condition that responds appropriately to recombinant human erythropoietin. Hormone therapy is usually indicated when the hematocrit declines to less than 30 (when most patients become symptomatic). Subcutaneous injections, approximately 50 U/Kg, three times a week will usually result in a good response and the target hematocrit (35-40) can be reached and maintained by adjusting the frequency from thrice to twice or once weekly. Some patients will need greater amounts of rHuEpo to attain a near-normal hematocrit. Iron stores must be maintained with either oral or intravenous iron.

Blood pressure may increase requiring new or additional antihypertensive medication in approximately 1/3 of patients during the induction phase of rHuEpo therapy. Other adverse effects are infrequent. No antibody formation has been detected after 3-4 years of use. Therapy is urged to prevent patient debilitation and the need for red cell transfusions. Therapy results in a significant improvement in quality of life, and the ability to continue working, and when renal dysfunction progresses to an endogenous creatinine clearance of 5-6 ml/min, lack of significant anemia results in an easier transition to maintenance dialysis therapy.

REFERENCES

1. Horina JH, Horn S, Silly H, Winkler HM, Roob J, Kaufmann P, Pogglitsch H, Krejs GJ: Need for erythropoietin treatment in predialysis patients. Lancet, 337: 562, 1991 (Letter to Editor).
2. Kleinman KS, Schweitzer SU, Perdue ST, Bleifer KH, Abels RI: The use of recombinant human erythropoietin in the correction of anemia in predialysis patients and its effect on renal function: a double-blind, placebo-controlled trial. Am J Kidney Dis, 14: 486-495, 1989.
3. Self KG, Conrady MM, Eichner ER: Failure to diagnose anemia in medical inpatients. Am J Med, 81: 786-790, 1986.
4. Loge JP, Lange RD, Moore CV: Characterization of the anemia associated with chronic renal insufficiency. Am J Med, 24: 4-18, 1958.
5. Aherne WA: The "burr" red cell and azotemia. J Clin Pathol, 10: 252-257, 1957.
6. Lacombe C, DaSilva JL, Bruneval P, Fournier JG, Wendling F, Casadevall N, Camilleri JP, Bariety J, Varet B, Tambourin P: Peritubular cells are the site of erythropoietin synthesis in the murine hypoxic kidney. J Clin Invest, 81: 620-623, 1988.
7. Koury ST, Bondurant MC, Koury MJ: Localization of erythropoietin synthesizing cells in murine kidneys by *in situ* hybridization. Blood, 71: 524-527, 1988.
8. Chaplin H, Mollison PL: Red cell life-span in nephritis and in hepatic cirrhosis. Clin Sci, 12: 351-360, 1953.
9. Hocken AG: Haemolysis in chronic renal failure. Nephron, 32: 28-31, 1982.

10. Rabiner SF, Molinas F: The role of phenol and phenolic acids on the thrombocytopathy and defective platelet aggregation of patients with renal failure. Am J Med, 49: 346-350, 1970.
11. McGonigle RJS, Wallin JD, Shadduck RK, Fisher JW: Erythropoietin deficiency and inhibition of erythropoiesis in renal insufficiency. Kidney Int, 25: 437-444, 1984.
12. Delwiche F, Segal GM, Eschbach JW, Adamson JW: Erythropoietin inhibitors in chronic renal failure: Studies of clinical correlations and *in vitro* specificity. Kidney Int, 29: 641-648, 1986.
13. Mladenovich J, Eschbach JW, Garcia JF, Adamson JW: The anemia of chronic renal failure in sheep. Studies *in vitro*. Brit J Haematol, 58: 491-500, 1984.
14. Segal GM, Eschbach JW, Egrie JC, Stueve T, Adamson JW: The anemia of end-stage renal disease: Hematopoietic progenitor cell response. Kidney Int, 33: 983-988, 1988.
15. The US Recombinant Human Erythropoietin Predialysis Study Group: Double-blind, placebo-controlled study of the therapeutic use of recombinant human erythropoietin for anemia associated. Am J Kidney Dis, 18: 50-59, 1991.
16. Stone WJ, Graber SE, Krantz SB, Dessypris EN, O'Neil VL, Olsen NJ, Pincus TP: Treatment of the anemia of predialysis patients with recombinant human erythropoietin: a randomized, placebo-controlled trial. Am J Med Sci, 296: 171-179, 1988.
17. Lim VS, DeGowin RL, Zavala D, Kirchner PT, Abels R, Perry P, Fangman J: Recombinant human erythropoietin treatment in pre-dialysis patients. A double-blind, placebo-controlled trial. Ann Int Med, 110: 108-114, 1989.
18. Eschbach JW, Kelly MR, Haley NR, Abels RI, Adamson JW: Treatment of the anemia of progressive renal failure with recombinant human erythropoietin. N Engl J Med, 321: 158-163, 1989.
19. Frenken LAM, Verberckmoes R, Michielsen P, Koene RAP: Efficacy and tolerance of treatment with recombinant human erythropoietin in chronic renal failure (pre-dialysis) patients. Nephrol Dial Transplant, 4: 782-786, 1989.
20. Abraham PA, Opsahl JA, Rachael KM, Asinger R, Halstenson CE: Renal function during erythropoietin therapy for anemia in predialysis chronic renal failure patients. Am J Nephrol, 10: 128-136, 1990.
21. Schwartz AB, Kelch B, Terzian L, Prior J, Kim KE, Pequinot E, Kahn SB: One year of rHuEPO therapy prolongs RBC survival and may stabilize RBC membranes despite natural progression of chronic renal failure to uremia and need for dialysis. ASAIO Trans, 36: 691-696, 1990.
22. Brown CD, Friedman EA: Clinical and blood rheologic stability in erythropoietin-treated predialysis patients. Am J Nephrol, 10: 29-33, 1990.
23. Teehan BP, Sigler MH, Brown JM, Benz RL, Gilgore GS, Schleifer CR, Morgan CM, Gabuzda TG, Kelly JJ, Figueroa WG, Peterson DD: Hematologic and physiologic studies during correction of anemia with recombinant human erythropoietin in predialysis patients. Transpl Proc, 21: 63-66, 1989.
24. Eschbach JW, Haley NR, Egrie JC, Adamson JW: A comparison of the responses to recombinant human erythropoietin in normal and uremic subjects. Kidney Int (in press).
25. Moia M, Vizzotto L, Cattaneo M, Mannucci PM, Casati S, Ponticelli C: Improvement in the haemostatic defect of uraemia after treatment with recombinant human erythropoietin. Lancet, II: 1227-1229, 1987.
26. Van Geet C, Hauglustanine D, Verresen L, Vanrusselt M, Vermylen J: Haemostatic effects of recombinant human erythropoietin in chronic haemodialysis patients. Thromb Haemost, 61: 117-121, 1989.
27. Lim VS, Kirchner PT, Fangman J, Richmond J, DeGowin RL: The safety and the efficacy of maintenance therapy of recombinant human erythropoietin in patients with renal insufficiency. Am J Kidney Dis, 14: 496-506, 1989.
28. Onoyama K, Kumagai H, Takeda K, Shimamatsu K, Fujishima M: Effects of human recombinant erythropoietin in anaemia, systemic haemodynamics and renal function in predialysis renal failure patients. Nephrol Dial Transplant, 4: 966-970, 1989.
29. Frenken LAM, Wetzels JFM, Sluiter HE, Koene RAP: Evidence for renal vasodilation in pre-dialysis patients during correction of anemia by erythropoietin. Kidney Int, 41: 384-387, 1992.
30. Yoshimura N, Oka T, Ohmori Y, Aikawa I: Effects of recombinant human erythropoietin on the anemia of renal transplant recipients with chronic rejection. Transplantation, 48: 527-529, 1989.
31. Salmonson T, Danielson BG, Wikstrom B: The pharmacokinetics of recombinant human erythropoietin after intravenous and subcutaneous administration to healthy subjects. Br J Clin Pharmac, 29: 709-713, 1990.

32. Eschbach JW, Egrie JC, Downing MR, Browne JK, Adamson JW: Correction of the anemia of end-stage renal disease with recombinant human-erythropoietin: results of a combined phase I and II clinical trial. N Engl J Med, 316: 73-78, 1987.
33. Eschbach JW, Abdulhadi MH, Browne JK, Delano BG, Downing MR, Egrie JC, Evans RW, Friedman EA, Graber SE, Haley NR, Korbet S, Krantz SB, Lundin AP, Nissenson AR, Ogden DA, Paganini EP, Rader B, Rutsky EA, Stivelman J, Stone WJ, Teschan P, Van Stone JC, Van Wyck DB, Zuckerman K, Adamson JW: Recombinant human erythropoietin in anemic patients with end-stage renal disease. Results of a phase III multicenter clinical trial. Ann Int Med, 111: 992-1000, 1989.
34. Garcia DL, Anderson S, Rennke HG, Brenner BM: Anemia and its prevention with recombinant human erythropoietin worsens glomerular injury and hypertension in rats with reduced renal mass. Proc natl Acad Sci USA, 85: 6142-6146, 1988.
35. Schwartz AB, Mintz GS, Kim KE, Prior JE, Kahn B: Recombinant human erythropoietin (rHuEPO) increases MAP, TPRI and systolic and diastolic dysfunction with increased impedance to LV ejection due to increased HCT and RBC mass in PTS with CRF. Kidney Int, 35: 334, 1989 (Abstract).
36. Lim VS, Fangman J, Flanigan MJ, DeGowin RL, Abels RT: Effect of recombinant human erythropoietin on renal function in humans. Kidney Int, 37: 131-136, 1990.

DIALYSIS

Chapter 14

MALNUTRITION IN PATIENTS ON RENAL REPLACEMENT THERAPY

JONAS BERGSTRÖM

Department of Renal Medicine, Karolinska Institute, Huddinge University Hospital, Stockholm, S-141 86 Huddinge, Sweden

INTRODUCTION

Protein-energy malnutrition and wasting are present in a large proportion of patients with chronic renal failure. This may be a consequence of multiple factors, including disturbances in protein and energy metabolism, hormonal derangements, infections and other superimposed illnesses, and poor food intake because of anorexia, nausea and vomiting, caused by uremic toxicity. In addition, several iatrogenic factors may contribute to poor nutrition.

Low-protein diet, prescribed for conservative therapy of uremia, may be inadequate both with regard to total protein supply and content of essential amino acids. Long-term therapy may result in muscle-wasting and cachexia.

Multiple drug therapy may interfere with appetite and corticosteroids may enhance net protein catabolism. Frequent blood sampling in uremic patients contributes to loss of proteins and other vital compounds.

Finally, renal replacement therapy such as hemodialysis and peritoneal dialysis may induce catabolism and increase protein requirements above the baseline of non-dialyzed uremic patients.

These changes, superimposed on the metabolic abnormalities of uremia, may have serious consequences in the form of malnutrition, susceptibility to infection, and increased hospitalization and mortality.

In the following, an overview is given concerning the prevalence, clinical consequences and causes of malnutrition in patients with chronic renal failure who are treated with hemodialysis (HD) and continuous ambulatory peritoneal dialysis (CAPD), i.e., the most common methods of renal replacement therapy.

PROTEIN-ENERGY MALNUTRITION IN MAINTENANCE DIALYSIS

In order to diagnose malnutrition in maintenance dialysis patients, it is important to appropriately assess the nutritional status; see recent review articles (1, 2). Validation of nutritional status may be based on clinical evaluation, diet history, anthropometric measurements and various biophysical and biochemical methods.

Hemodialysis

Several reports have shown that malnutrition is frequently present in patients treated with maintenance HD therapy (3-18). The signs of malnutrition in regular dialysis patients include the following: reduced energy stores (subcutaneous fat stores) and muscle mass assessed by anthropometric methods, low total body nitrogen determined by *in vivo* neutron activation analysis (14, 16), low concentrations of albumin, transferrin, and other visceral proteins, low alkali-soluble protein in muscle in relation to dry fat-free weight and DNA (5, 10), as well as abnormal plasma amino acids and intracellular amino acid profiles (7, 9, 17).

In various studies of HD patients (10, 13, 15, 18), a low percent ideal body weight or low body mass index was found in 10-30%, a low triceps skinfold thickness in 20-60%, and low arm muscle circumference in 0-44%. Low serum albumin was observed in 13-70% and low transferrin in 30-60% of HD patients. The anthropometric data may suggest that energy malnutrition is more prevalent than protein malnutrition in HD patients. However, results of a recent study using total body N determination by neutron activation analysis indicate that anthropometric measurements may underestimate the degree of protein malnutrition in HD patients (16).

CAPD

There is also a high prevalence of protein energy malnutrition in CAPD patients, with 18-56% of CAPD patients showing anthropometric and biochemical evidence of malnutrition (12, 19-27). Some data provide evidence of an increased net anabolism during the first year of CAPD with weight gain and improvement in anthropometric parameters and a rise in plasma proteins (21, 28, 29). However, prospective studies of total body protein show a gradual deterioration in nutritional status, indicating that the body protein mass decreases, especially in male patients, with large protein stores at the beginning of treatment (21, 22, 30).

The most extensive evaluation of nutritional status in CAPD patients included 224 patients from six centers in Europe and North America. A subjective nutritional assessment was made using 21 variables, derived from history and clinical examinations (26). On the basis of the subjective global nutritional assessment, 33% of the patients were mildly to moderately malnourished and 8% were severely malnourished. Residual renal function correlated with muscle-wasting, suggesting that loss of renal function with a concomitant increase in uremic toxicity may have been an important cause of anorexia and wasting.

Marckmann (12), who studied 32 patients on HD and 16 patients on CAPD, found an equally high prevalence of malnutrition in both groups (54% and 52%, respectively). In a multicenter study, comparing 609 HD and 138 CAPD patients, Nelson et al (31) noted no difference in nutritional status between the two groups. However, Maiorca et al (32) reported that CAPD patients, unlike HD patients, failed to correct the slight hypoalbuminemia present at the beginning of treatment.

In conclusion, the prevalence of protein energy malnutrition is high both in HD and CAPD patients. No conclusions can be drawn from the data available in the literature as to which method is superior, regarding adequacy of nutrition, especially since the patient populations in the various studies differed with regard to age, incidence of complicating diseases, socioeconomic conditions, time on dialysis, dialysis dose, dietary recommendations, etc.

LOW PROTEIN INTAKE, MALNUTRITION AND CLINICAL OUTCOME

It is generally accepted that suboptimal nutritional status is associated with increased morbidity and may impair rehabilitation and the quality of life. Cutaneous energy and other immune alterations strikingly similar to those observed in malnutrition, which have been documented both in HD and CAPD patients (6, 23), suggest that protein energy malnutrition may entail the risk of infection and septicemia.

Hemodialysis

Several studies suggest that malnutrition is an important risk factor for morbidity and mortality in HD patients (12, 13, 18, 33-36). In the National Cooperative Dialysis Study, a nationwide multicenter study performed in U.S.A. with the aim of defining the adequacy of HD, the protein catabolic rate (PCR) was assessed by means of urea kinetic modeling and it was used to estimate the protein intake (36). It was observed that a PCR of <0.8 g/kg b.w./day was associated with treatment failure (36). Among 120 HD patients, Acchiardo et al (35) found that a subgroup with a mean protein intake of 0.63 g/kg b.w./day (estimated from the urea appearance rate) had a mortality rate of 14% per year, while groups of patients with higher intakes, 0.93, 1.02, and 1.29 g/kg b.w./day, had mortality rates of only 4%, 3%, and 0%, respectively. The number of hospitalizations per year was also much higher in the group of patients having the lowest intake of protein, with higher frequencies of heart disease, pericarditis, infections, and gastrointestinal manifestations than in the other patient groups.

Lowrie and Lew (13) found a strong association between a low serum protein concentration and mortality in a population of more than 12,000 HD patients. The annual risk of death was seven times higher in patients with an albumin level below 30 g/liter, than in those with an albumin level above 40 g/liter, and no less than 14 times higher when adjusted for other risk factors that influence mortality by using logistic regression analysis. The risk of death was inversely related to the predialysis serum creatinine level, which is a marker of size of the muscle mass. Patients with the lowest BUN levels also ran a considerably increased risk of death suggesting that a low protein intake is also a risk factor. An association between low BUN values and an increased mortality rate has also been observed in other studies (33, 34).

CAPD

In CAPD patients there is some evidence that malnutrition is an important risk factor. Teehan et al (37) retrospectively analyzed the clinical outcome in 51 CAPD patients, followed longitudinally for five years, and found a strong association between low serum albumin and increased mortality and number of hospitalisation. It was also observed that a low protein intake (low PCR) was associated with increased number of hospital admissions, and that low BUN, reflecting a low protein intake, was a risk factor for low serum albumin. However, in another retrospective study by Blake et al (38) concerning 76 new patients on CAPD, followed over an average of 20 months, there was no association between PCR and clinical outcome, although some of these patients had protein intakes clearly below the recommended intake. Obviously, prospective, randomized studies in larger patient groups are warranted.

It should be kept in mind that the relationship between malnutrition and increased morbidity and mortality is not necessarily a cause-effect one. In addition to renal failure, a large proportion of maintenance dialysis patients have complicating diseases, such as severe cardiovascular disease, diabetic vascular complications, gastrointestinal and liver diseases, and other systemic diseases with an unfavorable prognosis. Such sick patients may become anorectic and malnourished and malnutrition may be a marker of illness, but not the direct cause of death.

PROTEIN AND ENERGY REQUIREMENTS IN MAINTENANCE DIALYSIS PATIENTS

In order to maintain a satisfactory nutritional status the intake of protein and energy must be sufficient to meet the requirements. A low intake of protein is especially detrimental in case the protein requirements are increased, which seems to be the case in patients on renal replacement therapy. In normal adults the average minimum requirements for protein are about 0.6 g/kg b.w./day which, after correction for 25% variability to include 97.5% of the population of young adults, raises the safe level of intake to 0.75 g/kg b.w./day (39).

Protein requirements in HD patients

Results of nitrogen balance studies in patients on HD twice a week suggested that approximately 0.75 g/kg b.w./day of high biological value protein is necessary to maintain nitrogen equilibrium (40) or a slightly positive nitrogen balance (41). However, according to more recent long-term studies, this amount of protein may not be adequate. Signs of malnutrition have been observed in many apparently well-rehabilitated patients on maintenance HD, who had a daily protein intake of about 1 g/kg b.w. /day (42). On the basis of clinical results with protein and energy supplements to the diet, it was suggested that 1.2 g of protein, primarily of high biological value, and an energy intake of 35 kcal/kg b.w./day should be prescribed for HD patients (42).

Protein catabolic rate (PCR), estimated from the urea appearance rate, reflects the protein intake in metabolically stable patients (43, 44). In the National Cooperative Dialysis Study, a PCR >1.0 was associated with a low morbidity, provided that the blood urea concentration was adequately controlled (45). Gotch and Sargent (46) performed a "mechanistic" analysis of the National Cooperative Dialysis data resulting in a nomogram which is now widely accepted for assessing the adequacy of dialysis. This nomogram expresses the relationship between the mid-week BUN, PCR and Kt/V with a region labeled adequate, within which the patient data should fit if the patient is adequately treated. According to this nomogram, the lower limit for an adequate PCR is 0.8 g/kg b.w./day.

However, it should be pointed out that the study period for patients in the National Cooperative Dialysis Study was only 24-52 weeks, which may have been too short to detect the long-term consequences of a marginally low protein intake on the mortality, which is the most tangible parameter for evaluating outcome. Moreover, strict inclusion criteria were used, excluding patients over 70 years of age, and those with diabetes, heart disease, uncontrolled hypertension, excessive weight gain and other pathological conditions (47). It is questionable whether the criteria for adequacy of nutrition based on an analysis of the data base of the National Cooperative Dialysis Study are applicable to such patients who constitute a large proportion of the dialysis patients today.

Protein requirements in CAPD patients

In CAPD patients the protein requirements also appear to be increased, compared to normal individuals.

The results of nitrogen balance studies, in a group of CAPD patients, using two levels of protein intake, 0.8 and 1.5 g protein/kg b.w./day, suggest that the protein requirements for CAPD patients are considerably higher than those for normal individuals (48). On the basis of these results a protein intake of ≥1.2 g/kg b.w./day was recommended for patients treated with CAPD to ensure nitrogen equilibrium or a positive nitrogen balance.

However, in another study, in which nitrogen balance was measured in CAPD patients receiving a diet that closely corresponded to their spontaneous daily intake of protein and energy, some of the patients were in neutral or positive nitrogen balance with a protein intake as low as 0.7 g/kg b.w./day (49).

The energy requirements

The energy requirements depend on the level of physical activity, an intake of 35-40 kcal/kg b.w./day being recommended for individuals not performing heavy physical exercise.

There is no evidence that the energy requirements of maintenance dialysis patients are usually different from those of normal subjects. Monteon et al (50) measured energy expenditure in normal subjects, non-dialyzed patients with chronic renal failure and maintenance HD patients and found no difference among the three groups with the subjects sitting, exercising or in the post-prandial state. This finding suggests that during a given physical activity the energy expenditure of chronic HD patients does not differ from that in normal subjects. Nor is there any evidence that the energy requirements in patients on CAPD differ from normal.

LOW NUTRITIONAL INTAKE AND ANOREXIA IN MAINTENANCE DIALYSIS PATIENTS

Considering all evidence that requirements for protein are increased in HD and CAPD patients and that an adequate energy supply is mandatory for maintaining the energy stores and optimizing utilization of ingested protein, low protein and energy intakes must be especially harmful in such patients. It may be difficult to fulfil the nutritional requirements since some dialysis patients seem to lose their appetite and reduce their protein and energy intakes spontaneously.

Nutritional surveys indicate that the mean intake of protein in HD patients is less than 1 g/kg b.w./day in a large proportion of maintenance HD patients (10, 12, 15). Jacob et al (15) noted in 61 HD patients that 45% had a protein intake less than 1 g/kg b.w./day.

The energy intake is also low in groups of HD patients, with a mean intake of 26-29 kcal/kg b.w./day (8, 12, 15), i.e. much less than the 35 kcal/kg b.w./day generally recommended. This is in keeping with observations that a high proportion of HD patients show signs of energy depletion.

A large proportion of CAPD patients also ingest considerably lower amounts of protein than the recommended intake of 1.2 g/kg b.w./day (10, 51). Lysaght et al (51) observed that the protein intake (PCR) was about 18% lower in CAPD compared to HD patients (0.91 and 1.13 g/kg b.w./day, respectively) and that some CAPD patients had as low PCR as 0.4-0.5 g/kg b.w./day. Retrospective observations by our group also demonstrate that the protein intake in CAPD patients is generally lower than in HD patients (Figure 1).

The energy intake in CAPD patients has been reported to be low in spite of the additional supply of energy as glucose by the peritoneal route (53, 54). There is also a decrease of protein and energy intake with time which is paralleled by a fall in nitrogen balance (22, 49, 55). The reduced nutritional intake with time during CAPD seems to be caused by anorexia with a reduced nutritional intake as a consequence, probably because CAPD patients become underdialyzed as the total solute clearance falls, due to a decrease in residual renal function.

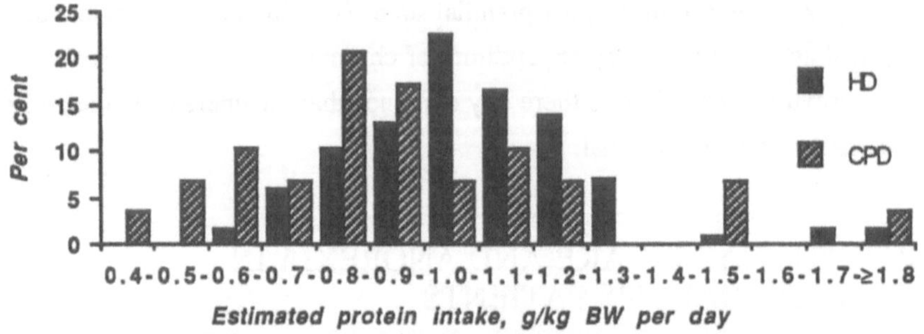

Figure 1. Percent distribution of estimated protein intake in 115 HD patients and 29 continuous peritoneal dialysis (CPD) patients (23 on CAPD and 6 on CCPD). Estimated protein intake was assumed to be equal to protein catabolic rate (PCR) in the HD patients, calculated from urea appearance according to the equation of Borah et al (43) and in the CPD patients from urea appearance by using an equation derived from data in 34 N-balance studies on 19 CAPD patients, adding the total protein losses (52). Estimated protein intake, HD: 1.10±0.23, CAPD: 1.00±0.34 ($p<0.001$).

Some factors which may contribute to a low intake of protein and energy are listed in Table 1. Anorexia may be due to unpalatable or inadequate diets, gastropathy (in diabetic patients with autonomic neuropathy), medications, psychosocial and socioeconomic factors such as loneliness, depression, ignorance and poverty, especially in elderly patients, and those with alcohol and drug problems. Nausea and vomiting, during and immediately after HD, which are frequently associated with cardiovascular instability and post-dialysis fatigue, may lead to a reduction in food intake during the dialysis days. In CAPD patients abdominal distension may lead to feelings of fullness and discomfort and the glucose uptake may suppress appetite. However, by far the most important anorectic factor, common to both HD and CAPD patients, is persistent uremia due to underdialysis.

An adaptive decrease in protein intake in HD patients dialyzed for a short time and with low efficacy was observed in the National Cooperative Dialysis Study (8). More recently, Lindsay and Spanner (56) reported a correlation between the dose of dialysis (Kt/V_{urea}) and the protein catabolic rate (PCR), which, in metabolically stable patients, reflects the protein intake. They increased the dose of dialysis (Kt/V) in individual patients and observed that the protein intake (PCR) increased spontaneously. The relationship between Kt/V and PCR seemed to vary with the type of membrane, so that with a more permeable and biocompatible membrane, AN 69, PCR increased more for the same increase in Kt/V than with cuprophane (56).

There is also evidence that the daily dose of dialysis is of critical importance for the intake of protein in CAPD patients, based on recent reports demonstrating a correlation between Kt/V_{urea} and protein intake, as assessed from the urea appearance rate (51, 56, 57). In general, CAPD patients have a lower weekly dialytic clearance of urea than do HD patients. The dietary protein intake has been reported to decrease in patients after switching from HD to CAPD, and to increase in patients after switching from CAPD to HD (58). This suggests that a less efficient removal of critical uremic toxins in CAPD may have suppressed appetite. However, a positive factor in favor of CAPD as compared to HD, is that the residual renal function seems to be better preserved in CAPD patients than in HD patients after starting dialysis (59).

Table 1. Causes of anorexia in maintenance dialysis patients.

Uremic toxicity (underdialysis)	
Unpalatable or inadequate diets	
Gastropathy (diabetic patients)	
Inflammation, infection, sepsis	
Medications	
Psychosocial and socioeconomic factors	
Loneliness	
Depression	
Ignorance	
Poverty	
Alcohol and drug abuse	
Effects of the HD procedure	Effects of the PD procedure
Cardiovascular instability	Abdominal discomfort
Nausea, vomiting	Glucose absorption
Post-dialysis fatigue	Peritonitis

We performed a retrospective analysis of Kt/V and PCR in a group of 115 unselected HD patients and a group of 29 patients on continuous peritoneal dialysis (CPD) and found that the relationship between Kt/V and PCR in the CAPD patients differed from than in the HD patients, most of whom were treated with cellulosic membrane (57). At the same low Kt/V levels the protein intake (PCR) in the CAPD patients was higher than in the HD patients and the protein intake increased more for the same increase in Kt/V in the CAPD than in the HD patients.

An attractive hypothesis for explaining the different relationships between Kt/V and PCR in CAPD patients and HD patients might be that the anorectic factor(s) are molecules of larger size than urea, which are relatively more efficiently dialyzed by the peritoneal route than by the cellulosic membranes in the artificial kidney. This hypothesis is supported by the challenging observation by Lindsay and Spanner mentioned earlier (56), indicating that with a permeable membrane (AN 69) protein intake increases proportionally more with the same increase in Kt/V_{urea} than with cellulosic membranes. The peak concentration hypothesis, recently presented by Keshaviah et al (60) affords an alternative explanation, namely that the periodic peak concentrations of urea and other toxins in HD patients, is more important than the time average concentration. Accordingly, a higher Kt/V_{urea} is required in intermittent HD patients than in CAPD patients for dialysis to be adequate. Today there is no proof that any of these hypothesis are more true than the other.

PROTEIN CATABOLIC FACTORS IN MAINTENANCE DIALYSIS PATIENTS

The observation that HD and CAPD patients seem to have a diminished utilization of ingested protein and increased protein requirements, compared to normal individuals, indicates that metabolic factors, not fully corrected for by dialysis treatment, as well as the treatment *per se*, may enhance net protein catabolism and impair the utilization of dietary protein. Many patients on renal replacement therapy are physically inactive for various reasons such as fatigue, anemia, skeleto-muscular disease, and psychological factors. Physical inactivity may result in muscle-wasting and a negative nitrogen balance (61).

In maintenance HD patients, investigated by ^{13}C leucine kinetics immediately before a routine thrice-weekly HD treatment, the protein breakdown was the same as that in controls, but the protein oxidation rate was higher and net the protein synthesis was lower, which was thought to contribute to muscle-wasting (62). In contrast, kinetic leucine studies in CAPD patients showed that the protein turnover and the rate of protein oxidation were lower than in controls and that the balance between synthesis and breakdown was higher before the start of dialysis and after three months on CAPD suggesting protein anabolism (25).

Low energy intake

Metabolic studies indicate that the utilization of protein is greatly dependent on the energy intake, so that a low energy intake reduces utilization, whereas a high energy intake has a protein-saving effect (63). Slomowitz et al (64) demonstrated that this also applies to HD patients. In six patients on a constant protein intake, averaging 1.13 g/kg desirable b.w./day, the nitrogen balance, adjusted for unmeasured losses, was negative when the energy intake was 25 kcal/kg b.w./day, but neutral or positive when the energy intake was 35 or 45 kcal/kg b.w./day.

In CAPD patients also, the nitrogen balance is strongly correlated to the total energy intake (49). Glucose is absorbed from the dialysate, averaging 8 kcal/kg b.w./day and varying between 5-20 kcal/kg b.w./day. Despite glucose uptake, many CAPD patients have a total energy intake below 35 kcal/kg b.w./day (1, 49, 53, 54).

Considering that many patients on maintenance dialysis ingest less than 35 kcal/kg b.w./day, energy deficiency may be an important factor contributing to poor utilization of dietary protein.

Metabolic acidosis

It has become increasingly evident that metabolic acidosis is an important stimulus for net protein catabolism. In non-dialyzed chronic uremic patients the correction of metabolic acidosis improves the nitrogen balance (65). A study of leucine kinetics in normal subjects during acute acidosis and alkalosis showed that total body protein breakdown as well as apparent leucine oxidation increase more during acidosis than during alkalosis (66).

In the aforementioned studies of leucine kinetics in HD patients (62), demonstrating an increased protein oxidation and reduced protein synthesis, the patients were acidotic with a plasma bicarbonate pre-dialysis averaging 18 mmol/l, suggesting that acidosis might have been a factor of importance.

In rats with chronic renal failure, acidosis, rather than uremia *per se,* appears to enhance protein catabolism (67). This effect seems to be mediated by the stimulation of skeletal muscle branched-chain keto acid decarboxylation, which increases the catabolism of the branched-chain amino acids (valine, leucine and isoleucine), which are mainly metabolized in muscle tissue (68). It was recently reported that metabolic acidosis also elicits the transcription of genes for proteolytic enzymes in muscle (69).

Our group has recently reported that the intracellular valine concentration in the muscle of patients treated with maintenance HD is low (70). The concentration showed a correlation with the pre-dialysis blood standard bicarbonate level which varied between 18 and 24 mmol/l, suggesting that even slight and intermittent acidosis may have stimulated the catabolism of valine in muscle, resulting in a valine depletion that may be a limiting factor for protein synthesis.

In our experience, acidosis is common in HD patients, despite the use of bicarbonate as the buffer in the dialysis fluid. In a group of 129 HD patients, we observed that 41% of the HD patients had pre-dialysis plasma bicarbonate concentrations ≥21 mmol/l and 17% ≥19 mmol/l (unpublished observations). We therefore speculate whether the intermittent acidosis in HD patients with a nadir concentration of plasma bicarbonate before each dialysis may act as an intermittent stimulus for protein catabolism.

It should be pointed out that acidosis is today the only identified uremic "toxic" factor, which induces catabolism and impairs nitrogen utilization. Full correction of acidosis is consequently an obvious goal for treatment both in HD and CAPD patients.

Loss of metabolizing renal tissue

The normal kidneys actively take part in the metabolism of amino acids where, among other processes, phenylalanine hydroxylation to tyrosine (71, 72) and glycine conversion to serine take place (73). In patients with chronic renal failure the concentration of free tyrosine is low and the phenylalanine/tyrosine ratio is increased in plasma and muscle, serine in plasma is low and glycine increased (74, 75). We observed that HD patients exhibit a more severe serine depletion with significantly reduced intracellular levels in muscle than do controls, non-dialyzed chronic uremic patients and CAPD patients (70). One possible explanation is that the non-dialyzed patients and CAPD patients still had some functioning renal tissue left, by means of which serine conversion could take place.

Infections

Uremia leads to disturbances in the immune response, with cutaneous anergy and impaired granulocyte function, thus increasing the susceptibility to infections. A severe infection is an important stimulus for protein catabolism. HD patients are especially at risk for developing sepsis from infections in arteriovenous fistulas, grafts and in-dwelling venous catheters.

Recurrent peritonitis

Recurrent peritonitis is one of the most serious complications of CAPD. Adverse effects of recurrent peritonitis on nutritional status were demonstrated by Rubin et al (76, 77), who observed that changes in total body potassium correlated negatively with the number of episodes of peritonitis per month and that patients with a high incidence of peritonitis had a lower arm muscle circumference and lower plasma protein than did patients with a lower incidence of peritonitis. Peritonitis is associated with increased losses of protein in the dialysate (*vide infra*). In addition the inflammatory response may be a strong catabolic stimulus superimposed on the enhanced protein losses.

DIALYSIS PROCEDURES AS STIMULI OF NET PROTEIN CATABOLISM

Some evidence suggests that the dialytic procedure *per se* induces net catabolism of protein. The mechanisms probably differ to some extent in HD and CAPD patients. Borah et al (43) in five HD patients on low and high protein intakes, respectively, observed that the nitrogen balance (corrected for changes in total body urea) was negative on the dialysis days, but less negative (with a protein intake of 0.5 g/kg b.w./day) or positive (with a protein intake of 1.4 g/kg b.w./day) on the days between the dialyses. Farrell, Ward and co-workers (78, 79) reported that the urea appearance rate is 30% higher during the HD procedure than in the interdialytic period. These results suggest that the dialytic procedure is a strong intermittent stimulus for net protein catabolism.

An increase in the urea appearance rate or a decrease in nitrogen balance may be due to reduced protein synthesis, enhanced breakdown of protein or a combination of both. With regard to the catabolic effect of the HD procedure the data suggest that both processes are involved.

Löfberg et al (80) performed percutaneous muscle biopsies before and after routine HD with acetate and found that the size distribution of ribosomes in muscle changed with a relative decrease in polyribosomes, suggesting that the protein synthetic capacity had decreased. Lim et al (81) studied leucine and alpha-keto-isocaproate kinetics by use of stable isotopes before, during and after cuprophane HD with acetate. They concluded that HD is a catabolic event, characterized not by enhanced protein degradation but by reduction in protein synthesis. However, there is also evidence that proteolysis is enhanced as a result of blood membrane interaction (see section on biocompatibility and protein catabolism). The mechanism by which HD elicits a reduction in protein synthesis remains unknown.

Loss of glucose

When a glucose-free dialysis fluid is used for HD about 28 g of glucose is removed during 4 h of HD (area 1 m^2), whereas the addition of glucose (11 mmol/l) to the dialysis fluid results in a gain of about 23 g of glucose by the patient (82). To avoid symptomatic hypoglycemia, glucose removed from the extracellular fluid by dialysis must be replaced by ingested carbohydrate, by breakdown of liver glycogen or by gluconeogenesis from amino acids; the latter should result in an enhanced protein breakdown and urea synthesis. Observations by Wathen et al (82) showing that pyruvate decreased during glucose-free dialysis, but was unchanged during glucose dialysis, indicate that gluconeogenesis may be stimulated by glucose-free dialysis. However, Ward et al (78) and Farrell and Hone (79) have reported that the urea appearance rate is stimulated to a similar extent by dialysis, whether glucose is present in the dialysis fluid or not.

CAPD patients are provided with glucose continuously by the peritoneal route, which is potentially beneficial by providing an additional energy supply. However, glucose uptake may also have negative metabolic effects, such as hyperglycemia, hyperinsulinemia, hyperlipidemia and obesity (1).

Loss of amino acids

During HD the average loss of free amino acids in the dialysis fluid has been reported to be 5-8 g/dialysis, of which about one third are essential amino acids (83-85). Moreover, 4-5 g of peptide-bound amino acids are lost per dialysis (83); thus, the total losses of amino acids are about 10-13 g/dialysis.

The losses of free amino acids into the dialysate during CAPD are of the same magnitude (per week) or smaller than with HD.

The reported average dialysate losses of free amino acids during CAPD vary between 1.2 and 3.4 g/24 h in different studies. About 30% of the amino acids lost into the dialysate are essential amino acids. Obviously, the losses of amino acids *per se* by dialysis are too small to fully account for the increased protein requirements in maintenance dialysis patients.

Protein losses during CAPD

Substantial loss of protein into the dialysate is a major drawback with peritoneal dialysis which is not present in HD.

In CAPD the reported average loss of protein into the dialysate varies between 5 and 15 g in different studies with large interindividual differences. Thus, dialysate protein loss may vary between 20 and 140 g/week in different patients.

In CAPD patients with mild peritonitis the dialysate protein losses increased by 50-100% to an average of 15.1±3.6 g/day (86), and remain elevated for several weeks (21, 87).

Biocompatibility and protein catabolism

The HD procedure may give rise to an inflammatory reaction, the intensity of which depends on the membrane material that is used, being more prominent with cellulosic than with synthetic membranes (88). Blood membrane contact elicits complement activation by the alternative pathway, with release of anaphylaxotoxins (C3a, C5a). Monocyte activation with increased release of monokines (IL-1, TNF) may result from direct membrane contact (89), activated complement (C5a) (90), endotoxin fragments passing through the membrane (91, 92) or acetate in the dialysis fluid (93). IL-1 and TNF may act in concert and induce *inter alia* lysosomal catabolism of muscle protein (94), an effect which is mediated by the release of prostaglandin E_2 (95). More recently it has been observed that IL-1, TNF and endotoxin may induce net catabolism of muscle protein by stimulating branched-chain keto acid dehydrogenase, which leads to an enhanced oxidation of branched-chain amino acids (96).

To determine whether blood membrane contact induces protein catabolism and whether the biocompatibility of the membranes plays a role we conducted a series of experiments with sham-dialysis in normal individuals (97, 98). Blood flow through the dialyzer was 100 ml/min and the duration of exposure 150 min. We found that blood membrane contact within a dialyzer with cuprophane membrane elicited an enhanced release of amino acids from the leg tissue (mainly skeletal muscle), corresponding to an enhanced protein breakdown of 15-20 g. By giving indomethacin before and during the procedure this catabolic response was abolished, a finding which suggests that the catabolic effect is mediated by prostaglandins. With a more biocompatible membrane (AN 69®, Hospal) there was no increase in amino acid release (97, 98). These studies demonstrate that *in vivo* blood membrane interaction in a dialyzer without dialysate stimulates net protein catabolism, especially when the membrane has a low biocompatibility.

It was also observed that sham-dialysis with cuprophane, but not with more biocompatible membranes, elicited an increased release from the leg musculature and an elevation in the plasma concentration of 3-methylhistidine (98). This amino acid is formed post-translationally by the irreversible methylation of histidine in actinomyosin proteins and cannot be reutilized after being released during protein degradation (99). The increase in leg efflux and elevated arterial concentration of 3-methylhistidine following sham-hemodialysis using cuprophane dialyzers therefore indicates that increased protein breakdown plays an important part in the net catabolic process induced by blood-membrane contact.

It is conceivable that in clinical HD with loss of glucose and amino acids, higher blood flow, longer exposure time and presence of endotoxins and acetate in the dialysate, the net catabolic effect is far more extensive than in sham HD and involves both reduced synthesis and increased breakdown of protein. Whether these stimuli altogether may explain the increased protein requirements in HD patients is still an open question.

PREVENTION AND TREATMENT OF MALNUTRITION

Since malnutrition may entail increased risk of morbidity and mortality in maintenance dialysis patients, measures should be taken to minimize or eliminate factors that result in inadequate nutritional intake (see Table I) aiming at a protein intake of ≥1.2 g/ kg b.w./day and an energy intake of ≥35 kcal/kg b.w./day.

Underdialysis, when present or suspected, should be corrected by increasing the dose of dialysis, in HD patients by prolonging the dialysis time and/or increasing the dialyzer clearance (higher blood flow, larger dialyzer surface area), in CAPD patients by increasing the number of daily exchanges and/or the exchange volumes. CAPD patients who remain underdialyzed in spite of these measures may have to be switched over to HD, which is less limitated regarding weekly dialysis dose. Metabolic acidosis should be corrected by oral medication with sodium bicarbonate or other alkaline salts, or by increasing the base concentration in the dialysis fluid. Whether HD with biocompatible, synthetic membranes, combined with sterile and pyrogen-free dialysis fluid, will prove to be advantageous compared to conventional HD by minimizing protein catabolism is still an open question. If severe malnutrition develops despite dialysis being adequate and measures having been taken to eliminate various anorectic and catabolic factors, enteral or parenteral nutritional supplementation with energy and amino acids may be warranted (100, 101). Intradialytic parenteral nutrition, i.e. intravenous supply of amino acids, glucose and lipids during the HD sessions, has become increasingly popular in recent years for treatment of malnourished HD patients (18, 102-105) and favourable effects on nutritional status have been recorded in some of these studies (18, 102, 103). However, the long-term impact on rehabilitation and survival remains open. Parenteral nutrition has been used successfully in infected HD an CAPD patients (103, 106). In CAPD patients amino acids have been used instead of glucose as osmotic agents with the dual purpose of acting as a glucose-free osmotic agent and for nutritional support to correct protein malnutrition and amino acid abnormalities (107). Although promising results have been recorded, suggesting a future role of AA solutions in malnourished CAPD patients, the experiences are still limited and untowards effects such as nausea, increase in BUN and enhanced metabolic acidosis have been observed.

GENERAL CONCLUSIONS

Malnutrition is common in maintenance dialysis patients, irrespectively whether they are treated with HD or CAPD, and it is strongly associated with increased morbidity and mortality. Contributing factors are increased protein requirements and low supply of energy and protein in relation to the needs. Anorexia with low protein and energy intake results from a variety of factors of which underdialysis with insufficient control of uremic toxicity seems to be a major one. CAPD patients have on average a lower protein intake than HD patients. The dialysis procedure *per se* seems to be a strong, intermittent catabolic stimulus in HD patients, whereas in CAPD patients the continuous protein loss in the dialysate is a recognized risk factor for protein malnutrition, which is far enhanced during episodes of peritonitis.

REFERENCES

1. Lindholm B, Bergström J: Nutritional management of patients undergoing peritoneal dialysis. In: "Peritoneal dialysis" (Ed KD Nolph), Kluwer Academic Publishers, Boston, 1989, pp 230-260.
2. Steinman TI, Mitch WE: Nutrition in dialysis patients. In: "Replacement of renal function by dialysis" (Ed MF Maher), Kluwer Academic Publishers, Boston, 1989, pp 1088-1106.
3. Sengar DPS, Rashid A, Harris JF: *In vitro* cellular immunity and *in vivo* delayed hypersensitivity in uremic patients maintained on hemodialysis. Archs Allergy Appl Immun, 47: 829, 1974.
4. Schaeffer G, Heinze V, Jontofsohn R, Katz N, Rippich TH, Schäfer B, Sudhoff A, Zimmerman W, Kluthe R: Amino acid and protein intake in RDT patients. A nutritional and biochemical analysis. Clin Nephrol, 3: 228-233, 1975.
5. Delaporte C, Bergström J, Broyer M: Variations in muscle cell protein of severely uremic children. Kidney Int, 10: 239-245, 1976.
6. Bansal VK, Popli S, Pickering J, Ing TS, Vertuno LL, Hano JE: Protein-calorie malnutrition and cutaneous anergy in hemodialysis maintained patients. Am J Clin Nutr, 33: 1608-1611, 1980.
7. Young GA, Swanepoel CR, Croft MR, Hobson SM, Parsons FM: Anthropometry and plasma valine, amino acids, and proteins in the nutritional assessment of hemodialysis patients. Kidney Int, 21: 492-499, 1982.
8. Schoenfeld PY, Henry RR, Laird NM, Roxe DM: Assessment of nutritional status of the National Cooperative Study population. Kidney Int, 23 (Suppl 13): 80-88, 1983.
9. Bergström J, Alvestrand A, Fürst P: Plasma and muscle free amino acids in maintenance hemodialysis patients without protein malnutrition. Kidney Int , 38: 108-114, 1990.
10. Guarnieri G, Toigo G, Situlin R, Faccini L, Coli U, Lannini S, Bazzato G, Dardi F, Campanacci L: Muscle biopsy studies in chronically uremic patients: evidence for malnutrition. Kidney Int, 24 (Suppl 16): 187-193, 1983.
11. Wolfson M, Strong CJ, Minturn D, Gray DK, Kopple JD: Nutritional status and lymphocyte function in maintenance hemodialysis patients. Am J Clin Nutr, 37: 547-555, 1984.
12. Marckmann P: Nutritional status and mortality of patients in regular dialysis therapy. J Intern Med, 226: 429-432, 1989.

13. Lowrie EG, Lew NL: Death risk in hemodialysis patients: the predictive value of commonly measured variables and an evaluation of death rate differences between facilities. Am J Kidney Dis, 15: 458-482, 1990.
14. Allman MA, Allen BJ, Stewart PM, Blagojevic N, Tiller DJ, Gaskin KJ, Truswell AS: Body protein of patients undergoing hemodialysis. Eur J Clin Nutr, 44: 123-131, 1990.
15. Jacob V, Le Carpentier JE, Salzano S, Naylor V, Wild G, Brown CB, El Nahas AM: IGF-I, a marker of undernutrition in hemodialysis patients. Am J Clin Nutr, 52: 39-44, 1990.
16. Rayner HC, Sroud DB, Salamon KM, Strauss BJG, Thomson NM, Atkins RC, Wahlqvist ML: Anthropometry underestimates body protein depletion in hemodialysis patients. Nephron 59: 33-40, 1991.
17. Oksa H, Ahonen K, Pasternack A, Marnela KM: Malnutrition in hemodialysis patients. Scand J Urol Nephrol, 25: 157-161, 1991.
18. Bilbrey GL, Cohen TL: Identification and treatment of protein calorie malnutrition in chronic hemodialysis patients. Dial Transplant, 18: 669-677, 1989.
19. Kopple JD, Blumenkrantz MJ, Jones MR, Moran JK, Coburn JW: Plasma amino acid levels and amino acid losses during continuous ambulatory peritoneal dialysis. Am J Clin Nutr, 36: 395-402, 1982.
20. Dombros N, Oren A, Marliss EB, Anderson GH, Stein AN, Khanna R, Petit J, Brandes L, Rodella H, Leibel BS, Oreopoulos D: Plasma amino acid profiles and amino acid losses in patients undergoing CAPD. Perit Dial Bull, 2: 27-32, 1982.
21. Williams P, Kay R, Harrison J, McNeil K, Petit J, Kellman B, Mendez M, Klein M, Ogilvie R, Khanna R, Carmichael D, Oreopoulos DG: Nutritional and anthropometric assessment of patients on CAPD over one year: Contrasting changes in total body nitrogen and potassium. Perit Dial Bull, 1: 82-87, 1981.
22. Heide B, Pierratos A, Khanna R, Petit J, Ogilvie R, Harrison J, McNeil K, Siccion Z, Oreopoulos DG: Nutritional status of patients undergoing continuous ambulatory peritoneal dialysis (CAPD). Perit Dial Bull, 3: 138-141, 1983.
23. Young GA, Young JB, Young SM, Hobson SM, Hildreth B, Brownjohn AM, Parsons FM: Nutrition and delayed hypersensitivity during continuous ambulatory peritoneal dialysis in relation to peritonitis. Nephron, 43: 177-186, 1986.
24. Fenton SSA, Johnston N, Delmore T, Detsky AS, Whitewell J, O'Sullivan R, Cattran DC, Richardson RMA, Jeejeebhoy KN: Nutritional assessment of continuous ambulatory peritoneal dialysis. Trans Am Soc Artif Intern Organs, 33: 650-653, 1987.
25. Goodship THJ, Lloyd S, Clague MB, Bartlett K, Ward MK, Wilkinson R: Whole body leucine turnover and nutritional status in continuous ambulatory peritoneal dialysis. Clin Sci, 73: 463-469, 1987.
26. Young GA, Kopple JD, Lindholm B, Vonesh EF, De Vecchi A, Scalamogna A, Castelnova C, Oreopoulos DG, Anderson GH, Bergström J, DiChiro J, Gentile D, Nissenson A, Sakhrani L, Brownjohn AM, Nolph KD, Prowant BF, Algrim CE, Martis L, Serkes KD: Nutritonal assessment of continuous ambulatory peritoneal dialysis patients: An international study. Am J Kidney Dis, 27: 462-471, 1991.
27. Lindholm B, Alvestrand A, Fürst P, Bergström J: Plasma and muscle free amino acids during continuous ambulatory peritoneal dialysis. Kidney Int, 35: 1219-1226, 1989.
28. Nolph KD, Sorkin MN, Rubin J, Arfania D, Prowant BF, Fruto L, Kennedy D: Continuous ambulatory peritoneal dialysis. Three-year experience at one center. Ann Intern Med, 92: 609-613, 1980.
29. Kurtz SB, Wong VH, Anderson CF, Vogel JP, McCarthy JT, Mitchell JC: Continuous ambulatory peritoneal dialysis. Three years' experience at the Mayo Clinic. Mayo Clin Proc, 58: 633-639, 1983.
30. Schilling H, Wu G, Petit J, Harrison J, McNeil M, Siccion Z, Oreopoulos DG: Nutritional status of patients on long-term CAPD. Perit Dial Bull, 5: 12-18, 1985.
31. Nelson EE, Hong CD, Pesce AL, Peterson DW, Singh S, Pollak VE: Anthropometric norms for the dialysis population. Am J Kidney Dis, 16: 32-37, 1990.
32. Maiorca R, Cancarini GC, Camerini C, Brunori G, Manili L, Movilli E, Feller P, Mombelloni S: Is CAPD competitive with haemodialysis for long-term treatment of uraemic patients? Nephrol Dial Transplant, 4: 244-253, 1989.
33. Degoulet P, Legrain M, Reach I, Aime F, Devries C, Rojas P, Jacobs C: Mortality risk factors in patients treated by chronic hemodialysis. Nephron, 31: 103-110, 1982.

34. Shapiro JI, Argy WP, Rakowski TA, Chester A, Siemsen AS, Schreiner GE: The unsuitability of BUN as a criterion for prescription dialysis. Trans Am Soc Artif Intern Organs, 29: 129-134, 1983.
35. Acchiardo SR, Moore LW, Latour PA: Malnutrition as the main factor in morbidity and mortality of hemodialysis patients. Kidney Int, 24 (Suppl 16): 199-203, 1983.
36. Harter HR: Review of significant findings from the National Cooperative Dialysis Study and recommendations. Kidney Int, 23 (Suppl 13): 107-112, 1983.
37. Teehan BP, Schleifer CR, Brown JM, Sigler MH, Raimondo J: Urea kinetic analysis and clinical outcome on CAPD. A five year longitudinal study. Adv Perit Dial, 6: 181-185, 1991.
38. Blake PG, Sombolos K, Abraham G, Weissgarten J, Pemberton R, Lian Chu G, Oreopoulos DG: Lack of correlation between urea kinetic indices and clinical outcomes in CAPD patients. Kidney Int, 39: 700-706, 1991.
39. FAO/WHO. Energy and protein requirements. Report of a joint FAO/WHO ad hoc Expert Committee. Tech Rep Ser No 522, Geneva, World Health Organization, 1973.
40. Ginn HE, Frost A, Lacy WW: Nitrogen balance in hemodialysis patients. Am J Clin Nutr, 21: 385-393, 1968.
41. Kopple JD, Shinaberger JH, Coburn JW, Sorensen MK, Rubini ME: Optimal dietary protein treatment during chronic hemodialysis. Trans Am Soc Artif Organs, 15: 302-308, 1969.
42. Kluthe R, Lüttgen FM, Capetianu T, Heinze V, Katz N, Südhoff A: Protein requirements in maintenance hemodialysis. Am J Clin Nutr, 31: 1812-1820, 1978.
43. Borah MF, Schoenfeld PY, Gotch FA, Sargent JA, Wolfson M, Humphreys MH: Nitrogen balance during intermittent dialysis therapy of uremia. Kidney Int, 14: 491-500, 1978.
44. Maroni BJ, Steinman TI, Mitch WE: A method for estimating nitrogen intake of patients with chronic renal failure. Kidney Int, 27: 58-65, 1985.
45. Laird NM, Berkey CS, Lowrie EG: Modeling success or failure of dialysis therapy: The National Cooperative Dialysis Study. Kidney Int, 23 (Suppl 13): 101-106, 1983.
46. Gotch FA, Sargent JA: A mechanistic analysis of the National Cooperative Dialysis Study. Kidney Int, 28: 526-534, 1985.
47. Parker TF, Reed RB, Lowrie EG: Description of the participating centers and the patient population in the National Cooperative Dialysis Study. Kidney Int, 23 (Suppl 13): 37-41, 1983.
48. Blumenkrantz MJ, Kopple JD, Moran JK, Coburn JW: Metabolic balance studies and dietary protein requirements in patients undergoing continuous ambulatory peritoneal dialysis. Kidney Int, 21: 849-861, 1982.
49. Lindholm B, Alvestrand A, Fürst P, Tranaeus A, Bergström J: Efficacy and clinical experience of CAPD - Stockholm, Sweden. In: "Peritoneal Dialysis" (Eds R Atkins, N Thomson, PC Farrell), Churchill Livingstone, Edinburgh, 1981, pp 147-161.
50. Monteon FJ, Laidlaw SA, Shaib JK, Kopple JD: Energy expenditure in patients with chronic renal failure. Kidney Int, 30: 741-747, 1986.
51. Lysaght MJ, Pollock CA, Hallet MD, Ibels LS, Farrell PC: The relevance of urea kinetic modeling to CAPD. Trans Am Soc Artif Intern Organs, 35: 784-790, 1989.
52. Bergström J, Alvestrand A, Lindholm B, Tranæus A, Fürst P: Urea appearance (UAR), protein catabolic rate (PCR) and dialysis efficacy (Kt/V) in CAPD patients. Abstract 6th Int Congr on Nutrition and Metabolism in Renal Disease, Harrogate, England, 1991.
53. Marckmann P: Dialysepatienters kost bestemt ved 7 dages kostregistrering. Ugeskr Laeger, 152: 317-320, 1990.
54. von Baeyer H, Gahl GM, Riedinger H, Borowzak R, Averdunk R, Schurig R, Kessel M: Adaptation to CAPD patients to the continuous peritoneal energy uptake. Kidney Int, 23: 29-34, 1983.
55. Oreopoulos DG, Marliss E, Anderson GH, Oren A, Dombros N, Williams P, Khanna R, Rodella H, Brandes L: Nutritional aspects of CAPD and the potential use of amino acid containing dialysis solutions. Perit Dial Bull, 3: 10-15, 1983.
56. Lindsay RM, Spanner E: A hypothesis: The protein catabolic rate is dependent upon the type and amount of treatment in dialyzed uremic patients. Am J Kidney Dis, 13: 382-389, 1989.
57. Bergström J, Alvestrand A, Lindholm B, Tranæus A: Relationship between Kt/V and protein catabolic rate (PCR) is different in continuous peritoneal dialysis (CPD) and haemodialysis (HD) patients. J Am Soc Nephrol, 2: 358, 1991.
58. Farrell PC, Randerson DH: Comparison of CAPD with HD and IPD. In: "Advances in Peritoneal Dialysis" (Eds GM Gahl, M Kessel, KD Nolph), Excerpta Medica, Amsterdam, 1981, pp 131-137.

59. Lysaght MJ, Vonesh EF, Gotch F, Ibels L, Keen M, Lindholm B, Nolph KD, Pollock CA, Prowant B, Farrell PC: The influence of dialysis treatment modality on the decline of remaining renal function. Trans Am Soc Artif Intern Organs, 37: 598-604, 1991.
60. Keshaviah PR, Nolph KD, Van Stone JC: The peak concentration hypothesis: A urea kinetic approach to comparing the adequacy of continuous ambulatory peritoneal dialysis (CAPD) and hemodialysis. Perit Dial Int, 9: 257-260, 1989.
61. Schoenheyder F, Heilskov NSC, Olsen K: Isotopic studies on the mechanism of negative nitrogen balance produced by immobilization. Scand J Clin Lab Invest, 6: 178-188, 1954.
62. Berkelhammer CH, Baker JP, Leither LA, Uldall PR, Whittall R, Slater A, Wolman SL: Whole-body protein turnover in adult hemodialysis patients as measured by ^{13}C-leucine. Am J Clin Nutr, 46: 778-783, 1987.
63. Kishi K, Miytani K, Inoue G: Requirement and utilization of egg protein by Japanese young men with marginal intakes of energy. J Nutr, 198: 658-669, 1978.
64. Slomowitz LA, Monteon FJ, Grosvenor M, Laidlaw SA, Kopple JD: Effect of energy intake on nutritional status in maintenance hemodialysis patients. Kidney Int, 35: 704-711, 1989.
65. Papadoyannakis NJ, Stefanidis CJ, Mcgeown M: The effect of the correction of metabolic acidosis on nitrogen and potassium balance of patients with chronic renal failure. Am J Clin Nutr, 40: 623-627, 1984.
66. Straumann E, Keller U, Küry D, Bloesch D, Thélin A, Arnaud MJ, Stauffacher W: Effect of acute acidosis and alkalosis on leucine kinetics in man. Clin Physiol, 12: 39-51, 1992.
67. Hara Y, May RC, Kelly RC, Mitch WE: Acidosis, not azotemia, stimulates branched-chain, amino acid catabolism in uremic rats. Kidney Int, 32: 808-814, 1987.
68. May RC, Hara Y, Kelly RA, Block KP, Buse M, Mitch WE: Branched-chain amino acid metabolism in rat muscle: Abnormal regulation in acidosis. Am J Physiol, 252: E712-718, 1987.
69. Mitch WE, Greiber S, Medina R, Goldberg AL: Cellular mechanisms of muscle protein breakdown in uremia. Abstract. 6th Int Congress on Nutrition and Metabolism in Renal Disease, Harrogate, U.K., 1991.
70. Bergström J, Alvestrand A, Fürst P: Plasma and muscle free amino acids in maintenance hemodialysis patients without protein malnutrition. Kidney Int, 38: 108-114, 1990.
71. Tizianello A, Deferrari G, Garibotto G, Gurreri G, Robaudo C: Renal metabolism of amino acids and ammonia in subjects with normal renal function and in patients with chronic renal insufficiency. J Clin Invest, 65: 1162-1173, 1980.
72. Fukuda S, Kopple JD: Uptake and release of amino acids by the kidney of dogs made chronically uremic with uranyl nitrate. Min Electr Metab, 3: 248-260, 1980.
73. Pitts RF, Macleod MB: Synthesis of serine by the dog kidney *in vivo*. Am J Physiol, 222: 394-398, 1972.
74. European Dialysis and Transplant Association-European Renal Association, EDTA/ERA Registry Report, Demography of Dialysis and Transplantation in Europe, 1984. Nephrol Dial Transplant, 1: 1-8, 1986.
75. Excerpts from United States Renal Data System, 1991 Annual Data Report, V. Survival probabilities and causes of death. Am J Kidney Dis, 18 (Suppl 2): 49-60, 1991.
76. Rubin J, Flynn MA, Nolph KD: Total body potassium - a guide to nutritional health in patients undergoing continuous ambulatory peritoneal dialysis. Am J Clin Nutr, 34: 94-98, 1981.
77. Rubin J, Kirchner K, Barnes T, Teal N, Ray R, Bower JD: Evaluation of continuous ambulatory peritoneal dialysis. Am J Kidney Dis, 3: 199-204, 1983.
78. Ward RA, Shirlow MJ, Hayes JM, Chapman GV, Farrell PC: Protein catabolism during hemodialysis. Am J Clin Nutr, 32: 243-2449, 1979.
79. Farrell PC, Hone PW: Dialysis-induced catabolism. Am J Clin Nutr, 33: 1417-1422, 1980.
80. Löfberg E, Wernerman J, Noree LO, Decken A, Vinnars E: Ribosome and free amino acid content in muscle during hemodialysis. Kidney Int, 39: 984-989, 1991.
81. Lim VS, Bier DM, Flanigan M, Symreng T: The effect of hemodialysis on protein metabolism. J Am Soc Nephrol, 1: 366, 1990.
82. Wathen RL, Keshaviah P, Hommeyer P, Cadwell K, Comty CM: The metabolic effects of hemodialysis with and without glucose in the dialysate. Am J Clin Nutr 31: 1870-1875, 1978.
83. Kopple JD, Swendseid ME, Shinaberger JH, Umezawa CY: The free and bound amino acids removed by hemodialysis. Trans Am Soc Artif Intern Organs, 19: 309-313, 1973.
84. Wolfson M, Jones MR, Kopple JD: Amino acid losses during hemodialysis with infusion of amino acids and glucose. Kidney Int, 21: 500-506, 1982.

85. Tepper T, Hem GK, van der Klip HG, Donker AJM: Loss of amino acids during hemodialysis: effect of oral essential amino acid supplementation. Nephron, 29: 25-29, 1981.
86. Bannister DK, Acchiardo SR, Moore LW, Kraus AP: Nutritional effects of peritonitis in continuous ambulatory peritoneal dialysis (CAPD) patients. J Am Diet Ass, 87: 53-56, 1987.
87. Verger C, Larpent L, Dumontet M: Prognostic value of peritoneal equilibration curves (EC) in CAPD patients. In: "Frontiers in peritoneal dialysis" (Eds JF Maher, JF Winchester), Field, Rich and Assoc., Inc., New York, 1986, pp 88-93.
88. Cheung AK: Biocompatibility of hemodialysis membranes. J Am Soc Nephrol, 1: 150-161, 1990.
89. Betz M, Haensch GM, Rauterberg EW, Bommer J, Ritz E: Cuprammonium membranes stimulates interleukin-1 release and arachidonic acid metabolism in monocytes in the absence of complement. Kidney Int, 34: 67-73, 1988.
90. Haeffner-Cavaillon N, Cavaillon MJ, Laude M, Kazatchkine MD: C3a/C3adesArg induces production and release of interleukin-1 (IL-1) by cultured human monocytes. J Immunol, 139: 794-799, 1987.
91. Lonnemann G, Bingel M, Floege J, Koch KM, Shaldon S, Dinarello CA: Detection of endotoxin-like interleukin-1-inducing activity during *in vitro* dialysis. Kidney Int, 33: 29-35, 1988.
92. Evans RC, Holmes CJ: *In vitro* study of the transfer of cytokine-inducing substances across selected high-flyx hemodialysis membranes. Blood Purif, 9: 92-101, 1991.
93. Bingel M, Lonnemann G, Koch KM, Dinarello CA, Shaldon S: Enhancement of *in vitro* human interleukin-1 production by sodium acetate. Lancet, 1: 14-16, 1987.
94. Flores EA, Bistrian BR, Pomposelli JJ, Dinarello CA, Blackburn GL, Istfan NW: Infusion of tumor necrosis factor. Cachectin promotes muscle catabolism in the rat. J Clin Invest, 83: 1614-1622, 1989.
95. Baracos V, Rodeman HP, Dinarello CA, Goldberg AL: Stimulation of muscle protein degradation and prostaglandin E_2 release by leukocytic pyrogen (interleukin-1). N Engl J Med, 308: 553-558, 1983.
96. Nawabi MD, Block KP, Chakrabarti MC, Buse MG: Administration of endotoxin, tumor necrosis, or Interleukin 1 to rats activates skeletal muscle branched-chain alpha-keto acid dehydrogenase. J Clin Invest, 85: 256-263, 1990.
97. Gutierrez A, Alvestrand A, Wahren J, Bergström J: Effect of *in vivo* contact between blood and dialysis membranes on protein catabolism in humans. Kidney Int, 38: 487-494, 1990.
98. Gutierrez A, Bergström J, Alvestrand A: Protein catabolism in sham hemodialysis: The effect of different membranes. Clin Nephrol, 1992 (in press).
99. Young VR, Munro HN: Methylhistidine and muscle protein turnover: an overview. Fed Proc, 37: 2291-2300, 1978.
100. Bergström J, Alvestrand A: Therapy with branched chain amino acids and keto acids in chronic uremia. In: "Branched chain amino and keto acids in health and disease" (Eds SA Adibi, W Fekl, U Langenbeck, P Schaunder), S. Karger, Basel, 1984, pp 391-422.
101. Alvestrand A: Nutritional requirements of hemodialysis patients. In: "Nutrition and the kidney" (Eds WE Mitch, S Klahr), Little, Brown and Company, Boston, 1989, pp 180-196.
102. Cano N, Labastie-Coeyrehourq J, Lacombe P, Stroumza P, di Costanzo-Dufetel J, Durbec JP, Coudray-Lucas C, Cynober L: Perdialytic parenteral nutrition with lipids and amino acids in malnourished hemodialysis patients. Am J Clin Nutr, 52: 726-730, 1990.
103. Vehe KL, Brown RO, Moore LW, Acchiardo SR, Luther RW: The efficacy of nutrition support in infected patients with chronic renal failure. Pharmacotherapy, 11: 303-307, 1991.
104. Snyder S, Bergen C, Sigler MH, Teehan BP: Intradialytic parenteral nutrition in chronic hemodialysis patients. ASAIO Trans, 37: M373-M375, 1991.
105. Toigo G, Situlin R, Tamaro G, Del Bianco A, Giuliani V, Dardi F, Vianello S, Toffoletto P, Faccini L, Guarnieri G: Effect of intravenous supplementation of a new essential amino acid formulation in hemodialysis patients. Kidney Int, 27: S278-S281, 1989.
106. Rubin J: Nutritional support during peritoneal dialysis-related peritonitis. Am J Kidney Dis, 15: 551-555, 1990.
107. Lindholm B, Bergström J: Amino acids in CAPD solutions: lights and shadows. In: "Peritoneal dialysis" (Eds G La Greca, C Ronco, M Feriani, S Chiaramonte, P Conz), Wichtig Editore, Milano, 1991, pp 139-143.

[illegible]
95. [illegible]
96. [illegible]
101. [illegible]

Chapter 15

REUSE OF DIALYZERS. ADVANTAGES AND DRAWBACKS

ROBERT J. WINEMAN AND NORMAN DEANE

National Nephrology Foundation, South Bronx Kidney Center, 1834 Webster Avenue, New York, N.Y. 10457, USA

The present paper reviews recent research, discussing factors which are relevant to advantages and drawbacks of hemodialyzer reuse. For earlier literature the reader is referred to other sources (1, 2). An especially useful document for any practitioner, when considering reuse of hemodialyzers, is the "Recommended Practice for Reprocessing Hemodialyzers", developed by a committee of the American Association for Advancement of Medical Instrumentation (AAMI), chaired by Ronald Easterling (3). With respect to the technology of reuse procedures, little new research has been reported on the various steps such as rinsing, cleaning, dialyzer evaluation, etc. Significant new information is available on sterilization, where new developments indicate a strong advantage for reuse. Recent research has also led to a more detailed understanding of biocompatibility of membranes, and the influence of reuse processes on the biocompatibility of reprocessed dialyzers.

More extensive information is now available on the experiences of nephrologists, in the practice of reuse since the United States Centers for Disease Control (CDC) maintains a continuing surveillance of dialysis associated diseases. Selected findings, relative to the merits of dialyzer reprocessing, are discussed.

RECENT DEVELOPMENTS IN HEMODIALYZER STERILIZATION FOR REUSE

Thermal sterilization

A major advancement in hemodialyzer reprocessing for subsequent use by the same patient is the development of a modified thermal process for dialyzer sterilization, reported by Frinak (4). Fresenius F80 and F60 polysulfone hollow fiber dialyzers were studied in a sterilization cycle using a lower temperature, (105 degrees C) and longer time cycle, than for conventional thermal sterilization (121 degrees C) for 15 minutes. Such longer time-lower temperature cycles are more suitable for the heat labile materials of the dialyzer. A ten hour time is required for the 105 degree C sterilization to be equivalent to 15 minutes at 121 degrees C. Biological challenge studies conducted with two organisms, Bacillus stearothermophilus and indigenous Pseudomonas sp., resulted in no growth after 10 and 15 hours.

Following reprocessing, using the Seratronics DRS-4 machine, F-80 dialyzers were filled with water and sterilized at 105 degrees C for 24 hours. Mouse fibroblast cytotoxicity tests and USP XXII rabbit whole blood hemolysis tests were negative. Dialyzer performance tests after 6, 14, and 20 sterilization cycles showed that the F80 and F60 dialyzer clearances decreased by a maximum of 3.5%.

The reprocessing procedure used for clinical studies consisted of: rinsing the dialyzer with AAMI standard quality water; filling the dialyzer with water, capping, bagging, and labeling with heat sensitive tape; placing the dialyzer in a 105 degree C oven for 24 hours; storing the dialyzer at room temperature until the next use; setting up the dialyzer for the next use and pressure testing it for leaks prior to the start of treatment. Records of oven temperature are made, and verification, before use, of the dialyzer sterilization process is accomplished by recording the condition of the temperature indicator strip. With respect to biocompatibility, studies of complement activation were made in four patients using F80 dialyzers, new as controls, and heat sterilized, reprocessed dialyzers. Complement (C3a des arg) levels were determined predialysis, 15 and 30 minutes into dialysis, and post dialysis. No significant difference was found in complement activation between new and heat sterilized, reprocessed dialyzers.

In this initial study of 16 patients, receiving a total of 420 treatments, the minimum reuse factor was 6.7. In October of 1991, a total of 250 patients in 5 centers were reusing dialyzers sterilized by this procedure.

Frinak (4) concludes that sterilization at 103-105 degrees C does not affect the integrity or clearance properties of the dialyzers, does not alter the biocompatibility of the polysulfone dialyzers, eliminates patient and staff exposure to chemical sterilants, and promises to be a safe and economical advance in dialyzer reprocessing technology.

Deterioration of dialyzer membranes by germicides

Previous epidemiological studies of bacteremia in dialysis patients conducted by the United States Centers for Disease Control (CDC) noted an association with dialyzers reprocessed with a specific germicide. As a result, a collaborative study was conducted by the Centers for Disease Control and the U.S. Food and Drug Administration on the effects of dialyzer disinfectants on five dialysis membranes. In the report of this study, Bland and associates (5) noted that all cellulosic membranes (cuprophan, cellulose acetate and cuprammonium rayon) were degraded by one active chlorine disinfectant, Warexin (Guardian Chemical), and failed all tests after 2-9 reprocessings. Other disinfectants studied were: 4% formaldehyde; Renalin (peroxyacetic acid), Minntech/Renal Systems; two glutaraldehyde formulations, (Cidex Dialyzer, Surgikos; Sporicidin HD, Sporicidin Co.) and RenNew-D, another active chlorine disinfectant. The latter has been withdrawn from the market by its manufacturer. Dialyzers studied included the Travenol 12:11 (Cuprophan), the CD Medical C-DAK 3500 (cellulose acetate), and the Terumo Clirans TAF 10M (cuprammonium rayon). Non-cellulosic dialyzers were the Asahi PAN 150 (polyacrylonitrile) and the Fresenius Hemoflow F-60 (polysulfone).

Following reprocessing and chemical disinfection, dialyzers were subjected to an air-pressure leak test and a microbiologic challenge test. Dialyzers were reprocessed 15 times or until failure of the air-pressure leak test. At that time dialyzers were subject to the microbiologic test, by circulating sterile saline on the blood side while dialysate contaminated with a known challenge organism was recirculated at 500 ml/min. After 15 minutes the blood side saline was assayed for the challenge organism. If the dialyzer failed either the air-pressure test or the microbiologic challenge test, the membrane was determined to be compromised. In the air-pressure leak test, other than the failures of the cellulosic dialyzers with Warexin, already cited, a single PAN Asahi 150 dialyzer, also disinfected with Warexin, failed on retest. In the microbiologic test, other than the cellulosics treated with Warexin, 3 cellulose acetate CD 3500 dialyzers, disinfected by Sporicidin, failed after 15 reprocessings. One polysulfone Fresenius 60, sterilized with formaldehyde, failed after 15 reprocessings, and one Fresenius 60, treated with RenNew-D, failed upon retest. To lessen the risk of bacteremia, the authors recommend inclusion of an air-pressure leak test in all dialyzer reprocessing systems.

Ishak et al (6) reported an outbreak of pyrogenic reactions and septicemia in 6 patients during dialysis using reprocessed dialyzers disinfected with Warexin. The identity of the dialyzer and membrane were not given. The center had recently changed from formaldehyde to Warexin, generically consisting of monoxychlorosene, an active chlorine disinfectant. Upon investigation by scanning electron microscopy, membranes from dialyzers exposed to 1.25% Warexin for 8 days at room temperature, were found to have distorted membranes, with longitudinal cracks, after 10-12 days 25 micron wide fissures were seen. Fibers immersed in formaldehyde or distilled water showed no deterioration. A high level of bacterial contamination of the dialysate was another key factor in the problem. The authors recommend evaluating a disinfectant's interaction with biomaterials as well as antimicrobial activity, and the testing of membrane integrity, after contact with disinfectant.

Influence of removable header-caps

High flux dialyzers with removable header-caps and O-rings, such as the Fresenius Hemoflow F-80 hollow fiber dialyzer, have been reported to be involved with cases of bacteremia of dialysis patients.

The U.S. Centers for Disease Control conducted a study of the likelihood of bacteria contaminating the blood compartment when such dialyzers were reused, after disinfection (7). Dialyzer header spaces and O-rings were exposed to aqueous bacterial suspensions, replaced on the dialyzers, which were reprocessed manually using 4% formaldehyde, 2.5% and 4% Renalin or sterile water as a control, or 3.25% Renalin with an automated reprocessor. After 48 hour storage the blood compartment was drained, rinsed twice and cultured. Dialysis was simulated by circulating sterile water in both the blood side and dialysate side for 15 min then culturing the former, as well as O-rings, header caps and fiber ends. In one of 38 tests (2.6%), one test organism was detected in the blood compartment circulate during simulated dialysis; and one test organism was recovered from blood compartment effluent or rinses in 4 of 113 assays (3.5%). Bland et al (7) conclude that microorganisms on sealed header caps and O-rings did not effectively contaminate the blood compartment of reprocessed dialyzers.

Bacterial biofilms

Bacterial biofilms experimentally produced in *in vitro* studies, have been shown by Vincent et al (8) to lower the effectiveness of disinfectant activity of sodium hypochlorite, formaldehyde and hydrogen peroxide.

In experiments using a Nephross lento, Cuprophan dialyzer (Organon Teknika), the production of a biofilm required the circulation of a bacterial suspension having a concentration of organisms in excess of 1000 bacteria/ml, which is far in excess of the AAMI, Canadian, and French standards of 200/ml. The observation that disinfectant activities are lower in the biofilm is of interest, but is not directly applicable to practical dialyzer reprocessing conditions.

Peracetic acid formulations

Peroxyacetic acid, as a commercially available solution, Dialox (L' Air Liquide), was evaluated for germicidal effectiveness in the reuse of HF80 (Fresenius) dialyzers.

Canaud and associates (9) used 3 test organisms at concentrations of $1.2\text{-}5.1 \times 10^{+7}$ to contaminate the high flux polysulfone dialyzers.

Reprocessing was conducted using the standard cycle of the Renatron (Minntech/Renal Systems), including two quality control tests, an airpressure membrane integrity test, and a blood compartment volume test. Five minutes after the reprocessing, no dialyzer showed any bacterial growth.

Use of a faulty mixing technique for dilution of the Renalin germicide, a peracetic acid formulation (Minntech/Renal Systems), was determined to be the cause of nine pyrogenic reactions and five gram-negative bacteremias occurring in eleven patients of a hemodialysis center (10).

The manual reprocessing technique specified concentrations of Renalin of 2.5%. Germicide concentrations found in 12 stored dialyzers, studied in the epidemic period, varied from 0.9 to 4.2%. Failure to properly mix the concentrated germicide during dilution apparently caused low levels of disinfectant, which in turn resulted in high bacteria and endotoxin levels. The latter were associated with outbreaks of pyrogenic reactions and bacteremias in the dialysis patients.

Fleming and coworkers (11) recently conducted a six-month prospective study of the use of Renalin to reprocess hemodialyzers over 2,759 dialyses on 59 patients. Dialyzers were reused up to a maximum of 6 times, with the average number of uses being 4.5. *In vivo* clearances of urea, creatinine and phosphate were similar to values for the new dialyzers. A small decrease in ultrafiltration characteristics was noted. Blood pressure was better preserved with the used dialyzers, and fewer intradialytic symptoms occurred.

A study of reuse and reuse sterilants on the "first-use syndrome" (12) was conducted over a 4 year period with 98 patients.

Vanholder and Ringoir (12) found that 5 patients developed symptoms of this syndrome. Marked improvement was noted when new dialyzers were automatically reprocessed using either formaldehyde or peracetic acid. No episodes of the syndrome occurred in patients using reused dialyzers. Formaldehyde sterilization was associated with the development of anti-N-like antibodies in the blood of four (8%) of 50 patients in a 14 month period. Two patients on formaldehyde reuse experienced itching on dialysis, which resolved when the sterilant was changed to peracetic acid.

Glutaraldehyde formulations

Parker and associates (13) conducted a comprehensive study of a glutaraldehyde formulation, Nephrex (Surgikos, Inc.), comparing it to formaldehyde as a dialyzer disinfectant. Three dialyzers were included in the study: Travenol 2308, Tri-Ex 3 (Extracorporeal), and the SCE-135 (Cordis Dow). Generally 2% formaldehyde was compared to 0.8% glutaraldehyde. Both disinfectants were effective against two Pseudomonas species in one hour; M chelonei required 12 hour exposure, and B subtilis spores needed 24 hours for complete kill. Glutaraldehyde performed better than formaldehyde against a species of waterborne Mycobacterium. Neither disinfectant affected membrane integrity, and biocompatibility tests were similar. Formaldehyde permitted a greater number of reuses (13.9), compared to 8.2 for glutaraldehyde. Dialyzers reprocessed with either germicide showed similar clearances and ultrafiltration rates.

BIOCOMPATIBILITY, IMMUNE RESPONSE AND REUSE

New dialyzer syndrome

Cheung (14) has pointed out that there is no concensus on the definition of biocompatibility for dialyzer membranes, and offers an operational definition of biocompatibility as the lack of any perturbation of blood constituents. Cordonnier and Foret (15) define biocompatibility as the sum of specific and non-specific interactions between blood and biomaterials. Over the years, a variety of symptoms, associated with membrane biocompatibility, have been observed in dialysis patients. Some, such as an acute respiratory distress syndrome, are very serious and can be life threatening. Ogden (16) coined the term "new dialyzer syndrome" for such severe reactions most often observed with new cuprophan dialyzers. Other reactions cause moderate to minor symptoms, and occur with more frequency (17).

With respect to dialyzer reuse, the biocompatibility of the reprocessed dialyzer is clearly dependent on the basic compatibility of the membrane and other biomaterials used to manufacture the dialyzer originally. Upon reuse, the compatibility of the dialyzer also is a function of the particular reuse process employed. With relatively bioincompatible membranes, such as cuprophan and other cellulosics, the reprocessed dialyzer can possess a level of compatibility superior to that of the new dialyzer. When the inherent biocompatibility of the new dialyzer increases, as with PAN and polysulfone membranes, the likelihood of the reprocessed dialyzer having better biocompatibility is less. In the latter cases the objective of the reprocessing is to restore the functionality and biocompatibility of the new dialyzer.

Cordonnier and Foret (15) review a number of biological criteria for biocompatibility, and both short and long term patient consequences of bioincompatibility.

Allergic reactions upon reuse

In a January, 1990 survey of 1290 dialysis centers in the USA, the Centers for Disease Control found that 38 centers (4%) reported clusters of acute allergic reactions with reused dialyzers. The clusters were defined as two or more patients experiencing acute reactions that occurred within the first 10 minutes of dialysis using reprocessed dialyzers (18). The clinical response was said to be similar to that of the "first-use syndrome".

Such clusters were not found to be associated with the type of disinfectant, the reprocessing method, or type of dialysate used. The risk for clusters was found to be associated with use of a specific heparin product, and with washing the blood compartment with either bleach or hydrogen peroxide. The data analysis has not been successful in identifying a specific allergenic substance. Such reports may represent a drawback in dialyzer reuse. The problem needs further study to determine the causative agent, or specific defect in methodology which led to these incidents.

Membranes, reuse and biocompatibility

Wauters and associates (19-21) have studied a number of critical factors concerning membrane biocompatibility, protein adsorption, and the effects of dialyzer reprocessing on dialysis induced neutropenia, complement activation and related effects. Upon reuse, neutropenia with cuprophan dialyzers improved markedly, but no improvement occurred with reuse of cellulose acetate, polysulfone, polycarbonate or polyacrylonitrile dialyzers. Monocytopenia was marked when using cuprophan and improved with reuse. Cellulose acetate and polycarbonate gave similar values of monocyte reduction on both first and second use. Polysulfone showed no reduction of monocytes on first use, but did on the second. Polyacrylonitrile produced substantial monocytopenia on first use, which disappeared on reuse. Platelet counts on first use fell only with cuprophan. Upon reuse, both cellulose acetate and polycarbonate caused significant reductions of platelets. Thrombocyte changes were relatively small compared to neutrophil changes. The reuse procedure consisted of water rinses, and disinfection with 3% formaldehyde, during storage at 4 degrees C, for all membranes. In the case of polyacrylonitrile, a pre-rinse with 1% sodium hypochlorite was used. In another study of membranes and reuse methods (22), three reuse procedures, formaldehyde, formaldehyde-hypochlorite, and peracetic acid were compared using cuprophan, cellulose acetate and polysulfone. Use of hypochlorite abolished the improvements in leucopenia and complement activation on cuprophan. Peracetic acid storage improved leucopenia, complement activation and thrombocyte count on the three membranes. From these studies it is clear that reprocessed membranes may not always be more biocompatible. The specific reuse method and membrane are the determinants of the biocompatibility properties of the reprocessed membranes.

Churchill and coworkers (23) conducted a multiple crossover study with random allocation of order of treatment to determine whether there were any advantages or disadvantages to reused dialyzers. The study design consisted of six cross-over periods of four weeks each on either single use or reuse with a week's wash-out period in between. In the wash-out period, single use of the dialyzers was employed. Dialyzers studied included cuprophan (GF 120 and GF180, Gambro), cellulose acetate (CD 3500 and CD 4000, Althin/CD Medical). Physicians, patients and nurses were blinded to dialyzer allocation and the dialyzers were covered with an opaque jacket. The analysis of data was done by comparing paired data on individual patients rather than use of group statistics. Reprocessing was conducted using automated equipment, the Seratronics DRS-4. The average number of reuses achieved was 4.4 for cuprophan dialyzers and 3.8 for cellulose acetate dialyzers. Intradialytic symptoms observed included pruritus, cramps, nausea, headache, chestpain, backache, and fatigue. Complement activation and neutropenia were similar in patients using new and reused dialyzers in this study. There were no clinically important or statistically significant differences for any symptom studied, with the possible exception of mild backache favoring single use. Other analysis revealed no effect of the number of uses on any symptom at any level of severity. Longer term effects were not addressed in this study. The authors cite other references for the economic benefits of dialyzer reprocessing.

First use reactions and ACE inhibitors

Verresen and associates (24, 25) conducted a retrospective study of 236 patients over the time period from April, 1986 to February, 1990 and determined that patients who were treated with a high flux parallel plate dialyzer, AN 69, and an acetate dialysate were likely to have anaphylactoid reactions if the patients were being treated with angiotensin-converting-enzyme (ACE) inhibitors. The dialyzers were reprocessed with 0.45% sodium hypochlorite. Nine of the 236 patients experienced anaphylactoid reactions. Such reactions were not due to hemodialyzer reuse as all nine of the patients had anaphylactoid reactions after first use of the membrane. Ethylene oxide hypersensitivity was excluded by a negative RAST test and persistence of reactions despite reuse. Heparin hypersensivity was excluded because of the disappearance of anaphylactoid reactions after interruption of the ACE inhibitor therapy without any change in the heparin treatment. The authors hypothesize that the ACE inhibitors may cause anaphylaxis when the first use of high flux membranes occurs, possibly by increased sensitivity to bacterial substances in the dialysate.

Caruana (26) reported three instances of hypersensitivity reactions occurring within 20 minutes of starting dialysis using new, non-reprocessed, cuprophan or cellulose acetate hemodialyzers. In each instance the chronic dialysis patient had been transferred from a facility which reprocessed cuprophan dialyzers, including new ones, prior to first use. The referred patients had no history of "first use reactions" though they had been on dialysis for 18-24 months. Thus, the patient's experience with a given dialyzer and its reuse may be a critical piece of information to communicate upon referral to another facility.

Dialysis amyloidosis and reuse

In recent years the importance of dialysis associated amyloidosis has been recognized as a potential complication of long term hemodialysis. The characteristics of the specific membrane used for hemodialysis determines whether stimulation of precursors to amyloidosis occurs and whether the membrane itself is capable of permitting the mass transfer of the precursors across the dialysis membrane to the dialysate.

The membrane characteristics are also influenced by the reuse procedure, if such a procedure is employed.

Goldman and coworkers (27) have studied the adsorption of the major precursor, beta-2-microglobulin (B2M) on dialysis membranes and the effects of reuse procedures on this process. In brief, cuprophan membranes were found not to adsorb B2M, while AN69, high flux polysulfone, and modified polyamide were found to adsorb average amounts of 49, 17 and 38 mg respectively. Upon reuse of AN69 membranes, use of sodium hypochlorite did not affect the adsorption of B2M, but use of peracetic acid reduced the adsorption to 20 mg. This study also confirmed that when using cuprophan membranes, no removal of B2M occurred either by transport (because of small pore size) or by adsorption.

Di Raimondo and Pollak (28) studied the kinetics of B2M removal in dialysis and the effects of dialyzer reuse. Studies of each dialyzer (cuproammonium rayon, Terumo TAF 12M, and polysulfone, Fresenius Hemoflow F80) were done on the first and third uses. Dialyzers were reprocessed with an automated device (the Seratronics DRS 4), using bleach and 1.5% formaldehyde. The mean predialysis levels of B2M decreased (post dialysis) 16.6% with cuproammonium rayon, and 57.1% with polysulfone. After reprocessing the respective decreases were 21.8% for cuproammonium rayon and 58.9% for polysulfone. Differences between new and reprocessed membrane values were not significant for either membrane type. Adsorption of B2M was not changed by reuse status of either membrane type. Polysulfone adsorbed about 30% of B2M in an *in vitro* phosphate buffer, compared to 2% for cuproammonium rayon.

In a study of several factors on reuse of cuproammonium dialyzers up to 6 times, Chan and Lau (29) observed pre to post reductions of 5-20% of the predialysis B2M concentrations in six patients in a 6-hr dialysis. The values were not corrected for ultrafiltration. The intradialytic changes in neutrophil count, platelet count, and serum C3 decrease as the number of reuses rises, indicating an advantage for reuse.

Anti-N-like antibodies

For more than a decade, it has been recognized that when dialyzers are reprocessed and sterilized with formaldehyde, inadequate removal of the sterilant prior to the next use may induce the formation of anti-N-like antibodies. Since there has been uncertainty concerning the lower limit of residual formaldehyde, below which formation of anti-N-like antibodies would not occur, Vanholder and coworkers carried out a prospective study of the problem (30). Ninety-eight patients were studied: 50 were treated with 4% formaldehyde-sterilized reprocessed dialyzers, and 48 were treated with first use dialyzers or those reprocessed with peracetic acid. Dialyzers of the formaldehyde group were rinsed on the dialysate side for 30 min at a flow of 500 ml/min, followed by blood-side rinsing single pass with saline at 150 ml/min for 15 min, while rinsing is continued on the dialysate side. Residual formaldehyde in the venous effluent was controlled to be at or below 1 ppm. At the start of the study no patient had a positive titer for anti-N-like antibodies. Five of the fifty patients of the formaldehyde group developed positive anti-N-like antibody titers. Gotch and Keen (31) studied the kinetics of formaldehyde removal from reprocessed dialyzers, using higher temperatures (37 degrees C), lower initial formaldehyde concentration, and recirculation of the saline on the blood-side. Their technique permitted reduction of formaldehyde to 1-5 ppm, in 15-45 minutes based on the initial storage concentration (1.5-4%) used. With formaldehyde dialyzer disinfection, removal of residual disinfectant is a critical requirement of the reuse process. Assuring its proper removal is important to avoid potential adverse effects, such as formation of anti-N-like antibodies.

Other allergic responses

The United States Centers for Disease Control reported that in the period from July 18 to November 27, 1989 nine patients had 12 acute allergic reactions during hemodialysis at one center. The reactions occurred within 10 minutes of the start of dialysis, and were characterized by sensations of warmth (75%), fullness in the mouth or throat (58%), tingling paresthesias (50%), nausea (33%) and tightness in the chest (33%). All reactions occurred with patients using mechanically reprocessed dialyzers which had been rinsed with hydrogen peroxide and filled with peracetic acid. Dialysis of the same patients with unused dialyzers were without incident. There was no specific cause identified for the reactions (32).

Pollak and associates (33) studied the incidence rates of intradialytic symptoms during first and subsequent reuses. In the first time period dialyzers were processed by a manual method both before first use and subsequent uses. In the second period automated reprocessing replaced the manual method. In the first period, they observed that the symptom of chest pain occurred 2.8 times more frequently during first use than subsequent uses. Back pain was 6 times, and concurrent chest and back pain, 42 times more prevalent in first use than other uses, characterizing a "first-use syndrome". When automated reprocessing replaced the manual method, increased numbers of symptoms were no longer observed on first use. The results are interpreted to show that use of automated reprocessing before first use can markedly reduce the incidence of "first-use syndrome". An alternative interpretation is that dialyzer manufacturers corrected some problems with new dialyzers, so that the symptom incidence was reduced by the second time frame. Taken at face value, observations of this study demonstrate an advantage for reuse, especially automated reuse.

In a study in which hemodialysis patients' intradialytic symptoms, complement activation, and Limulus amebocyte lysate reactive material (LAL-RM) were measured during dialysis on either cuprophan or cellulose acetate membranes, the role of the

LAL-RM in complement activation was found to be minor (34). Both membrane dialyzers were reprocessed on an automated device, Renatron, using Renalin, a formulation of peracetic acid of Minntech/Renal Systems. Complement levels (C3a) reached their peak 15 min into dialysis, with means for cuprophan about twice the values for cellulose acetate. Cuprophan membranes were found to release LAL-RM into the patients' blood, reaching levels of 2.8 ng/ml. Cellulose acetate essentially released no LAL-RM. There was no correlation between complement activation and LAL-RM level. Patients' symptoms were less with cellulose acetate than with cuprophan. This study confirmed the beneficial effect of dialyzer reuse on reducing the complement activation of cuprophan membranes.

REUSE EFFECTIVENESS: ADVERSE AND BENEFICIAL EFFECTS

For the last 15 years the United States Centers for Disease Control have conducted surveillance of various aspects of dialysis-associated diseases. Since 1982 the centers have made an annual survey of all dialysis providers in the country to study trends in the practice of hemodialyzer reuse for the same patient. The percentage of centers practicing reuse increased markedly from the mid 70's to the mid 80's. In 1989 68% of the 1867 centers reused dialyzers, serving 73% of the patient population (Table 1). Trends of the average number of reuses and the mean maximum number of uses are given for '86-'89 (35-38). The following are statistics from the 1988 report (37); 55% of the centers reported using only an automated system for reprocessing, and 45% reported only a manual system. Fifty-four percent of the centers used formaldehyde as the germicide for reprocessing, 40% peracetic acid, and 6% glutaraldehyde. Seventy-seven percent of the centers reported using only conventional membranes, mainly cuprophan or cellulose acetate. Centers practicing high flux dialysis were more likely to report pyrogenic reactions than centers that did not use high flux, whether dialyzers were reused or not. For centers reusing high flux dialyzers, the likelihood of pyrogenic reactions increased in direct relationship to the number of reuses, regardless of manual or automated reprocessing. Sixteen percent of the centers which reused dialyzers reported pyrogenic reactions compared to 11% of centers which did not reuse. When adjusted for the size of the centers, the difference is not significant. Comparing only centers that used conventional membranes, centers that reused dialyzers were more likely to report pyrogenic reactions occurring either sporadically or in clusters when dialyzers were manually reprocessed. In contrast, in the 1989 report, this increased risk was associated only with centers that use peracetic acid or glutaraldehyde for reprocessing (not formaldehyde) and occurred with both manual and automated systems. Septicemia was reported with a similar frequency in centers that reused dialyzers compared to centers that did not. New dialyzer syndrome was reported by 40% of the centers, a similar frequency to previous years. Use of high flux dialyzer membranes was associated with reported pyrogenic reactions, occurring both sporadically and in clusters, even in centers that did no reuse. The risk of pyrogenic reactions associated with reuse of high flux dialyzers was much greater than the risk with conventional dialyzer membrane reuse. Reuse of dialyzers has never been associated with an increased risk of acquiring hepatitis B infection among patients or staff. Most centers, however, do not reprocess dialyzers from HBsAg-positive patients.

Table 1. Extent of reuse practice in the United States from Centers for Disease Control surveys, 1986-89 (35-38).

Year	Facilities surveyed	% of centers reusing	% of dialysis patients	Number of patients reusing	Average number reuses
1986	1350	63	69	60,315	10
1987	1630	64	70	67,678	11
1988	1734	67	72	77,127	11
1989	1867	68	73	89,596	12

In an editorial accompanying the publication of the CDC report cited above, Victor Pollak (39) observed: "Practiced carefully, dialyzer reuse is safe and is associated with excellent care while containing costs".

Shusterman et al (40) conducted an extensive review of hemodialyzer reprocessing, concluding that additional studies of a variety of designs are needed to understand the impact of dialyzer reuse.

Various investigators have observed that reprocessed dialyzers, especially those based on cellulosic membranes, had improved biological properties compared to new dialyzers. Such observations provided a medical as well as an economic basis for reuse. The potential drawbacks of reuse cited are: possible inadequate dialysis due to loss of membrane surface area, infectious disease hazards if disinfection is inadequate, the risk of use of the dialyzer on the wrong patient, and the long term risks of exposure to small amounts of sterilant. The first drawback of reuse cited, potential underdialysis, is currently a topic of high priority for discussion among U.S. nephrologists. Dialyzer reuse may contribute to the risk of underdialysis, if the center does not measure residual cell volume of the dialyzer with each use, in accord with the AMMI recommended practice (3), and compensate for any loss of clearance, by revision of the patient's dialysis prescription. Aside from reuse, other factors which may be even more important in avoiding underdialysis are providing an adequate dialysis prescription initially, and assuring that the prescribed dialysis is indeed delivered to the patient. The risk of infection, if the disinfection step of the reuse process is inadequate, is a valid concern. Care in consistently following validated procedures is necessary in dialyzer reprocessing, as in any other medical procedure. Generally, use of automated equipment has been shown to provide a higher degree of reliability in reprocessing than manual procedures (35-38). Careful observance of validated steps (especially assuring correct concentrations and identities of all chemicals of the process) is essential even with automated equipment. Quality control and quality assurance are essential to reduce risks (3). The chance of use of the reused dialyzer on the wrong patient is low, because most centers have a second person, often the patient, confirm the patient's name on the dialyzer. As pointed out by Shusterman et al (40) no untoward outcome has ever been reported from this cause. Finally, the risk of long term consequences of infusion of small amounts of residual sterilant has continued to be a concern up to the present time. When formaldehyde is used, current removal techniques, involving recirculation of saline on the blood side while dialysate or purified water is circulated on the dialysate side, are capable of reducing the concentration to below 1-2 ppm. The recommended practice (3) requires each dialyzer to be tested before use, thus minimizing the risk of infusion of appreciable amounts of sterilant. With the advent of thermal sterilization of hemodialyzers (4) now possible with one make of polysulfone dialyzer, this risk is eliminated entirely, as well as the risk of sterilant release to the environment.

Gordon et al (41) report a study of an outbreak of 18 pyrogenic reactions occurring in 16 long term hemodialysis patients at one center. The investigation by the Centers for Disease Control (CDC) showed that the pyrogenic reactions were associated with reuse of hemodialyzers. The concentrations of bacteria and endotoxins in the tap water used to rinse the reused dialyzers and in the product water used to dilute the germicide were greater than 10,000 CFU/ml and greater than 6 ng/ml respectively. These levels of contamination exceed the AAMI maximum recommended concentrations for water used to rinse dialyzers and to prepare germicides for disinfecting dialyzers (<200 CFU/ml and <1 ng/ml of endotoxin, respectively) (3). The investigators conclude by providing some general recommendations, which have been demonstrated by practitioners, experienced in dialyzer reuse, to give good results: [1]

Processed water used to prepare dialysate, dilute germicide or rinse dialyzers should be cultured monthly, and should conform to AAMI standards. [2] An active surveillance system for adverse reactions in hemodialysis patients should be routine in all centers. [3] A dialyzer membrane integrity test should be made on all reprocessed dialyzers prior to subsequent use, and a detailed log book kept of key reprocessing data. [4] Monthly or more frequent disinfection of the water distribution system should be conducted. [5] The source of the product water used to dilute germicide and rinse dialyzers should be delivered through an integral part of the water system with a faucet outlet which is routinely disinfected. Plastic or rubber hoses should be eliminated or replaced frequently.

Careful attention to dialyzer function, when patients are treated with reprocessed dialyzers, is recommended by Delmez and associates (42). In one manufacturer's lot of hollow fiber dialyzers, the authors observed a marked decline in clearances, as routine urea kinetics were measured, despite monitoring of each dialyzer's cell volume and ultrafiltration rate. Further investigation revealed that upon injection of methylene blue into the dialysate port, the dialyzers showed non-uniform dialysate flow. *In vitro* studies showed that clearances of one lot of dialyzers, subjected to daily reprocessing but no patient exposure, declined about 50%, with 15 reprocessings; but dialyzers of another lot showed no decline. While the magnitude of the problem and its cause could not be demonstrated in this study, the admonition to carefully monitor reprocessed dialyzer performance is well taken, and is a potential drawback of reuse.

Noting that dialyzer reuse remains a contentious issue, Garred et al (43) focused their study on the possible deleterious effect of repeated reuse on dialyzer performance. The study was conducted over a nine month period on all 21 patients of one shift in a satellite dialysis unit. Patients were dialyzed on Fresenius F60 or HF80 polysulfone dialyzers, which were reprocessed on a Renatron machine (Minntech/Renal Systems) using peracetic acid as cleansing and sterilizing agent. Once each month, blood side and dialysate side clearances for urea and creatinine were measured. Average blood and dialysate flows were 345 ml/min and 498 ml/min, respectively. Dialyzers were used an average of 14.4 times. A blood compartment loss of about 1% occurred over a 5 week/15 use period. The dialyzer mass transfer coefficient declined about 3% over the same period for urea and creatinine. No allergic or pyrogenic reaction was observed in the study. The authors conclude that polysulfone dialyzers, reprocessed with peracetic acid, may be used for a 5 week/15 session period with negligible loss of dialyzer performance on small molecule transport. When effective performance is demonstrated, and coupled with clear economic benefits in lowering the per treatment cost of the dialyzer, a strong advantage is shown for dialyzer reuse.

Levin and Striker (44), in a recent editorial concerning research on problems of the dialysis patient, noting the increased use of new, more porous membranes, point out the need for high standards in the reprocessing of dialyzers. With the newer, more biocompatible, more porous, and more costly dialyzers, effective dialyzer reprocessing with high standards becomes a necessity if costs are to be contained.

HEMODIALYZER REUSE AND PATIENT SURVIVAL

In the earlier literature, two studies on the effect of reuse on survival of hemodialysis patients have been done by the European Dialysis and Transplant Registry (45-47). In the 1977 study, the Registry compared one year survival of patients, starting dialysis in the year of the study, and found that there was no significant difference between the two groups: 93.2% of reusers vs 91.2% for non-reusers. Another study compared survival in countries with relatively high reuse practice to countries with low reuse practice. Except for patient age, which was controlled, there are other variables, which were not possible to control in these studies, making general conclusions difficult.

Held et al (48) conducted a retrospective survival analysis of 4,661 dialysis patients who began treatment in 1977 and were followed for 4.5 years through 1981. The primary variables of this study were attributes of the patient (diagnoses, race, sex, age) and characteristics of the patient's coordinating dialysis center (type of center: transplant center, hospital center, hospital facility, free-standing unit, size of center, for-profit or not for profit, whether the center was a long time reuser of dialyzers before 1980, whether the dialysis unit had open staffing or not, and the number of physicians staffing the unit). A patient had to have more than 85% of his/her dialyses in the coordinating dialysis center to be entered in the study. The findings of the study, with respect to reuse of hemodialyzers, were that patients of centers who were long-time reusers of dialyzers had a relative risk of dying of 0.88 compared to patients of centers that never reuse, whose relative risk for this comparison was 1.00. Patients of centers who recently started to reuse dialyzers had a relative risk of dying of 1.01 compared to centers that never reused. The authors point out that the findings of this study with respect to reuse, focus specifically on mortality and not on other issues concerning reuse. They do comment that the estimated coefficient for long-term reuse was "robust".

Held et al (49) recently completed another study of mortality and various factors in hemodialysis treatment, focusing on the duration of each dialysis session as the key factor in the analysis. In this study a covariate applied to each patient was dialyzer reuse, and for each center, the dialyzer reuse policy was a covariate: 597 patients from 36 dialysis centers were studied. Short time dialysis (less than 3.5 hr) was found to carry higher mortality risks. Patients in the shorter time treatment group were more likely to be in a dialysis center that had just begun dialyzer reuse (within 2 yrs), and were more likely to be treated with a reused dialyzer. Unfortunately, this study did not isolate or measure the effect of dialyzer reuse on patient mortality.

CONCLUDING COMMENTS

Assuming there are no regulatory barriers against reprocessing hemodialyzers for repeated use by the same patient, the decision to reuse or not is clearly the responsibility of the medical director of each facility.

The potential economic benefits and in some cases, improved biocompatibility of reused dialyzers must be weighed against the added requirements for the facility in staff, equipment, and expertise to carry out a technically demanding process with a high level of quality control and assurance.

Current experience shows that automated reprocessing is less likely to have problems than a manual process, but care and quality control remain essential. The specific dialyzer(s) and reuse process(es) must be validated in the center initiating a dialyzer reuse program.

The economic benefits of dialyzer reprocessing increase in proportion to the initial cost of the dialyzer being reused. The higher flux, more biocompatible dialyzers, capable of shorter treatment times, are generally more expensive, hence more likely to be reprocessed.

As discussed above, experience has shown that with more porous membranes, the risk of pyrogenic reactions is greater. When such membranes are used, higher standards need to be applied to all aspects of the dialysis process: water treatment, dialyzer reprocessing, microbial content of the dialysate, etc. Thus a high quality dialyzer reuse program can facilitate cost containment. This enables more expensive dialyzers to be broadly utilized for shorter time, more biocompatible treatments.

Two of the most attractive, practical advances in the reports summarized above are: the availability on the market of a dialyzer which can be thermally sterilized, and the validation of a suitable, lower temperature sterilization process. The two contributions make possible a more simple reuse process, which eliminates chemical sterilants, sterilant residues, and sterilant environmental problems. Because of its simplicity, this process should facilitate high standards of reliability and process quality. Such a development contributes to a better quality of care for all participating patients.

REFERENCES

1. Deane N, Wineman RJ, Bemis JA (Eds): Guide to reprocessing of hemodialyzers. Martinus Nijhoff Publishing, Boston, 1986.
2. Deane N, Wineman RJ: Multiple use of hemodialysers. In: "Replacement of renal function by dialysis" (Ed JF Maher), Kluwer Academic Publishers, Boston, 1989, pp 400-416.
3. AAMI: Recommended practice for reuse of hemodialyzers. Association for Advancement of Medical Instrumentation, Arlington, VA, 1986.
4. Frinak S: Heat sterilization of dialyzers. Paper presented at Seventh Annual Advanced Dialysis Symposium, 18 October, 1991, Toledo, Ohio, U.S.A.
5. Bland LA, Favero MS, Oxborrow GS, Aguero SM, Searcy BP, Danielson JW: Effect of chemical germicides on the integrity of hemodializer membranes. Trans Am Soc Artif Intern Organs, 34: 172-175, 1988.
6. Ishak M, Laverdiere M, Baron C, Nolin L, Labrecque L: Pseudomonas aeruginosa septicemia related to structural damage to hemodializer membranes following disinfection with monoxychlorosene. Canada Diseases Weekly Report, 16-6: 27-28, 1990.
7. Bland LA, Arduino MJ, Aguero SM, Favero MS: Recovery of bacteria from reprocessed high flux dialyzers after bacterial contamination of the header spaces and o-rings. Trans Am Soc Artif Intern Organs, 35: 314-316, 1989.
8. Vincent FC, Tibi AR, Darbord JC: A bacterial biofilm in a hemodialysis system, assessment of disinfection and crossing of endotoxin. Trans Am Soc Artif Intern Organs, 35: 310-313, 1989.
9. Canaud B, Nguyen QV, Garred LJ, Nicolle R, Mion C: Germicidal effectiveness of Dialox, a new stable peroxyacetic acid solution, in the reuse of high-flux dialyzers. Nephrol Dial Transplant, 4: 1000-1002, 1989.
10. Beck-Sague CM, Jarvis WR, Bland LA, Arduino MJ, Aguero SM, Verosic G: Outbreak of a gram-negative bacteremia and pyrogenic reactions in a hemodialysis center. Am J Nephrology, 10: 397-403, 1990.
11. Fleming SJ, Foreman K, Schanley K, Mihrshahi R, Siskind V: Dialyzer reprocessing with Renalin. Am J Nephrology, 11: 27-31, 1991.
12. Vanholder R, Ringoir S: Influence of reuse and of reuse sterilants on the first-use syndrome. Artificial Organs, 11: 137-139, 1987.
13. Husni L, Kale E, Climer C, Bostwick B, Parker TF: Evaluation of a new disinfectant for dialyzer reuse. Amer J Kidney Dis, 14: 110-118, 1989.
14. Cheung AK: Biocompatibility of hemodialysis membranes. J Am Soc Nephrology, 1: 150-161, 1990.
15. Cordonnier DJ, Foret M: Biocompatibility criteria in hemodialysis. In: "Present-day concepts in the treatment of chronic renal failure". Contrib Nephrol (Eds J Traeger, F Cantarovich, M Olmer), Karger, Basel, 1989, 71, pp. 30-35.
16. Ogden DA: New dialyzer syndrome. N Engl J Med, 302: 1262-1263, 1980.
17. Villarroel F, Ciarkowski AA: A survey of hypersensitivity reactions in hemodialysis. Artif Organs, 9: 231-238, 1985.
18. Miller GB, Wilber J: Acute allergic reactions associated with reprocessed hemodialyzers - United States, 1989-1990, From the Centers for Disease Control. JAMA, 265: 1511, 1991.
19. Heierli C, Markert M, Lambert PH, Kuwahara T, Wauters P: On the mechanisms of hemodialysis-induced neutropenia: a study with five new and reused membranes. Nephrol Dial Transplant, 3: 773-783, 1988.
20. Markert M, Heierli C, Kuwahara T, Frei J, Wauters JP: Dialyzed polymorphonuclear neutrophil oxidative metabolism during dialysis: a comparative study with 5 new and reused membranes. Clinical Nephrology, 29: 129-136, 1988.

21. Kuwahara T, Markert M, Wauters JP: Proteins adsorbed on hemodialysis membranes modulate neutrophil activation. Artificial Organs, 13: 427-431, 1989.
22. Kuwahara T, Markert M, Wauters JP: Biocompatibility aspects of dialyzer reprocessing: a comparison of 3 re-use methods and 3 membranes. Clinical Nephrology, 32: 139-143, 1989.
23. Churchill DN, Taylor DW, Shimizu AG, Beecroft ML, Singer J, Barnes CC, Ludwin D, Wright N, Sackett DL, Smith EKM: Dialyzer reuse- a multiple crossover study with random allocation to order of treatment. Nephron, 50: 325-331, 1988.
24. Verresen L, Waer M, Vanrenterghem Y, Michielsen P: Angiotensin-converting-enzyme inhibitors and anaphylactoid reactions to high-flux membrane dialysis. Lancet, 336: 1360-1362, 1990.
25. Verresen L, Waer M, Vanrenterghem Y, Michielsen P: Anaphylactoid reactions, hemodialysis and ACE inhibitors. Lancet, 337: 1294, 1991.
26. Caruana RJ: First-use reactions: a potential hazard for referral centers. Int J Artif Organs, 12: 688-691, 1989.
27. Goldman M, Lagmiche M, Dhaene M, Amraoui Z, Thayse C, Vanherweghem JL: Adsorption of beta-2-microglobulin on dialysis membranes: comparison of different dialyzers and effects of reuse procedures. Int J Artif Organs, 12: 373-378, 1989.
28. Di Raimondo CR, Pollak VE: Beta-2-microglobulin kinetics in maintenance hemodialysis: a comparison of conventional and high flux dialyzers and the effects of dialyzer reuse. Am J Kidney Diseases, 13: 390-395, 1989.
29. Chan MK, Lau N: Optimal reuse of cuprammonium rayon hollow-fiber dialyzers. Int J Artif Organs, 12: 223-228, 1989.
30. Vanholder R, Noens L, De Smet R, Ringoir S: Development of anti-N-like antibodies during formaldehyde reuse in spite of adequate predialysis rinsing. Am J Kidney Dis, 11: 477-480, 1988.
31. Gotch F, Keen, M: Formaldehyde kinetics in reused dialyzers. Trans Am Soc Artif Intern Organs, 29: 396-401, 1983.
32. Miller GB, Sikes RK: Acute allergic reactions associated with reprocessed hemodialyzers - Virginia, 1989. JAMA, 263: 501, 1990.
33. Charoenpanich R, Pollak VE, Kant KS, Robson MD, Cathey M: Effect of first and subsequent use of hemodialyzers on patient well-being: the rise and fall of a syndrome associated with new dialyzer use. Artif Organs, 11: 123-127, 1987.
34. Moss AH, Hamrick RM, Shen SH: Limulus Amebocyte lysate reactivity, complement activation, and patients' symptoms; comparison of dialyzer membranes. Trans Am Soc Artif Intern Organs, 35: 812-815, 1989.
35. Alter MJ, Favero MS, Miller JK, Coleman PJ, Bland LA: Reuse of hemodialyzers - results of nationwide surveillance for adverse effects. JAMA, 260: 2073-2076, 1988.
36. Alter MJ, Favero MS, Miller JK, Moyer LA, Bland LA: National surveillance of dialysis-associated diseases in the United States, 1987. Trans Am Soc Artif Intern Organs, 35: 820-831, 1989.
37. Alter MJ, Favero MS, Moyer LA, Miller JK, Bland LA: National surveillance of dialysis-associated diseases in the United States, 1988. Trans Am Soc Artif Intern Organs, 36: 107-118, 1990.
38. Alter MJ, Favero MS, Moyer LA, Bland LA: National surveillance of dialysis-associated diseases in the United States,1989. Trans Am Soc Artif Intern Organs, 37: 97-109, 1991.
39. Pollak VE: Adverse effects and pyrogenic reactions during hemodialysis. JAMA, 260: 2106-2107, 1988.
40. Shusterman NH, Feldman HI, Wasserstein A, Strom BL: Reprocessing of Hemodialyzers: a critical review. Amer J Kidney Dis, 14: 81-91, 1989.
41. Gordon SM, Tipple M, Bland LA, Jarvis WR: Pyrogenic reactions associated with reuse of disposable hollow-fiber hemodialyzers. JAMA, 260: 2077-2081, 1988.
42. Delmez JA, Werts CA, Hasamear PD, Windus DW: Severe dialyzer dysfunction undetectable by standard reprocessing validation tests. Kidney Int, 36: 478-484, 1989.
43. Garred LJ, Canaud B, Flavier JL, Poux C, Polito-Bouloux C, Mion C: Effect of reuse on dialyzer efficacy. Artif Organs, 14: 80-84, 1990.
44. Levin NW, Striker GE: Research on problems of the dialysis patient. J Am Soc Nephrology, 1: 1055-1056, 1991.
45. Challah S, Wing AJ, Brunner FP, Brynger HOA, Oules R, Selwood NH: Use and reuse of dialyzers in Europe. In: "Guide to reprocessing of hemodialyzers"(Eds N Deane, RJ Wineman, JA Bemis), Martinus Nijhoff Publishing, Boston,1986, pp 99-106.

46. Jacobs C, Brunner FP, Chantler C, Donckerwolcke RA, Gurland HJ, Hathway RA, Jacobs C, Selwood NH, Wing AJ: Combined report on regular dialysis and transplantation in Europe, VII. Proc Eur Dial Transplant Assoc, 14: 3-69, 1977.
47. Wing AJ, Brunner FP, Brynger H, Chantler C, Donckerwolcke RA, Gurland HJ, Jacobs C, Selwood NH: Mortality and morbidity of reusing dialyzers. Br Med J, 2: 853-855, 1978.
48. Held PJ, Pauly MV, Diamond L: Survival analysis of patients undergoing dialysis. JAMA, 257: 645-650, 1987.
49. Held PJ, Levin NW, Bovbjerg RR, Pauly MV, Diamond LH: Mortality and duration of hemodialysis treatment. JAMA, 265: 871-875, 1991.

Chapter 16

PRACTICAL ISSUES IN PRESCRIBING PERITONEAL DIALYSIS

ZBYLUT J. TWARDOWSKI

Division of Nephrology, Department of Medicine, University of Missouri, Harry S. Truman Veterans Administration Hospital, Dalton Research Center, Columbia, Missouri, U.S.A.

HISTORICAL PERSPECTIVE

Intermittent peritoneal dialysis (IPD) regimen for chronic renal failure was introduced in the early 1960s (1) and gained popularity after two crucial improvements made by Tenckhoff: a safe and permanent chronic peritoneal access (2) and an automated sterilization and delivery system of dialysis solution that allowed therapy at home (3). The method, however, could not compete successfully with hemodialysis because of low efficiency, resulting in inadequate dialysis and a shorter technique survival than on other forms of renal replacement therapy. All efforts to increase the efficiency of dialysis to shorten the time of dialysis proved unsuccessful and peritoneal dialysis for chronic renal failure began to decline in the early 1970s.

A revival of peritoneal dialysis resulted from the concept of portable/wearable equilibrium peritoneal dialysis, using several long-dwell exchanges each day (4). Assuming that the urea equilibrates between plasma and dialysate at the end of the long dwell exchange and that the urea nitrogen generation rate equals 8.2 g/day (5), simple calculations indicated that five 2-liter exchanges plus 1.8 liter of ultrafiltration would yield 11.8 liter of urea clearance per day, which would keep BUN below 70 mg/dl in anuric patients. Initial clinical studies confirmed that adequate steady state control of azotemia, sodium and water balance, hyperkalemia and acidosis could be achieved in patients with end-stage renal failure using five 2-liter volume exchanges per day and the technique was renamed continuous ambulatory peritoneal dialysis (CAPD) (6). However, five exchanges per day appeared to be cumbersome for the majority of patients, so four 2 liter exchanges were recommended (7). This schedule seemed to be adequate, particularly for patients with preserved residual function. The concept and practice of CAPD are contrary to the objectives of IPD over the years - delivery of large amounts of fluid intraperitoneally to increase efficiency and sophisticated automation. CAPD utilizes a manual method of fluid delivery and drainage, and overcomes inefficiency of IPD by a continuous dialysis regimen in the sense that the dialysis is performed around the clock every day while the patient is ambulatory or asleep.

During the 1980s the number of patients on CAPD has steadily increased. With increased patient population, it has become increasingly evident that there is interindividual and intraindividual variation in peritoneal transport kinetics of CAPD patients (8-12). The metabolite generation rate varies with dietary protein intake, body weight, and catabolic rate, while residual renal function tends to decrease with the duration of dialysis. Renal function decline rates vary among patients, but after 2 - 5 years of dialysis the urine output becomes negligible in almost every patient (13-15). In many patients a dialysate to plasma equilibrium, even for urea, is not attained during long dwell exchanges (16).

In hemodialysis the efficiency of dialysis depends on blood and dialysis solution flow rates as well as the kind of dialyzer and may be relatively easily manipulated.

Peritoneal transport kinetics depend mainly on peritoneal membrane resistance, vary widely among patients, and are difficult to manipulate. Thus, individualized dialysis schedules appeared necessary to ensure that CAPD patients with different dialysis requirements and peritoneal transport rates receive adequate dialysis (16).

Although CAPD proved to be remarkably superior to IPD in efficiency and long term survival, the need of performing several exchanges during the daytime appeared cumbersome to some patients, particularly those requiring helpers because of poor manual dexterity due to disease or age (children and/or elderly). The possibility of combining positive features of CAPD and IPD with a reduction of the negative aspects was predicted by Scribner in 1979 (17). Soon thereafter, Diaz-Buxo et al (18, 19) and Price and Suki (20) introduced continuous cyclic peritoneal dialysis (CCPD). Unlike CAPD, where short dwell exchanges are performed during the daytime and one long dwell exchange overnight, with original CCPD short dwell exchanges took place at night with an automatic cycling machine and one long dwell exchange was performed during the day.

During the early 1980s it became evident that the presence of intraperitoneal fluid in the upright position was an undesirable feature of both CAPD and CCPD in a subset of patients with complications related to high intra-abdominal pressure. Also, patients with rapid glucose absorption had poor ultrafiltration during long dwell exchanges. For these patients nightly peritoneal dialysis (NPD) was introduced (21).

GLOSSARY

A confusing peritoneal dialysis terminology developed throughout the years, particularly in relation to the terms continuous and intermittent, which have been used to describe regimens and techniques (22, 23). The term regimen refers to the overall systematic plan of dialysis. The term technique refers to the peritoneal dialysis procedure by which a regimen is accomplished, particularly to the method of dialysis solution flow during a single dialysis session.

In intermittent flow peritoneal dialysis, during a fluid exchange, three distinctive periods occur - inflow, dwell, and outflow. After the outflow, before the next inflow and during the dwell, the flow of fluid is interrupted, hence the term intermittent. When, in the early 1960s, Boen et al (1) introduced peritoneal dialysis for the treatment of chronic renal failure, the dialysis sessions were performed periodically, several times per week, consequently the term "periodic peritoneal dialysis" was applied to this regimen. Single dialysis sessions were performed with the intermittent flow technique and gradually the term "intermittent" became synonymous with "periodic" and the latter term was abandoned.

In continuous flow peritoneal dialysis, during a single dialysis session, dialysis solution flows continuously between two single lumen peritoneal catheters or between two lumens of the double lumen catheter, hence the term continuous. In the late 1970s, after the introduction of continuous ambulatory peritoneal dialysis, the term continuous was applied to the regimen and meant that the dialysis was performed around the clock with only brief, insignificant interruptions for infrequent exchanges. As a matter of fact, continuous ambulatory peritoneal dialysis is performed with intermittent flow technique. In this chapter when describing regimens performed periodically, the term intermittent peritoneal dialysis will be used. However, when describing techniques, the term intermittent flow peritoneal dialysis will be used in its original meaning.

A recently introduced technique, tidal peritoneal dialysis (TPD), may be considered as a hybrid of continuous and intermittent flow techniques. After an initial fill of the peritoneal cavity, only a portion of dialysate is drained and replaced by fresh dialysis fluid with each cycle, leaving the majority of dialysate in constant contact with the peritoneal membrane until the end of the dialysis session when the fluid is drained as completely as possible.

Peritoneal dialysis method is a means or manner in which peritoneal dialysis procedure is attained. Three methods are in use: manual, assisted manual, and automated. The last one is performed without active participation of a person but by a preset peritoneal dialysis machine (cycler). It is becoming customary to use a term automated peritoneal dialysis (APD) for any regimen employing a cycler.

Peritoneal dialysis prescription is a term which encompasses a peritoneal dialysis regimen combined with a technique and method of peritoneal dialysis. A dose of dialysis and an infusion volume further define the prescription. A dose of dialysis is the amount of dialysis solution used in a specified time. Infusion volumes in adults ranges from 1.5 to 3 liters.

OPTIMAL AND ADEQUATE DIALYSIS

Optimal dialysis may be defined as the amount of dialysis yielding results which cannot be further improved. The results would be measured by comparison of longevity, morbidity, and general wellness in dialysis patients to those in the general population. In this approach, the overall measure of the dialysis amount includes the efficiency of dialysis (average weekly clearance/standard body surface area or weekly Kt/V or some other efficiency measure), and the weekly distribution of dialysis sessions (continuous, infrequent intermittent, daily, nightly, or twice daily). Because of "cost and time" limitations, no attempt has been made to provide optimal dialysis, rather the efforts are directed to provide merely adequate dialysis. According to Webster, "optimal" means most desirable or satisfactory; "adequate" means sufficient for a specific requirement, especially barely sufficient or satisfactory. This latter term has two usages: [a] a dialysis prescription fulfilling certain criteria and [b] the condition of a patient achieved with a particular prescription. This condition constitutes a criterion of dialysis adequacy.

During the early years of chronic hemodialysis, a definition of adequate dialysis was based on clinical grounds, particularly on the absence of symptoms and signs of uremia (24). In the early 1970s the definition was based on a mixture of clinical symptoms and laboratory data. These definitions used *a priori* criteria of adequacy and were supposed to predict long term results of dialysis (25, 26). The National Institutes of Health (NIH)-sponsored National Cooperative Dialysis Study (NCDS) used overall morbidity and mortality as decisive objective criteria for the relative values of different dialysis prescriptions (27). This approach used an *a posteriori* (from the actual results) criterion of dialysis adequacy. A dialysis prescription was based on Kt/V index, developed by Gotch and Sargent (28). This index is a dimensionless parameter defining the fractional clearance of the solute distribution volume. Most commonly the measured solute is urea, K is dialyzer clearance, t is the treatment time and V is urea distribution volume, which equals the total body water. With the use of "conventional" dialyzers, it has been established that Kt/V of less than 0.8 per treatment with 3 times weekly dialysis (less than 2.4/wk) was associated with high morbidity. It was found also that shorter dialysis on "conventional" dialyzers was associated with higher mortality (29). The impact of high flux or high efficiency dialyzers on mortality and morbidity has not been yet studied on a large patient population. Several groups showed better survival with urea Kt/V higher than 1.25 with 3 times weekly dialysis (30-32). All these results indicate that more dialysis is better than less dialysis, but no attempt has been made to establish the optimal prescription.

The adequacy of peritoneal dialysis prescription has never been tested in well controlled prospective studies. By default, the adequacy of peritoneal dialysis must be judged mainly by selected clinical and laboratory criteria, which are presumed to predict long term results (33, 34).

The adequately dialyzed patient "feels well and looks good", has stable lean body mass, well controlled blood pressure, perfect fluid balance, and does not exhibit even subtle uremic symptoms such as anorexia, asthenia, dysgeusia, insomnia, nausea, and/or emesis.

Manifestations of inadequate dialysis often develop insidiously. Most commonly, inadequate dialysis results in decreased appetite leading to poor nutrition with wasting and loss of lean body weight. Blood urea nitrogen may be low because of poor protein intake, but creatinine level is usually high. With long term inadequate dialysis, the serum creatinine may ultimately decrease due to diminished generation with reduced muscle mass. A well dialyzed patient has normal electrolytes, maintains hematocrit above 25% (without anabolic steroids or erythropoietin), serum albumin above 3.5 g/dl, and serum creatinine below 0.08 mg/dl/cm height. With the use of erythropoietin, the hematocrit cannot be used as a sign of dialysis adequacy. It may be predicted that the weekly erythropoietin requirement to keep hematocrit at the certain level may serve the same purpose in the future.

A controversial issue is whether other symptoms and signs of uremia should indicate inadequate dialysis.

Control of serum phosphorus to prevent secondary hyperthyroidism by dialysis alone without phosphate binders is unrealistic, thus hyperphosphatemia and hyperparathyroidism are not considered as indicating inadequate dialysis. Serositis may occur in otherwise adequately dialyzed patients and generally is not considered as indicating inadequate dialysis; however, more intensive dialysis is indicated to treat serositis.

MASS TRANSFER AREA COEFFICIENT

Dialysate to plasma ratios of solute concentrations change at different rates in different patients on peritoneal dialysis and peritoneal clearances measured during standard intermittent peritoneal dialysis vary from patient to patient (35-41). The mass transfer area coefficient (MTAC) was introduced to separate influences of dialysate flow rate and convective transport on solute transfer (42-46). This coefficient, based on kinetic models of the solute mass transfer process, is the inverse of peritoneal diffusion resistance and represents the clearance rate which would be realized in the absence of both ultrafiltration and solute accumulation in the dialysate.

The MTAC measurement is not used in routine clinical practice because of the complexity of calculations. Hiatt et al (47) published a nomogram to calculate MTAC from a single measurement of solute dialysate to plasma ratio (D/P) at 4, 5, or 6 hour dwell time; however, such a recalculation does not have any advantage over a presentation of the result as a simple D/P ratio.

ULTRAFILTRATION

In peritoneal dialysis, ultrafiltration is osmotically induced and the predominant transperitoneal osmotic pressure gradient is produced by the glucose concentration of the dialysis solution. Consequently the net transcapillary ultrafiltration rate is maximal at the beginning of the exchange and decreases exponentially as the glucose concentration gradient is dissipated by a combination of transperitoneal glucose absorption and dilution by the ultrafiltrate (48). The intraperitoneal volume increases until a maximum is reached when the net transcapillary ultrafiltration rate equals the peritoneal cavity lymphatic absorption rate (49). Transcapillary ultrafiltration during exchanges using the same dialysis solution is primarily dependent on differences in peritoneal MTAC. Transperitoneal osmotic pressure is equal to the sum of the products of the osmotic gradient and peritoneal reflection coefficient of each solute. Because glucose creates most of the osmotic driving force, high peritoneal MTAC reduces cumulative transcapillary ultrafiltration by two related mechanisms: [A] at any given osmotic gradient the lower peritoneal reflection coefficient for glucose generates reduced osmotic driving force and diminished ultrafiltration and [B] rapid absorption of glucose from the dialysate dissipates the transperitoneal osmotic gradient more quickly during the dwell time.

Transcapillary ultrafiltration into the peritoneal cavity is negated by a variable rate of lymphatic drainage from the peritoneal cavity, but lymphatic absorption is independent of transcapillary MTAC for glucose (50). Consequently, in patients with high peritoneal MTAC, peak ultrafiltration occurs earlier during dwell time and net positive ultrafiltration lasts shorter compared to patients with low MTAC.

PERITONEAL EQUILIBRATION TEST (PET)

The peritoneal equilibration test (PET) was introduced as a simpler measurement of peritoneal membrane performance in individual patients. It may be compared to the hemodialyzer clearance as provided by a manufacturer and measured under standard conditions (blood flow, dialysate flow) and depending on dialyzer design, kind of membrane, its thickness, and surface area. In peritoneal dialysis the peritoneal membrane ("dialyzer") surface area, thickness, pore size and density, as well as blood flow are given by nature and the efficiency of the "dialyzer" needs to be found to adjust time of dialysis and dose of dialysis solution.

In an unabridged test, the peritoneal transfer rates of urea, creatinine, glucose, protein, potassium, and sodium as well as drain and residual volumes were measured during a 4 hour dwell exchange with 2 liters of 2.5% Dianeal® solution. Excellent reproducibility was seen after tests were standardized for length of preceding exchange, inflow volume, inflow position, inflow rate, dwell time, dwell position, drain time, drain position, methods of obtaining and processing samples, and laboratory assays. Wide variations of the results were found in the study population. Drain volume after a 4 hour dwell, the dialysate to plasma ratio of creatinine at 2 and 4 hours of dwell time, as well as the ratio of dialysate glucose at 2 and 4 hours of dwell time to dialysate glucose at 0 dwell time proved to be most valuable for prognostic and diagnostic purposes (51, 52). As the consequence of several years' experience with the results of the unabridged equilibration test, a simplified, abridged, equilibration test was developed (53).

To achieve a satisfactory reproducibility of results, the procedure must be standardized including the exchange preceding the equilibration test. According to the protocol, the preceding exchange must dwell for 8-12 hrs. This pre-test exchange is completely drained over 20 min in the vertical position and 2 liters of 2.5% dialysis solution (Dianeal® 2.5%) is infused at a rate of 400 ml per 2 min over a total of 10 min. The patient is in the supine position during infusion and rolls from side to side after each 400 ml is infused for better mixing of residual volume and infused solution. Exactly 10 min after the start of infusion, at the completion of infusion (0 dwell time), 200 ml of solution is drained into the bag, mixed well, a 10 ml sample of dialysate is taken and the remaining 190 ml reinfused. The patient is ambulatory during the dwell period. After 120 min of dwell time, a sample of dialysate is taken with the same technique as at 0 dwell time and a blood sample is obtained. After a 4 hr dwell time, the dialysate is drained over 20 min with the patient in the vertical position, total volume is measured and a sample taken. The total time of the equilibration exchange is 270 min.

Concentrations of creatinine and glucose are measured in the dialysate and blood samples. Chemistries should best be run immediately after samples are taken or within a few days for refrigerated samples. If dialysate is frozen, the samples have to be thoroughly thawed, preferably at 37°C for at least 2 hrs and very well mixed before runs. Glucose interferes with the Jaffe reagent for creatinine, thus creatinine values in dialysate are overestimated and are adjusted downward from the falsely high values. Omitting this adjustment will result only in a modest error (about 6%) in the D/P creatinine ratio at 4 hours. However, to compare the results to those we have reported or to use the D/P creatinine ratio for determination for dialysis clearance values with short dwell exchanges, the adjustment for glucose is recommended. The exact adjustment for glucose will undoubtedly vary between laboratories since many methods of creatinine determination are in use.

In our laboratory, when we used ABA 200 Bichromatic Analyzer, Abbott, the adjustment was 0.053 mg/dl of creatinine for each 100 mg/dl glucose; now, we use Perspective Analyzer, American Monitor, and the adjustment is 0.033 mg/dl for each 100 mg/dl glucose.

A simple method of determining the correction factor is to have the glucose and creatinine measured on an aliquot of fresh bag of 2.5% dextrose dialysis solution. Dividing the creatinine value obtained by the measured glucose value provides an approximate adjustment assuming, as we have found, a linear relationship between dialysate glucose level and the extent of the false elevation in creatinine.

Even the abridged protocol is designed to provide a maximal level of reproducibility, accuracy, and internal control. However, the PET protocol is still labor intensive, requiring measurement of glucose and creatinine in 3 dialysate samples and in one blood sample.

Therefore, a further simplification of the PET was established by using only one dialysate sample for glucose and creatinine from the total drained dialysate after 4 hour dwell and a blood sample taken at the end of the test exchange - the Fast PET (FPET) (54). After an overnight dwell of 8-12 hours, the patient is instructed to drain completely over at least 20 min while in the upright position, then infuse 2 liters of 2.5% dextrose dialysis solution over ten minutes. The exact time infusion ends should be noted. The patient then arranges to be at the dialysis center in sufficient time to allow supervision of the complete draining of the abdomen over 20 min in the upright position starting exactly four hours after inflow ended. The volume of drained dialysate is measured and an aliquot sent for glucose and creatinine determinations. A blood sample is obtained for creatinine and glucose measurement (and other laboratory tests, as indicated). The laboratory phase is the similar to that for an abridged test. Glucose should be measured with the hexokinase method preferably. The ratio of dialysate to plasma (D/P) creatinine is calculated; glucose is reported as a concentration.

In our center we prefer the abridged test because it is more reliable as performed by nurses in the center, whereas the Fast PET relies on the patients' strict adherence to the protocol. A baseline test is performed soon after patients begin CAPD and the test is repeated as needed for diagnostic purposes. Results are compared to those in Table 1.

Table 1. Transport categorization according to abridged PET (APET) and Fast PET (FPET) results.

Transport Classification	Dialysate glucose 2 hr/0 hr	Dialysate glucose 4 hr/0 hr	Dialysate/ plasma creatinine after 2 hr	Dialysate/ plasma creatinine after 4 hr	Drain volume after 4 hr (ml)	Dialysate glucose after 4 hr (mg/dl)
	APET	APET	APET	APET FPET	APET FPET	FPET
Low	0.78-0.67	0.61-0.50	0.23-0.34	0.34-0.49	2651-3326	945-1214
Low Average	0.66-0.56	0.49-0.39	0.35-0.47	0.50-0.64	2369-2650	724-944
Mean	0.55	0.38	0.48	0.65	2368	723
High Average	0.54-0.44	0.37-0.26	0.49-0.62	0.66-0.81	2085-2367	502-722
High	0.43-0.24	0.25-0.12	0.63-0.87	0.82-1.03	1580-2084	230-501

PET = Peritoneal Equilibration Test

If the test is performed properly, the values for glucose, creatinine, and drain volume should fall within the same or neighboring category.

In diabetics with high serum glucose levels (>300 mg/dl), the results of glucose equilibration and drain volume are not useful for patient categorization and inconsistent with creatinine values.

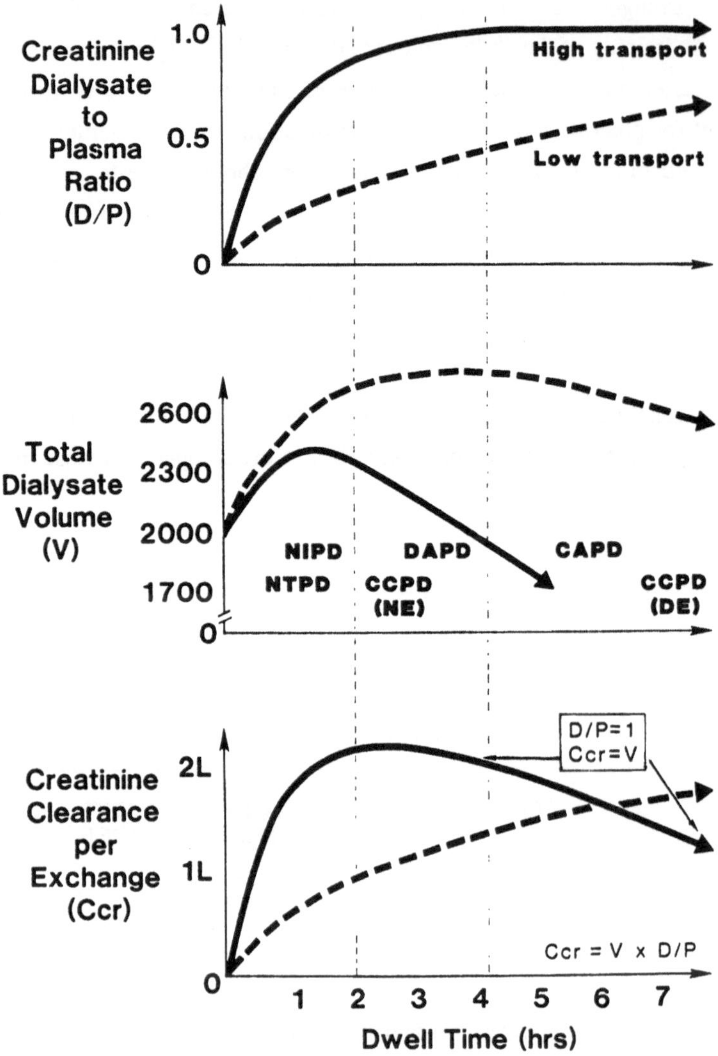

Figure 1. Idealized curves of creatinine and water transport during exchange with 2 liters of 2.5% glucose dialysis solution in patients with extremely low and high peritoneal transport characteristics. Upper panel shows dialysate to plasma ratio (D/P), middle panel total dialysate volume (V), which is the sum of infusion volume and ultrafiltration, and lower panel creatinine clearance per exchange (Ccr). The curves in the lower panel are derived from those of the upper and middle panels. NIPD - nightly intermittent peritoneal dialysis - and NTPD - nightly tidal peritoneal dialysis - utilize short dwell exchange and are more suitable for high peritoneal transport patients. CAPD - continuous ambulatory peritoneal dialysis - and CCPD(DE) - diurnal exchanges of continuous cyclic peritoneal dialysis - utilize long dwell exchanges and are more suitable for low peritoneal transport patients. DAPD - daytime ambulatory peritoneal dialysis - and CCPD(NE) - nocturnal exchanges of continuous cyclic peritoneal dialysis - usually operate within an intermediate range of dwell times (2-4 hours) and are also suitable for patients with high peritoneal solute transport rates. Diurnal exchanges (DE) of CCPD are not suitable for patients with high transport rates (Reproduced with permission from: Twardowski ZJ: Nightly peritoneal dialysis (why? who? how? and when?). ASAIO Transactions, 36: 8-16, 1990) (55).

Table 2 Choice of dialysis prescription depending on the baseline PET results in patients with well functioning catheter after break-in.

Peritoneal solute transport	Drain volume	Predicted long term response to standard dose CAPD[1] or CCPD[2] after loss of residual renal functions		Preferred dialysis prescription after loss of residual renal functions
		Ultrafiltration	Dialysis	
High	Low	Poor	Adequate	DAPD[3], NIPD[4], NTPD[5]
High average	Low average	Adequate	Adequate	Standard dose PD[6]
Low average	High average	Good	Adequate or inadequate[7]	Standard dose PD[6] High dose PD[8]
Low	High	Excellent	Inadequate	High dose PD[8] or hemodialysis[9]

[1] CAPD = Continuous ambulatory peritoneal dialysis.
[2] CCPD = Continuous cyclic peritoneal dialysis.
[3] DAPD = Daytime (diurnal) ambulatory peritoneal dialysis = peritoneal dialysis performed only during daytime using 3-4 exchanges.
[4] NIPD = Nightly (nocturnal) intermittent peritoneal dialysis = Intermittent peritoneal dialysis performed every night for 8-12 hours using 10.0-20.0 liters of dialysis solution (the higher the peritoneal transport rate the shorter time of dialysis is required for adequate clearances).
[5] NTPD = Nightly tidal peritoneal dialysis = periodic peritoneal dialysis performed every night with tidal flow technique for 8-12 hours using 15-35 liters of dialysis solution. Time of dialysis sessions have much greater influence on clearances than the dose of dialysis solution.
[6] Standard dose PD = standard dose CAPD or CCPD.
Standard dose CAPD = CAPD with 7.5-9.0 liters of dialysis solution used per 24 hours.
Standard dose CCPD = CCPD with 6.0-8.0 liters of dialysis solution used overnight and 2.0 liters daytime.
[7] Inadequate dialysis likely in patients with body surface area >2.00 m^2.
[8] High dose PD = high dose CAPD or CCPD.
High dose CAPD = CAPD with >9.0 liters of dialysis solution used per 24 hours.
High dose CCPD = CCPD with >8.0 liters of dialysis solution used overnight and/or >2.0 liters daytime.
[9] Hemodialysis may be needed in patients with body surface area >2.00 m^2.

ULTRAFILTRATION AND CLEARANCE PATTERNS IN RELATION TO SOLUTE TRANSPORT

Figure 1 portrays creatinine dialysate to plasma ratios, dialysate volumes, and creatinine clearances (Ccr) versus dwell time in patients with extremely low and high transport rates using dialysis solution with a 2.5% glucose concentration. In patients with low transport rates, peak ultrafiltration occurs late during dwell time and net ultrafiltration is still obtained after a long dwell time. Also, D/P ratios increase almost linearly during the dwell; consequently clearances per exchange also increase almost linearly throughout the long dwell exchange. In these patients time of dialysis is crucial for adequate clearances and they benefit from continuous regimens such as CAPD or CCPD with diurnal exchanges. Because of a well maintained dialysate/plasma concentration gradient for an extended period during dwell, clearances per unit time are augmented relatively little by rapid exchange techniques such as IPD or TPD. Consequently, intermittent techniques require long treatment times for adequate clearances. Conversely, patients with high peritoneal transport rates have poor ultrafiltration on standard CAPD with dwell times exceeding 4 hours. In these patients peak ultrafiltration occurs early during the dwell time and is followed by dialysate absorption. If dialysate is drained after a 4 hour dwell, there is minimal or no net ultrafiltration. Also, the mass transfer of small molecular weight solutes in long-dwell exchanges decreases proportionately with the reduction in drain volume. After several hours of dwell, the clearance per exchange is less than in patients with low peritoneal transport rates. Reducing the dwell time in patients with high transport rates captures maximum ultrafiltration while maintaining near complete equilibration of small molecular weight solutes and so increases net solute removal. These patients benefit from techniques utilizing rapid exchanges and may achieve adequate clearances with intermittent peritoneal dialysis regimens of relatively short duration. Patients with transport rates between these two extremes have intermediate patterns.

DIALYSIS PRESCRIPTION BASED ON THE EQUILIBRATION TEST

Table 2 summarizes the usefulness of the peritoneal equilibration test as a dialysis prescription guide. The patients with high peritoneal transport are ideal candidates for regimens with short dwell exchanges [Nightly Intermittent Peritoneal Dialysis (NIPD), Nightly Tidal Peritoneal Dialysis (NTPD), Daytime Ambulatory Peritoneal Dialysis (DAPD)]. The patients with high average transport are excellent candidates for any peritoneal dialysis prescription. Most patients with low average peritoneal transport can be maintained on the standard dose CAPD; however, many of them may require a modified prescription (high dose CAPD, high dose CCPD) when residual renal function becomes negligible, particularly if they have high body surface area. These patients have excellent ultrafiltration with moderate dialysis solution glucose concentrations.

Finally, patients with low peritoneal transport rates usually have excellent ultrafiltration with low dialysis solution glucose concentration and are very likely to develop symptoms of inadequate dialysis on standard CAPD when their residual renal function becomes negligible. These patients are not good candidates for regimens with short dwell exchanges.

Table 3. Formulas used to calculate solute (urea and creatinine) kinetic indices in peritoneal dialysis.

[1] $$Kt = Kt_p + Kt_r$$

where: Kt = total weekly solute clearance; Kt_p = weekly peritoneal solute clearance; Kt_r = weekly residual renal solute clearance

[2] $$Kt_p = (D/P \times Dvl) \times 7$$

where: D = solute concentration in total daily dialysate; P = solute plasma concentration; Dvl = daily dialysate volume

[3] $$Kt_r = (U/P \times Uvl) \times 7$$

where: U = solute concentration in total daily urine; Uvl = daily urine volume

[4] $$BSA(m)^2 = ht(m)^{0.725} \times wt(kg)^{0.425} \times 71.84$$

where: BSA = body surface area; ht = height; wt = weight

[5] $$V(l) = 9.787 + 27.4889 \times BSA(m^2) \text{ [males]}$$

[6] $$V(l) = 3.757 + 21.1104 \times BSA(m^2) \text{ [females]}$$

[7] $$V(l) = 2.447 - 1074 \times ht(m) + 0.3362 \times wt(kg) - 0.09516 \times Age(yr) \text{ [males]}$$

[8] $$V(l) = 2.097 - 10.69 \times ht(m) + 0.2466 \times wt(kg) \text{ [females]}$$

[9] $$V(l) = IBV(kg) \times 0.6 \text{ [males]}$$

[10] $$V(l) = IBV(kg) \times 0.55 \text{ [females]}$$

where: V = total body water (liters) = urea and/or creatinine distribution volume; IBW or ideal body weight was defined as the lowest weight at which the patient could be maintained without signs or symptoms indicative of volume depletion.

Formula [4] according to Du Bois and Du Bois (56), formulas [5] and [6] according to Humes and Wyers (57); formulas [7] and [8] according to Watson PE et al (58); formulas [9] and [10] according to Blake et al (59).

UREA KINETICS

With hemodialysis, traditional urea kinetics calculations are complex because of rapid changes in urea concentration during dialysis. Steady state BUN in CAPD renders these calculations easy.

Table 3 presents formulas used in urea kinetic calculations. Kt/V values may be reported as "hemodialysis equivalent" by dividing weekly value by 3. Even with CCPD and NPD, BUN is practically steady and the same formula may be used. It is important to have a complete collection of daily dialysate and urine.

Unlike hemodialysis, studies utilizing urea kinetics to predict outcome of peritoneal dialysis have provided conflicting results. First and foremost, the CAPD Kt/V values providing clinical results similar to hemodialysis are markedly lower.

Lysaght et al (60) compared urea Kt/V between hemodialysis and CAPD patients and found significantly lower values in the patients on CAPD despite similar clinical outcomes.

To explain this paradox, Keshaviah et al (61) proposed a peak concentration hypothesis. This hypothesis presumes that uremic toxicity is not dependent on average, but on peak urea concentrations. Invoking the single pool urea kinetic model and this hypothesis, they calculated that, to maintain the same peak BUN concentrations of 80 mg/dl, Kt/V of 2.6 in hemodialysis corresponds to 1.7 in CAPD.

Keshaviah et al (62) found a good correlation between the Kt/V urea index and protein catabolic rate (PCR) in 19 CAPD patients. There was also a correlation between clinical assessment of adequacy based on 12 parameter score and Kt/V urea in 74% of patients. Weekly Kt/V urea index below 1.2 was defined as inadequate, between 1.2 and 1.7 as marginal and over 1.7 as adequate.

Teehan et al (63) found that the Kt/V value was partially predictive for mortality and transfusion requirements and postulated, on theoretical grounds, the ideal weekly Kt/V of 2.29, but did not provide any clinical support for this value. Such a value would be difficult to achieve in the majority of anuric patients on CAPD.

Blake et al (59) found no predictive value of urea kinetics on clinical outcome. It appears that a higher Kt/V urea index is associated with better clinical condition of the patient; however, its correlation with mortality and morbidity has not yet been well documented.

If Kt/V is to be used as a measure of adequate prescription, the index has to be better standardized.

In one of my male patients with clinically adequate dialysis, urea clearances (Kt) from the same dialysate and urine collection, measured with 3 different instruments in 3 different laboratories, gave values from 71 - 78 liters/wk. Using 3 different formulas for estimation of total body water, the calculated Kt/V urea index ranged from 1.61-1.98. This exercise supports the notion that all reported values have to be taken with caution because the authors use a variety of instruments to measure solute concentrations and a variety of formulas to calculate Kt/V.

Teehan et al (63) included only patients with urea D/P ratio of 1.0 ± 0.1 in total daily dialysate (a ratio not attainable by a sizeable group of patients) and did not report their method of total body water calculation.

Others use various formulas shown in Table 3. Gotch (64) used formulas [5] and [6], Keshaviah et al used formulas [7] and [8], and Blake et al (59) used formulas [9] and [10].

CREATININE KINETICS

For adequate intermittent peritoneal dialysis, Boen et al (65) postulated a combined Ccr of 5.5 ml/min (7.92 liters/day, or 55.44 liters/wk) in a standard patient with body surface area (BSA) of 1.73 m^2. Our personal clinical experience (33) indicated that patients fulfilling criteria of adequate dialysis have at least a combined Ccr of 4.0 - 5.0 ml/min/1.73 m^2 (5.8 - 7.2 liters/day; 40 - 50 liters/wk). These values were derived by comparisons of dialysis adequacy clinical assessments with clearance measurements during several studies related to the efficiency of various peritoneal dialysis regimens and techniques (66-69). These were minimal values found in anuric patients fulfilling clinical criteria of dialysis adequacy. It is important to realize that not all patients require the same Ccr to achieve adequate dialysis. Body metabolic rates depend not only on protein intake but also on intrinsic variability characteristic of all living creatures, including humans. In animals of various sizes, basal metabolic rates per unit of body weight are higher in small animals, where body surface area to body mass ratios are higher. To satisfy energy demand, small animals, such as hummingbirds or shrews, have to consume the amount of food equal to or exceeding their body weights per day. This is in distinct contrast from large birds and/or mammals. Although the differences in metabolic rates in humans are not that large, there is a definitive variability. Metabolic rate variability depends also on differences in endocrine function (thyroid, parathyroid, adrenals) and central nervous system function; there may be other factors. Thus, some patients may require weekly Ccr of more than 50 liters/1.73 m^2 BSA, others may achieve clinically adequate dialysis with that of 40 liters/1.73 m^2 BSA or even less.

The contribution of residual renal Ccr to clinical status of the patient is important but is not an equivalent of the peritoneal clearance. This is not surprising because otherwise the patients with endogenous Ccr of 4 - 5 ml/min (40 - 50 liters/wk) per 1.73 m^2 BSA would not require commencement of peritoneal dialysis; however, it is a well established practice to start peritoneal (or hemodialysis) with Ccr slightly below 10 ml/min/1.73 m^2 BSA and in patients with diabetic nephropathy even markedly over 10 ml/min/1.73 m^2 BSA. One of the reasons is that creatinine is secreted in tubules and Ccr does not reflect true glomerular filtration rate. An even more important reason is that peritoneal clearance of 40 liters/wk is capable of correcting water, electrolyte, and acid/base disturbances, which poorly functional kidneys are not able to do, and which must be corrected to achieve adequate dialysis. It seems that the residual renal Ccr should be counted as 1/4-1/2 of peritoneal clearance. Ccr measurements seem to be more consistent than urea Kt/V because creatinine concentrations show less variability with various instruments.

Moreover, body surface area is calculated almost exclusively using formula [4]. Combined Ccr from the same collection as for Kt/V ranged only from 39.4-39.6 liters/wk/1.73 m^2 BSA.

Table 4. Formulas used to calculate efficacy number.

[11]
$$EN = {}^{cr}(D/P) \times \frac{V_{24}}{ACP_{PD}}$$

where: EN = efficacy number in l/g_{cr} (liters per gram of generated creatinine)
${}^{cr}(D/P)$ = creatinine dialysate to plasma ratio after 4 hour dwell
V_{24} = volume of prescribed exchanges in l/day
ACP_{PD} = adjusted creatinine production in g/day

[12]
$$ACP_{PD} = \frac{(D_{cr} \times V \times 6) + (0.4 \times S_{cr} \times LBW)}{1000}$$

where: D_{cr} = dialysate creatinine concentration in mg/dl at 4 hour dwell
V = dialysate volume after 4 hour dwell in dl
0.4 = constant extra renal clearance in dl/kg/day
S_{cr} = serum creatinine in mg/dl
LBW = lean body weight in kg

EFFICACY NUMBER (EN)

Brandes et al (70) introduced the efficacy number (EN) as a simple method to determine the amount of dialysis. This number represents a volume of dialysate per mass of generated creatinine.

Table 4 presents the formulas used in calculations.

Although the formula [11] does not include "urine" Ccr, such a correction can be made (70).

In the preliminary study, the authors found better clinical outcome as judged by uremic symptoms, hospitalizations, mortality, laboratory tests and transfer to hemodialysis with improvement in symptoms in patients with EN of 5.75 liters/g_{cr} or higher as compared to those with EN of 4.53 liters/g_{cr} or less (70). In a follow-up study the same group found that EN, normalized Ccr, and Kt/V urea correlated well with clinical outcomes (71).

In CAPD patients, good clinical outcomes were found with Ccr greater than 40-50 liters/wk/1.73 m^2 BSA, Kt/V over 1.7-1.8, and EN over 5.5 liters/g_{cr}.

WEEKLY CLEARANCES OF UREA AND CREATININE WITH LONG AND SHORT DWELL EXCHANGES

Urea equilibrates faster than creatinine so that the D/P creatinine to D/P urea ratio is lowest early during the dwell and increases with dwell time.

In the peritoneal equilibration study, the mean D/P creatinine after 1 hr dwell was 0.35 and the D/P urea was 0.55, thus the ratio of the ratios was 0.35/0.55 = 0.64. After 4 hour dwell the ratio reached 0.65/0.91 = 0.71 (51, 52).

In another study the ratio after 6 hr reached 0.65/0.91 = 0.77 and 0.87/1.0 = 0.87 after 12 hr (16).

Because weekly creatinine to urea clearance ratio is equal to the ratio of D/P creatinine divided by D/P urea (time and volume terms cancel out), then the main determinant of clearance ratios is also dwell time (72). This relationship should be kept in mind while switching a patient from CAPD or CCPD to NIPD or NTPD and *vice versa*. If after changing from CAPD to NIPD the same weekly Kt/V urea is preserved, then, depending on the transport rate on PET, weekly Ccr will decrease by approximately 15-25%; maintaining the same Ccr will increase Kt/V by approximately 20-30%. Lower Ccr is associated with lower clearances of substances with molecular size similar to creatinine; higher urea clearance is not harmful.

In our studies of tidal peritoneal dialysis on anuric patients, we elected to maintain Ccr while switching from CAPD to TPD and the mean urea clearance increased by 20% (67-69).

It seems safer, while switching from continuous (long dwell exchange) regimen to intermitted (short dwell exchange) regimen, to maintain the same Ccr and increase Kt/V urea instead of maintaining the same urea clearance and lowering Ccr.

PET VERSUS CLEARANCES FOR DETERMINING PERITONEAL DIALYSIS PRESCRIPTIONS

The PET is a simple and useful guide in choosing dialysis prescription in the majority of patients; however, it cannot replace clearance measurements. On the other hand, clearance alone is insufficient as a guide for choosing regimen and technique (intermittent vs continuous, short vs long dwell exchanges).

Moreover, PET is very useful in diagnosis of causes of insufficient dialysis or ultrafiltration (53). The PET and clearance measurements are complementary guides in dialysis prescription.

CHOICE OF PERITONEAL DIALYSIS

CAPD is the most popular regimen because of adequate clearances and ultrafiltration rates in the majority of patients, convenience, and low cost. On the other hand, the number of patients using automated peritoneal dialysis (CCPD, NIPD, and NTPD) is growing faster than that of CAPD. Table 5 provides the most important features of currently used peritoneal dialysis therapies.

Continuous cyclic peritoneal dialysis (CCPD)

The advantages of CCPD include (73):

[a] uninterrupted daytime activities;

[b] simplicity of adjusting a dialysis prescription contingent on the required efficiency by modifying the number of nightly exchanges; and

[c] a decreased burden on the partner, if one is required, because all technical assistance take place early in the morning and late in the evening.

Indications to CCPD are based on these advantages.

I consider CCPD particularly useful for medical reasons in patients with below normal peritoneal membrane permeability or area who are underdialyzed on CAPD even with five 2 liter exchanges per day and unable to use high volume exchanges. High overnight dialysate flow combined with two or even three exchanges per day provide adequate dialysis in these patients. The previously reported advantage of lower peritonitis rates on CCPD compared to CAPD (74) was made obsolete by current wide spread use of Y-set for CAPD. Psycho-social circumstances constitute an important incentive to CCPD instead of CAPD (75, 76). School children and employed patients frequently are unable or unwilling to perform exchanges during the day. When a partner is necessary, the convenience of CCPD becomes particularly attractive. Parents dialyzing children or relatives dialyzing elderly and debilitated patients usually prefer CCPD over CAPD. The compliance with a prescribed dialysis schedule seems to be improved on CCPD.

The main disadvantage of CCPD, reflected by the lower popularity compared to CAPD, is the higher cost of CCPD.

Travel is difficult with CCPD because of the need to transport a cycler; however, if CCPD is chosen because of psycho-social reasons, CAPD may be performed during travel and vacation.

For most patients CAPD is still more attractive because it does not require machines and there are no sleep interruptions related to machine alarms.

Table 5. Characteristics of CAPD, CCPD, DAPD, NIPD, and NTPD in adults (compiled on the basis of data from references # 16, 21-23, 51, 52, 55, 66-69, 72, 77-79).

	CAPD	CCPD	DAPD	NIPD	NTPD
Regimen	Continuous	Continuous	Intermittent	Intermittent	Intermittent
Flow technique	Intermittent	Intermittent	Intermittent	Intermittent	Tidal
Method	Manual	Automated	Manual	Automated	Automated
Interrupted day	Yes	No or Yes	Yes	No	No
Interrupted night with possible alarms	No	Yes	No	Yes	Yes
Helper convenience	No	Yes or No	No	Yes	Yes
Travel convenience	Yes	No	Yes	No	No
Intraabdominal pressure with fluid	High	High	High	Low	Low
Leaks/hernias	Common	Common	Common	Rare	Rare
Night (hr/24 hr)	8-10	8-10	0	8-12	8-11
Night (number of exchanges)	1	4-8	0	4-10	10-30
Night (exchange volume-l)	1.5-3.0	1.0-2.0	0	1.0-2.0	1.0-1.5
Night (reserve volume-l)	0	0	0	0	1.0-1.5
Daytime (hr/24 hr)	14-16	14-16	14-16	0	0
Daytime (exchange volume-l)	1.5-3.0	1.5-3.0	1.5-3.0	0	0
Daytime (number of exchanges)	3-4	1-3	3-4	0	0
Total volume (l/24 hr)	6.0-12.0	10.0-20.0	6.0-9.0	10.0-20.0	15.0-38.0
Preferred transport category	Average/low	Average/low	High	High/average	High/average
Glucose absorption/UF (g/l)	60-160	50-150	80-120	30-70	50-90
Na removal/UF (mEq/l)*	120-140	80-130	120-140	20-90	30-100
Blood pressure control	Easy	Easy	Easy	Less easy	Less easy
Preferred solution Na (mEq/l)	132	132	132	126-132	120-132
Minimum adequate Ccr ($l/wk/1.73\ m^2$)	40-50	40-50	40-50	40-50	40-50
Minimum adequate weekly Kt/V	1.4-1.7	1.5-1.8	1.6-1.9	1.8-2.2	1.8-2.2

° CAPD = Continuous ambulatory peritoneal dialysis. CCPD = Continuous cyclic peritoneal dialysis. DAPD = Daytime (diurnal) ambulatory peritoneal dialysis. NIPD = Nightly (nocturnal) intermittent peritoneal dialysis. NTPD = Nightly tidal peritoneal dialysis.

* with dialysis solution sodium concentration of 132 mEq/l.

Daytime (diurnal) ambulatory peritoneal dialysis (DAPD)

This is an intermittent regimen performed during the daytime. This regimen is suitable only for high peritoneal solute transport patients who do not want to be treated with nocturnal peritoneal dialysis but because of rapid glucose absorption cannot achieve adequate ultrafiltration on continuous regimens.

Nightly peritoneal dialysis (NPD)

NPD is an intermittent peritoneal dialysis performed every night or may be considered as CCPD without long dwell daytime exchanges. NPD was introduced in patients with recurrent abdominal leaks and hernias, bladder prolapse, rapid glucose absorption resulting in poor ultrafiltration on CAPD, abdominal discomfort, chronic hypotension, and patient preference (21, 55). NPD is the best choice in patients with: [a] complications related to elevated intraabdominal pressure and who cannot be on hemodialysis and [b] high peritoneal transport rates resulting in poor ultrafiltration on CAPD or CCPD and excellent dialysis efficiency on NPD (Figure 1).

NIPD treatments are performed overnight on a PD cycler with 1.5 to 2 liter fill volumes of commercial peritoneal dialysis solutions. Total dialysis time ranges from 8 to 12 hours per night (56-84 hrs/wk). A total volume of used dialysis solution per dialysis ranges from 8-20 liters (56-140 liters/wk). The time of dialysis and dialysate dose are adjusted according to the patient's peritoneal solute transport rate. The higher the transport rate, the shorter the time of sessions and lower the volume of dialysis solution used per treatment. Drain time is restricted to 12-15 minutes (1 min for 120 - 170 ml) to minimize the period when the peritoneal cavity is almost empty and dialysis efficiency is markedly reduced. If a low drain alarm is triggered during the initial one or two exchanges, the patients are instructed not to prolong drain time but to bypass cycles and thus create some sump volume in the peritoneal cavity. Low drain alarms usually do not occur during third or later cycles, unless the extension tubing is occluded. The principle of restricted outflow time to increase efficiency is fully optimized in a tidal peritoneal dialysis technique (NTPD). Tidal flow technique yields about 20% higher clearances compared to intermittent flow technique only with high dose of dialysis solution (67-69). Although the NTPD efficiency is not significantly higher compared to NIPD with usual dose of 8-20 liters per session, tidal technique is becoming popular because of better flow mechanics and comfort. The constant presence of a reserve volume allows for faster flow and less alarms, even with catheter tip outside the true pelvis. Also, patients with infusion pain, while using intermittent flow technique, have less discomfort on TPD.

The main disadvantages of NPD are bed confinement during treatment and the need for a cycler. In patients with low peritoneal transport rates, the duration of the dialysis session may be excessively long. In such patients the cost of dialysis is markedly higher than that of CAPD. The patients with low peritoneal solute transport may have inadequate sodium balance resulting in thirst and poor blood pressure control. This is due to the low sodium concentration in ultrafiltrate resulting from solute sieving (80). Convective net removal of sodium per liter of ultrafiltrate is usually well below extracellular fluid concentration. Thus, dialysate sodium concentration is initially reduced due to solute sieving with ultrafiltration and tends to increase later in the dwell time due to diffusion and diminished ultrafiltration rate. Dialysate sodium concentration decreases more in patients with low peritoneal solute transport (51, 52). Most NPD patients use dialysis solution with a standard sodium concentration of 132 mEq/l. In a few patients a sodium concentration of 120 - 126 mEq/l is used. For this purpose 5% glucose solution (D5W) is mixed with peritoneal dialysis solution in an appropriate proportion to achieve the desired sodium concentration (55).

STEPWISE APPROACH TO PD PRESCRIPTION

CAPD with four 2 liter exchanges is the most common initial prescription. In patients with well preserved residual renal function (Ccr >5.0 ml/min) a total dialysis solution inflow may be decreased to below 7.5 liters per day. Peritoneal equilibration test is recommended to serve as a prognosticator of a patient's response to various peritoneal dialysis regimens. The patient should be followed closely and the prescription should be modified when the residual renal function becomes negligible and/or criteria of adequate dialysis are not fulfilled. Although *a priori* criteria still remain a "gold standard", clearance measurements, despite of their drawbacks, are helpful in integrated assessment of dialysis adequacy. For example, in a patient with nausea, poor appetite, dysgeusia, and/or insomnia, a weekly Ccr under 40 liters/1.73 m^2 BSA or Kt/V less than 1.4 strongly support a diagnosis of inadequate dialysis, whereas the same symptoms in a CAPD patient with weekly Ccr over 50 liters/1.73 m^2 BSA or Kt/V more than 1.7 suggest other etiology, such as drug toxicity, depression, and/or peptic ulcer. However, if other etiology is not confirmed, a higher dose of dialysis is recommended. All peritoneal dialysis regimens, techniques, and methods should be offered and the patients switched among them as needs arise.

REFERENCES

1. Boen ST, Mulinari AS, Dillard DH, Scribner BH: Periodic peritoneal dialysis in the management of chronic uremia. Trans Am Soc Artif Intern Organs, 8: 256-262, 1962.
2. Tenckhoff H, Schechter H: A bacteriologically safe peritoneal access device. Trans Am Soc Artif Intern Organs, 14: 181-186, 1968.
3. Tenckhoff H, Shilipetar G, Van Paasschen WH, Swanson E: A home peritoneal dialysate delivery system. Trans Am Soc Artif Intern Organs, 15: 103-107, 1969.
4. Popovich RP, Moncrief JW, Decherd JF, Bomar JB, Pyle WK: The definition of a novel portable/wearable equilibrium dialysis technique. Am Soc Artif Intern Organs, 5: 64A, 1976 (Abstract).
5. Gotch FA, Sargent JA, Keen M, Prowitt M, Grady M: Solute kinetics in intermittent dialysis therapy. Proc Annu Contractor's Conf Artif Kidney-Chronic Uremia Prog (NIAMDD), 9: 98, 1976.
6. Popovich RP, Moncrief JW, Nolph KD, Ghods AJ, Twardowski ZJ, Pyle WK: Continuous ambulatory peritoneal dialysis. Ann Intern Med, 88: 449-456, 1978.

7. Oreopoulos DG, Robson M, Izatt S, Clayton S, de Veber CA: A simple and safe technique for continuous ambulatory peritoneal dialysis. Trans Am Soc Artif Intern Organs, 24: 484-489, 1978.
8. Smeby LC, Wideroe TE, Jorstad S: Individual differences in water transport during continuous peritoneal dialysis. ASAIO, J 4: 17-27, 1981.
9. Slingeneyer A, Canaud B, Mion C: Permanent loss of ultrafiltration capacity of the peritoneum in long-term peritoneal dialysis: An epidemiological study. Nephron, 33: 133-138, 1983.
10. Smeby LC, Wideroe TE, Mjaaland S, Dahl K: Changes in ultrafiltration and solute transport during CAPD. In: "Frontiers in Peritoneal Dialysis" (Eds JF Maher, JF Winchester), Field Rich and Associates Inc., New York, 1986, pp 68-74.
11. Spencer PC, Farrell PC: Solute and water kinetics in CAPD. In "Continuous Ambulatory Peritoneal Dialysis" (Ed R Gokal), Churchill Livingstone, Edinburgh, 1986, pp 38-55.
12. Verger C, Larpent L, Dumontet M: Prognostic value of peritoneal equilibration curves in CAPD patients. In: "Frontiers in Peritoneal Dialysis" (Ed JF Maher, JF Winchester), Field Rich and Associates Inc, New York, 1986, pp 88-93.
13. Ahmad S, Gallagher N, Shen FH: Intermittent peritoneal dialysis: Status reassessed. Trans Am Soc Artif Intern Organs, 25: 86-88, 1979.
14. Ghantous WN, Salkin MS, Adelson BN, Ghantous S, McGinnis K, Valenziano A, Cronin M: Limitations of peritoneal dialysis (PD) in the treatment of ESRD patients. Trans Am Soc Artif Intern Organs, 25: 100-103, 1979.
15. Schmidt RW, Blumenkrantz MJ: IPD, CAPD, CCPD, CRPD - Peritoneal dialysis: Past, present and future. Int J Artif Organs, 4: 124-129, 1981.
16. Twardowski ZJ: Individualized dialysis for CAPD patients. Uremia Invest, 8:35-43, 1984.
17. Scribner BH: A current perspective on the role of intermittent vs continuous ambulatory peritoneal dialysis. Proc NE Regional Meeting of Renal Physicians Assoc, 3: 76-81, 1979.
18. Diaz-Buxo JA, Walker PJ, Farmer CD, Chandler JP, Holt KR: Continuous cyclic peritoneal dialysis - a preliminary report. Artif Organs, 5: 157-161, 1981.
19. Diaz-Buxo JA, Walker PJ, Farmer DF, Chandler JT, Holt KL, Cox P: Continuous cyclic peritoneal dialysis. Trans Am Soc Artif Intern Organs, 27: 51-53, 1981.
20. Price CG, Suki WN: Newer modifications of peritoneal dialysis: options in the treatment of patients with renal failure. Am J Nephrol, 1: 97-104, 1981.
21. Twardowski ZJ, Nolph KD, Khanna R, Gluck Z, Prowant BF, Ryan LP: Daily clearances with continuous ambulatory peritoneal dialysis and nightly peritoneal dialysis. Trans Am Soc Artif Intern Organs, 32: 575-580, 1986.
22. Twardowski ZJ: Peritoneal dialysis glossary. II. Perit Dial Int, 8: 15-17, 1988.
23. Twardowski ZJ: Peritoneal dialysis glossary. III. Perit Dial Int, 10: 173-175, 1990.
24. Pendras JP, Erickson RV: Hemodialysis: A successful therapy for chronic uremia. Ann Intern Med, 64: 293-311, 1966.
25. De Palma JR, Abukurah A, Rubini ME: "Adequacy" of haemodialysis. Proc Europ Dial Transplant Assoc, 9: 265-270, 1972.
26. Twardowski Z: The adequacy of haemodialysis in treatment of chronic renal failure. Acta Med Pol, 15: 227-243, 1974.
27. Parker TF, Laird NM, Lowrie EG: Comparison of the study groups in the National Cooperative Dialysis Study and a description of morbidity, mortality, and patient withdrawal. Kidney Int, 23 (Suppl 13): S-42-S-49, 1983.
28. Gotch F, Sargent JA: A mechanistic analysis of the National Cooperative dialysis study (NCDS) Kidney Int, 28: 526-534, 1985.
29. Held PJ, Levin NW, Bovbierg RR, Pauly MV, Diamond LH: Mortality and duration of hemodialysis treatment. JAMA, 265: 871-875, 1991.
30. Charra B, Calemard E, Chazot C, Terrat JC, Vanel T, Ruffet M, Laurent G: Survival as an index of adequacy of dialysis. J Amer Soc Nephrol, 1: 351, 1991 (Abstract).
31. Shen F-H, Hsu K-T: Lower mortality and morbidity associated with higher Kt/V in hemodialysis patients. J Amer Soc Nephrol 1: 377, 1991 (Abstract).
32. Ahmad S, Cole JJ: Lower morbidity associated with higher Kt/V in stable hemodialysis patients. J Amer Soc Nephrol 1: 346, 1991 (Abstract).
33. Twardowski ZJ, Nolph KD: Opinion: Peritoneal dialysis - how much is enough? Seminars in Dialysis 1: 75-76, 1988.
34. Twardowski ZJ: PET - a simpler approach for determining prescriptions for adequate dialysis therapy. In: "Advances in Continuous Ambulatory Peritoneal Dialysis." Proceedings of the Tenth

Annual CAPD Conference, Dallas, Texas, February 1990. (Eds R Khanna, KD Nolph, BF Prowant, ZJ Twardowski, DG Oreopoulos) Peritoneal Dialysis Bulletin, Inc., Toronto, 1990, pp 186-191.
35. Odel HM, Ferris DO, Power MH: Peritoneal lavage as an effective means of extrarenal excretion. A clinical appraisal. Am J Med, 9: 63-77, 1950.
36. Maxwell MH, Rockney RE, Kleeman CR, Twiss MR: Peritoneal dialysis. I. Technique and applications. JAMA, 170: 917-924, 1959.
37. Boen ST: Kinetics of peritoneal dialysis. Medicine (Baltimore), 40: 243-287, 1961.
38. Frank HA, Seligman AM, Fine J: Further experiences with peritoneal irrigation for acute renal failure. Ann Surg, 128: 561-608, 1948.
39. Miller JH, Gipstein R, Margules R, Swartz M, Rubini ME: Automated peritoneal dialysis: Analysis of several methods of peritoneal dialysis. Trans Am Soc Artif Intern Organs, 12: 98-105, 1966.
40. Pirpasopoulos M, Lindsay RM, Rahman M, Kennedy AC: A cost-effectiveness study of dwell times in peritoneal dialysis. Lancet, 2: 1135-1136, 1972.
41. Kablitz C, Stephen RL, Duffy DP, Jacobsen SC, Zelman A, Kolff WJ: Technological augmentation of peritoneal urea clearance: past, present, and future. Dial Transpl, 9: 741-778, 1980.
42. Randerson DH: Continuous ambulatory peritoneal dialysis - A critical appraisal. PhD Thesis, University of New South Wales, Sydney, Australia, 1980.
43. Farrell PC, Randerson DH: Mass transfer kinetics in continuous ambulatory peritoneal dialysis. In: "Continuous Ambulatory Peritoneal Dialysis" (Ed M Legrain), Excerpta Medica, Amsterdam, 1980, pp 34-41.
44. Pyle WK: Mass Transfer in Peritoneal Dialysis. PhD Thesis, University of Texas, Austin, 1981.
45. Garred LJ, Canaud B, Farrell PC: A simple kinetic model for assessing peritoneal mass transfer in continuous ambulatory peritoneal dialysis. Am Soc Artif Intern Organs, J 6: 131-137, 1983.
46. Popovich RP, Moncrief JW, Pyle WK, Transport kinetics. In: "Peritoneal Dialysis." (Ed KD Nolph), Kluwer Academic Publishers, Dordrecht, Third Edition, 1989, pp 96-116.
47. Hiatt MP, Pyle WK, Moncrief JW, Popovich RP: A comparison of the relative efficacy of CAPD and hemodialysis in the control of solute concentration. Artificial Organs, 4: 37-43, 1980.
48. Mactier RA, Twardowski ZJ: Influence of dwell time, osmolality, and volume of exchanges on solute mass transfer and ultrafiltration in peritoneal dialysis. Seminar in Dialysis, 1: 40-49, 1988.
49. Mactier RA, Khanna R, Twardowski ZJ, Nolph KD: Role of peritoneal cavity lymphatic absorption in peritoneal dialysis. Kidney Int, 32: 165-172, 1987.
50. Mactier RA, Khanna R, Twardowski ZJ, Moore H, Nolph KD: Contribution of lymphatic absorption to loss of ultrafiltration and solute clearances in continuous ambulatory peritoneal dialysis. J Clin Invest, 80: 1311-1316, 1987.
51. Twardowski ZJ, Nolph KD, Khanna R, Prowant BF, Ryan LP, Moore HL, Nielsen MP: Peritoneal equilibration test. Perit Dial Bull, 7: 138-147, 1987.
52. Twardowski ZJ, Khanna R, Nolph KD: Peritoneal dialysis modifications to avoid CAPD dropouts. In: "Advances in Continuous Ambulatory Peritoneal Dialysis." Proceedings of the Seventh Annual CAPD Conference, Kansas City, Missouri, February 1987. (Eds R. Khanna, KD Nolph, BF Prowant, ZJ Twardowski, DG Oreopoulos) Perit Dial Bull Inc, Toronto, 1987, pp 171-178.
53. Twardowski ZJ: Clinical value of standardized equilibration tests in CAPD patients. Blood Purif, 7: 95-108, 1989.
54. Twardowski ZJ: The fast peritoneal equilibration test. Seminars in Dialysis, 3: 141-142, 1990.
55. Twardowski ZJ: Nightly peritoneal dialysis (why? who? how? and when?). ASAIO Transactions, 36: 8-16, 1990.
56. Du Bois D, Du Bois EF: A formula to estimate the approximate surface area if height and weight be known. Arch Int Med, 17: 863-871, 1916.
57. Hume R, Wyers E: Relationship between total body water and surface area in normal and obese subjects. J Clin Pathol, 24: 234-238, 1971.
58. Watson PE, Watson ID, Batt RD: Total body water volumes for adult males and females estimated from simple anthropometric measurements. Am J Clin Nutr, 33: 27-39, 1980.
59. Blake PG, Sombolos K, Abraham G, Weissgarten J, Pemberton R, Chu GL, Oreopoulos DG: Lack of correlation between urea kinetic indices and clinical outcomes in CAPD patients. Kidney Int, 39: 700-706, 1991.

60. Lysaght MJ, Pollock CA, Hallet MD, Ibels LS, Farrel PC: The relevance of urea kinetic modeling in CAPD. Trans Am Soc Artif Intern Organs, 35: 784-790, 1989.
61. Keshaviah PR, Nolph KD, Van Stone JC: The peak concentration hypothesis: A urea kinetic approach to comparing the adequacy of CAPD and hemodialysis. Perit Dial Int, 9: 257-260, 1989.
62. Keshaviah PR, Nolph KD, Prowant B, Moore H, Ponferrada L, Van Stone J, Twardowski ZJ, Khanna R: Defining adequacy of CAPD with urea kinetics. In: "Advances in Continuous Ambulatory Peritoneal Dialysis" Proceedings of the Tenth Annual CAPD Conference, Dallas, Texas, February 1990. (Eds R Khanna, KD Nolph, BF Prowant, ZJ Twardowski, DG Oreopoulos) Peritoneal Dialysis Bulletin, Inc., Toronto, 1990, pp 173-177.
63. Teehan BP, Schleifer CR, Brown JM, Sigler MH, Raimondo J: Urea kinetic analysis and clinical outcome on CAPD. A five year longitudinal study. In: "Advances in Continuous Ambulatory Peritoneal Dialysis." Proceedings of the Tenth Annual CAPD Conference, Dallas, Texas, February 1990. (Eds R Khanna, KD Nolph, BF Prowant, ZJ Twardowski, DG Oreopoulos) Peritoneal Dialysis Bulletin, Inc., Toronto, 1990, pp 181-185.
64. Gotch FA: Application of urea kinetic modeling to adequacy of CAPD therapy. In: "Advances in Continuous Ambulatory Peritoneal Dialysis." Proceedings of the Tenth Annual CAPD Conference, Dallas, Texas, February 1990. (Eds R Khanna, KD Nolph, BF Prowant, ZJ Twardowski, DG Oreopoulos) Peritoneal Dialysis Bulletin, Inc., Toronto, 1990, pp 178-180.
65. Boen ST, Haagsma-Schouten WAG, Birnie RJ: Long-term peritoneal dialysis and a peritoneal dialysis-index. Dial Transplant, 7: 377-380, 1978.
66. Twardowski ZJ, Nolph KD, Khanna R, Gluck Z, Prowant BF, Ryan LP: Daily clearances with continuous ambulatory peritoneal dialysis and nightly peritoneal dialysis. Trans Am Soc Artif Intern Organs, 32: 575-580, 1986.
67. Twardowski ZJ, Nolph KD, Khanna R, Prowant BF, Frock JT, Dobbie J, Kenley RS, Serkes KD, Witsoe DA, Garber JW: Tidal peritoneal dialysis. In: "Ambulatory Peritoneal Dialysis "- Proceedings of the IVth Congress of the International Society for Peritoneal Dialysis, Venice, Italy, June 29 - July 2, 1987, (Eds MM Avram, C Giordano) Plenum Publishing Corporation, New York, 1990, pp 145-149.
68. Twardowski ZJ, Prowant BF, Nolph KD, Khanna R, Schmidt LM, Satalowich RJ: Chronic nightly tidal peritoneal dialysis (NTPD). ASAIO Transactions, 36: M584-M588, 1990.
69. Twardowski ZJ: Tidal peritoneal dialysis - acute and chronic studies. European Dialysis and Transplant Nurses Association, European Renal Care Association. Journal XV, Sept 1990, pp 4-9.
70. Brandes JC, Piering WF, Beres JA: A method to assess efficacy of CAPD: Preliminary results. In: "Advances in Continuous Ambulatory Peritoneal Dialysis." Proceedings of the Tenth Annual CAPD Conference, Dallas, Texas, February 1990, (Eds R Khanna, KD Nolph, BF Prowant, ZJ Twardowski, DG Oreopoulos) Peritoneal Dialysis Bulletin, Inc., Toronto, 1990, pp 192-196.
71. Campbell D, Fritche C, Brandes J: A review of urea and creatinine kinetics in predicting CAPD outcome. In: "Advances in Continuous Ambulatory Peritoneal Dialysis." Proceedings of the Twelve Annual CAPD Conference, Seattle, WA, Febr 1992 (Eds R Khanna, KD Nolph, BF Prowant, ZJ Twardowski, DG Oreopoulos) Perit Dialysis Bulletin Inc., Toronto, 1992(in press).
72. Nolph KD, Twardowski ZJ, Keshaviah PR: Weekly clearances of urea and creatinine on CAPD and NIPD. Perit Dial Int, 12: 1992 (in press).
73. Diaz-Buxo JA: CCPD is even better than CAPD. Kidney Int, 28 (Suppl 17):S26-S28, 1985.
74. Diaz-Buxo JA: Incidence of peritonitis with CCPD. Perspectives Perit Dialysis, 3: 49-50, 1985.
75. Salusky IB, Davidson D, Hall T, Fine RN: Indications for CCPD in the child. Perspectives in Peritoneal Dialysis, 3: 48-48, 1985.
76. Nissenson AR: Indications for CCPD in the adult. Perspectives in Peritoneal Dialysis, 3: 46-47, 1985.
77. Twardowski Z, Ksiazek A, Majdan M, Janicka L, Bochenska-Nowacka E, Sokolowska G, Gutka A, Zbikowska H: Kinetics of continuous ambulatory peritoneal dialysis (CAPD) with four exchanges per day. Clin Nephrol, 15: 119-131, 1981.
78. Twardowski ZJ, Prowant BF, Nolph KD, Martinez AJ, Lampton LM: High volume, low frequency continuous ambulatory peritoneal dialysis. Kidney Int, 23: 64-70, 1983.
79. Twardowski ZJ, Khanna R, Nolph KD, Scalamogna A, Metzler MH, Schneider TW, Prowant BF, Ryan LP: Intraabdominal pressure during natural activities in patients treated with continuous ambulatory peritoneal dialysis. Nephron, 44: 129-135, 1986.
80. Nolph KD, Hano JE, Teschan PE: Peritoneal sodium transport during hypertonic peritoneal dialysis: Physiologic mechanisms and clinical implications. Ann Intern Med, 70: 931-941, 1969.

RENAL TRANSPLANTATION

Chapter 17

LIVING DONORS FOR RENAL TRANSPLANTATION: ETHICAL CONSIDERATIONS

PETER A. UBEL AND MARK SIEGLER

Department of Medicine, Center for Clinical Medical Ethics, University of Chicago, Chicago IL 60637-1470, USA

Living donor kidney transplantation occurs when a person willingly donates a kidney to a person in need. As such, it involves two values that medical ethicists look upon with great esteem: autonomy and altruism. Autonomy stands as one of the fundamental factors influencing ethical decisions. According to Beauchamp and Walters (1), the principle of autonomy can be formulated as follows: "Insofar as an autonomous agent's actions do not infringe on the autonomous actions of others, that person should be free to perform whatever action he or she wishes (presumably even if it involves considerable risk to himself or herself and even if others consider the action to be foolish)" (1). In medical ethics, this principle demands that health care providers either respect patient wishes or have very good reasons not to do so.

Altruism is also looked upon favorably by ethicists. Philosophers generally understand altruism as a counter to egoism, whereby altruistic actions are those actions that cannot be explained by self interest (2). Such actions are understood to be motivated not by concern for one's own interests, but by concern for others' interests. While many philosophers debate whether people can act without concern for their self-interest (3), most agree that if such altruistic acts exist, they are good things. Indeed, philosophers even have a special word for actions that are so good they go beyond the call of duty: supererogatory.

Wherever the boundary lies between dutiful action and supererogation, when a person autonomously volunteers to undergo the risks of a unilateral nephrectomy in order to donate a kidney to another person, that person has offered to do a morally laudable act. It seems that our respect for both altruism and autonomy would bow to this kind of action. Yet, despite the moral virtue of a person willing to donate a kidney to one in need, some transplant specialists question whether we should ever allow these people to donate

(4, 5). In what can only be understood as classic medical paternalism, they want to protect potential living donors from their own generosity.

This position should not be entirely surprising, because autonomy is not thought to extend so far that physicians must perform any procedure a patient demands (6). As Woodruff (7) stated in 1964: "The question is not whether the donor is right to offer to give up his kidney, but whether the doctor is right to allow him to do so". Physicians have a duty to determine whether a prospective donor should be allowed to donate.

In this chapter, we explore the ethical issues surrounding living donor renal transplantation. We argue that physicians have a legitimate right to refuse to accept kidneys from informed competent patients when they feel such actions would harm either the donor or recipient. We provide a framework for dealing with living donor renal transplantation that can maintain the delicate balance between protecting donors and respecting their autonomy. Finally, we discuss what physicians and ethicists should consider in deciding whether to accede to a living person's desire to donate a kidney to another person.

CHANGING VIEWS ON LIVE KIDNEY DONATION

Physicians deciding whether to use living kidney donors must consider at least five factors: [1] risks and benefits to the donor, [2] risks and benefits to the recipient, [3] possibility and validity of consent for donation, [4] issues regarding donor privacy and confidentiality and [5] best interests of society. Before discussing each of these factors, it will be helpful to see how their respective weights have changed over the last three decades.

Since patients began receiving living donor kidney transplants, changes in medical practice have created shifts in the procedure's acceptability. The first successful kidney transplant, in the mid 1950's, involved a genetically identical living donor (8). At that time, cadaver transplants were not a viable option, because there were no successful immunosuppressive regimens (9). Even when such regimens were developed (10), there were still compelling reasons to pursue living donor transplants: dialysis was scarce, and therefore recipients often needed kidney transplants to live (11). In addition, living donor transplants were significantly more likely to function one year after transplant than cadaver transplants (11). These undeniable recipient benefits were a great impetus for the start of living donor transplants.

Yet even under such favorable circumstances, some questioned the appropriateness of using living donors, because neither the risks nor benefits to the donor were known. The operative and long term risks of unilateral nephrectomy in healthy people had not been well studied. McGeown (11) argued that because donors could not possibly benefit from donating, such unknown risks could not be justified.

McGeown's concerns about risks and benefits to donors were alleviated in the early years of living donor kidney transplantation (12-17). Operative mortality and morbidity proved to be small - with an average of only one death in over 1500 operations and major temporary morbidity in 2-3% of donors (12-14, 18). In addition, McGeown's claim that there would be no donor benefits was proven wrong by psychological studies of donors (18-22).

With clear benefits to both donors and recipients and minimal risks to either, a strong case could be made throughout the 1970s for living donor kidney transplant. This case has weakened over the last 10-12 years. With the introduction of cyclosporine, cadaver kidney transplant has approached the success of living donor transplant (5). At the same time, the quality of life of dialysis patients is improving, both with refinement of dialysis techniques and with the introduction of new drugs like erythropoietin (23). Thus, the relative benefit of living donor transplant over both cadaver transplant and dialysis may have decreased. This has caused Starzl (5) to argue that "{I}f current trends continue, it may be hard to justify using living donors".

FACTORS RELEVANT TO APPROPRIATENESS OF LIVE DONATION

With Starzl's challenge in mind, we shall now look more closely at what issues one should consider to determine when living donation should be allowed. As listed above, there are at least five factors relevant to such a decision.

(1) Risks and benefits to the donors

If kidney donation carried no risk, few would debate the appropriateness of living donor transplant. But unlike practices such as blood donation, which carry little risk, kidney donation involves the risks of major surgery and the removal of an irreplaceable organ.

The most serious risk of kidney donation is death. Studies estimate that operative mortality in live kidney donation is approximately 1 death per 1600 nephrectomies (12, 24).

Others report on less serious operative complications. In a review of over 600 kidney donations at the University of Minnesota, 17% of donors were reported to experience at least minor surgical complications, but only 2.5% suffered serious complications (such as wound infection or pulmonary embolism) (14). In follow up, these patients experienced an 11.4% incidence of persistent incisional pain, but less than 1% had more than mild amounts of pain. There were no reports of death or renal failure associated with donation.

In other studies, researchers have examined long-term kidney function in donors up to twenty years after donation and found only mild increases of serum creatinine (15-17). In addition, they found only small increases in blood pressure and urine protein, neither of which exhibited any noticeable clinical significance. Thus, although donation carries real risks, large series show relatively low surgical morbidity and insignificant long term sequelae.

Although kidney donors take some risks, psychological studies show that they also receive important benefits. Fellner and Marshall (19) studied kidney donors 5 weeks to 18 months after surgery and found that most had significant increases in self-esteem. In a later study, the same authors described two overlapping phases in which donors improved their self-esteem (20). In the first phase, running immediately prior to donation and lasting approximately one month, donors received an outpouring of positive feedback from relatives, friends and strangers, causing marked improvements in self image. This led to a second phase, in which the donors began to look more positively at themselves independent of outside attention. By donating, they felt like they had become better people.

These psychological benefits remain intact over long periods of time and usually exist regardless of transplant outcome. The donors studied by Marshall and Fellner (22) continued to have improved self-esteem nine years after surgery. Many donors said they got through difficult moments in their lives by remembering their donations. Kamstra-Hennen et al (25) studied a separate group of donors five years after their operations and found that the success of the transplant had little impact on the donors' attitudes. Of those whose donation ended in a successful transplant, only five percent regretted their decision to donate or had any difficulty relating to the recipient. These regrets only increased a small amount in those who donated a kidney to a transplant that ultimately failed. In this group, ten percent regretted donating their kidney and eighteen percent had difficulty relating to the recipient. In both groups, then, the vast majority had no regrets about donating and most felt closer to the recipient whether or not the transplant was successful.

(2) Risks and benefits to the recipient

Patients with renal failure no longer depend on live donor transplant to remain alive, because of alternate forms of therapy. Thus, live donor transplants can only be justified if they confer benefits not achievable with cadaver transplant or dialysis, either in survival or quality of life.

Compared to dialysis, a number of studies indicate that transplant patients live longer (26-29). However, because there are no randomized trials comparing dialysis and transplant, it is not clear whether this longevity is a result of treatment or selection bias. In a retrospective study, Burton and Walls (30) made adjustments for nine independent variables influencing survival in end-stage renal disease (ESRD). They found no significant survival difference over ten years of treatment by either CAPD, hemodialysis or transplantation. In contrast, Silins et al (29) still found increased survival in transplant patients after adjusting for similar variables. In addition, Bradley et al (28) studied a group of patients and found that those transplanted only showed survival advantages compared to dialysis when both groups were followed longer than ten years.

Whether or not this survival advantage holds up to scrutiny, a number of researchers assert that transplant yields significant improvement in quality of life (27, 31-38). In general, these studies show that transplant patients rate higher in "objective" quality of life measures, such as activity level or employment (27, 31-34, 36-38). "Subjective" quality of life measures, such as perceptions of well being or general affect, yield more variable results, being more difficult to interpret (39). In addition, by some subjective criteria dialysis and transplant patients rate their quality of life higher than does the normal population, raising questions about whether these measures truly reflect the impact of serious illness on quality of life (32). Nonetheless, even with subjective measures transplant patients generally rate their quality of life higher than dialysis patients (32, 36-38, 40), although home dialysis patients often show similarly high ratings (33, 36, 37).

The higher quality of life ratings of both home hemodialysis and transplant patients is influenced in part by selection bias. Compared to other treatment groups, these two groups of patients tend to be younger and better educated, variables also associated with higher quality of life ratings. Efforts to reduce this bias have yielded disparate results, showing either a continued improvement in quality of life for these patients (31, 32, 37, 40) or, in a case-matched study, no significant differences among treatment groups (41).

To give a complete view of ESRD treatment, one must also compare living donor transplant to cadaver transplant. Cyclosporine has improved the success rate of cadaver transplant. There is no measurable difference in patient survival between living donor and cadaver transplantation (42). However, living donor kidneys have significantly better one and five year graft survival (26, 42, 43). This is relevant to measuring patient benefits, because graft failure is associated with a significant drop in patient quality of life measures, to the lowest ratings among all ESRD patients (35, 37).

In summary, it is difficult to sum up the risks and benefits to recipients of living donor transplants. Most successfully transplanted patients feel the transplants improved the quality of their lives (33, 34, 38). While they may have reasons to overstate the benefits they received from transplant, it is reasonable to expect transplant to remain the best treatment for many patients. For these patients, living donor organs offer decreased waiting time for available organs, increased graft survival, and perhaps an associated increase in recipient quality of life.

(3) Possibility and validity of consent

In general, before a physician treats or performs a procedure on a patient, it is important to determine whether the patient is able to provide informed consent. To do so, patients must be given relevant and sufficient information to make a rational decision and must be competent to understand this information (44). In order to reach informed decisions, patients must also have adequate time to make their decisions free of coercion. Can a potential kidney donor, under pressure to help another person, sufficiently understand the risks and benefits to reach an informed decision to donate without being unduly influenced by other considerations?

The answer to this question depends on what patients we are considering. For example, children and incompetent adult donors cannot, in general, meet the requirements of informed consent. Since any decision allowing such individuals to donate would violate the doctrine of informed consent, we must either deny them the opportunity to donate or find a way to justify allowing them to donate even though they cannot provide informed consent.

Courts have settled upon one way to justify donation from children and incompetent adults: they can donate a kidney when it is in their best interests (45). In most cases, this necessitates that the recipient be a relative whose continued health is important to the donor. In *Strunk vs. Strunk*, for example, the Kentucky Court of Appeals determined that the state could permit removal of a kidney from a mentally incompetent ward for transplantation into his brother, who provided him with companionship and care giving (46). Similarly, in *Hart vs. Brown* the court approved removal of a kidney from a seven year old for transplantation into her identical twin, arguing that it would be a very great loss to the donor if her sister died (47).

Although both these decisions were essentially decided on the grounds of the donor's best interests, in the *Hart* case the court based its opinion on the "doctrine of substituted judgment". When using this doctrine, courts try to decide what a person would have done were they competent to decide for themselves. Generally, this standard is used in decisions involving temporarily or permanently incompetent adults, whose previous wishes or attitudes can be considered. In the *Hart* case, this doctrine seems misplaced. It makes no sense to ask what a seven year old would decide to do if she were competent; seven year olds are simply not capable of making these kinds of decisions.

Two later courts, recognizing the misapplication of "substituted judgment" in *Hart*, clarified the standard upon which these types of cases would be resolved, basing their decisions squarely on the best interests of the potential donor. For example, in *Richardson* the Louisiana Court of Appeals used a best interests standard to deny procurement of a kidney from a seventeen year old with a mental age of three. They argued that the potential donor's mental impairment was so severe he would not have benefitted from his sister's good health (48). Similarly, in *Pescinski* the court denied approval for kidney donation from a thirty nine year old chronic, catatonic schizophrenic man for whom it found no benefits from donation (49).

As we have shown, courts do not require that all kidney donors meet standards of informed consent. Instead, incompetent patients are allowed to donate when it is in their best interests. While this legal standard is well established, those looking for moral guidance may want more. Law, after all, does not define morality. It is our opinion, however, that in this instance it is ethically appropriate to use a best interests standard to decide whether or not to use a kidney from an incompetent person.

Even with competent adults, some have questioned whether many donors reach their decisions to donate in ways that reflect genuine informed consent. Many patients do not take the time to reach an informed decision. Fellner and Marshall (20) found that a high percentage of competent adult donors made their decisions without any time to reflect on them, before even asking for information about risks and benefits. The potential donors knew immediately that they wanted to donate, and said that no amount of reflection could have changed their minds. They said such a decision process was unlike any other they normally used.

These findings are unacceptable to those demanding that competent kidney donors meet strict legal and ethical standards of informed consent. They would argue that the doctrine of informed consent was developed to protect patients. If patients cannot make rational, informed decisions, then we (the law or health care providers) have a duty to keep them from harming themselves.

Yet it is not clear that informed consent doctrine requires patients to make only "rational" decisions. Competent patients, with the ability to understand information pertinent to their decisions, may not choose to reflect upon the information or to come to their decisions in ways that we find "rational". Irrational decision making is only relevant to determination of informed consent when it suggests that the patient is incompetent. The doctrine of informed consent allows competent patients to make decisions others might regard as irrational. Thus, one can accept Fellner and Marshall's findings and still allow patients to donate. If patients are given sufficient time and information, law and morality should not demand that they make decisions in ways we always find rational. Kidney donation is a special kind of act, and does not always work in ways consistent with the standard of informed consent we require for many other medical procedures.

In discussing informed consent, one other group deserves our attention: adolescent donors. This group fits uncomfortably between the groups we have already discussed. For young children and incompetent adults, we accept donors based on what we think is in their best interests. For competent adults, we often accept donors who decide freely to donate even when they reach their decision hastily or irrationally. For adolescents, we want to protect their best interests while giving more weight to their reasons for donating than we do for children.

Like many competent adults, adolescent donors frequently decide to donate in irrational ways.

Bernstein and Simmons (50) studied a group of 16-20 year old kidney donors and found that they commonly made instantaneous decisions to donate. However, they were motivated to donate for troubling reasons. Many hoped that donating a kidney would bring them recognition as adults. One felt donation would bring more access to the family car, while others, who viewed themselves as "black sheep", hoped to become more accepted by their families.

The existence of such motives increases our need to not only listen closely to why adolescents want to donate but also to make sure that donation would truly be in their best interests.

(4) Issues regarding donor privacy and confidentiality

Transplant teams considering living donors often need to evaluate multiple members of potential recipient's families. This raises special concerns regarding the privacy and confidentiality of potential donors. It is frequently difficult for transplant teams to keep such information private (51).

Earlier we discussed the importance of assuring that potential donors decide to donate without being coerced. This freedom is compromised when families become privy to the decision the potential donor is contemplating. This can cut both ways. Some potential donors, unwilling to donate, receive significant pressure to change their minds. Others who wish to donate feel the opposite pressure, as spouses or close family members encourage them not to donate. On occasion, multiple members of a family wish to donate and they actually fight over who will be allowed (51).

(5) Benefits to society

Living donor transplants have an impact on not only the donors and recipients, but also on persons awaiting cadaver organs and on persons contributing money to ESRD treatment. Others awaiting transplant are benefitted because living donor organs decrease the number of people competing for cadaver organs.

In 1991, over 18,000 patients awaited cadaver kidney transplants in the US, with the waiting list growing at an annual rate of almost 1,000 people (52). The number waiting would have been even greater if not for living donor transplants, which made up over twenty percent of transplant reported to the UCLA Registry between 1984 and 1988 (43).

Live donor kidney transplants benefit other members of society as well. Because it costs less to care for transplant patients than for those on dialysis (53), all those who pay for the care of patients with ESRD, either through government or private insurance programs, save money.

We do not suggest that these social benefits are sufficient to justify pursuing living donor transplantation.

Rather, one cannot decide whether living donor transplants should be pursued without considering these consequences. For example, if living donor transplants offered minimal benefits to those involved but had disastrous social consequences, one could convincingly argue that society should not encourage such procedures. In reality, this is not the case, so there are no compelling social reasons not to pursue living donor transplantation.

SPECIAL GROUPS

In general, the five factors we discuss above can be used to evaluate the appropriateness of accepting most potential donors. However, there are several categories of potential living donors that, due to special problems of either biological status or informed consent, deserve special attention.

Anencephalic newborns

Amidst great controversy, anencephalic newborns have been proposed as potential sources of transplantable organs.

This controversy arises because anencephalic infants do not fit criteria for brain death, since those born with functioning vital organs (the only anencephalic newborns of interest in this debate) must therefore have functioning brain stems (54). They also do not fit criteria for persistent vegetative state (PVS). Persons in PVS generally lose cortical function after suffering some type of brain injury. After the injury, they often have stable neurologic function, living for years after the initial damage (55). Anencephalic newborns, on the other hand, never enjoy cortical function. They do not suffer damage to formerly normal brains, for they never develop normal brains in the first place (56).

Because of their unusual neurologic status, anencephalic newborns cannot be placed into conventional donor categories. Were they brain dead, their organs could be retrieved much as they are from other brain dead persons. Were they in PVS, they would presumably be grouped with other PVS persons from whom we do not presently retrieve vital organs. Were they like normal infants, with present or future interests, we could harvest kidneys from them under conditions in which it served their best interests.

Several authors have proposed ways to justify retrieving organs from anencephalic newborns.

At Loma Linda, Peabody et al (57) tried to provide life support to anencephalic newborns until they met criteria for brain death, at which point they could retrieve their vital organs. In this way they would avoid harvesting organs from anencephalic newborns before they were technically brain dead. After intensive support of twelve infants, only two met the criteria for brain death after one week and no vital organs could be retrieved from either. If we are to use anencephalic newborns as sources of kidneys, we shall have to find an alternative approach.

Others have provided alternative ways to justify organ retrieval, that would avoid Peabody's low harvesting rate.

Holzgreve et al (58) propose that anencephalic infants be placed in a special category of "brain absent" persons. With this special category, they would not have to meet brain death criteria, and could thus be used as sources of organs before losing all brain stem function.

Unfortunately, Holzgreve's nomenclature is no more appropriate for anencephalic infants than was the term "brain dead".

To be more accurate, Holzgreve would need to classify them as "cortically absent", but then this would still leave their donor status up in the air.

Finally, Truog and others (59) have argued that we should allow retrieval from anencephalics on the same grounds that we do for brain dead persons, namely that neither group has any real expectation for sentient life or survival apart from life support. Although this approach has merit, it has received little support from those who develop public policy.

This lack of support stems largely from the fact that retrieving hearts or livers from anencephalics could be construed as an act of homicide.

The situation would be different for kidney retrieval, for surgeons could avoid directly killing them by taking only one kidney from each newborn (60). Although this approach avoids some of the problems associated with heart and liver retrieval, few urge that we do this and no one expects that such a practice would do much to relieve kidney shortage.

Institutionalized persons

An additional category of vulnerable patients include those whose ability to provide informed consent is compromised by institutionalization, such as prisoners.

Starzl (61) used kidneys from prisoners serving long sentences for serious crimes, but later regretted this practice. Moore and colleagues (62) were faced with a similar situation at the Peter Bent Brigham Hospital in Boston. They refused to take kidneys from prisoners on the grounds that the prisoners might expect favorable treatment or reduced sentences in return.

For similar reasons, courts generally require stricter levels of informed consent from prisoners, because such people are especially vulnerable to undue coercion.

Women

Another category of potential living donors susceptible to coercion is women, who may disproportionately donate because of discrimination. In the United States, 64% of kidneys donated to children by their parents come from the child's mother even though kidneys donated by children's fathers have a longer average graft survival (63). There are a couple explanations for this inequality. First, mothers may disproportionately donate because they are more likely than men to be primary care givers for the children. Second, women on average have lower incomes than men and therefore, when they donate, families do not lose as much income. In either case, men would not be as likely to donate unless they were significantly closer immunologically to the child, perhaps accounting for their improved graft survival.

The problem for transplant teams is deciding when a mother's choice to donate is a result of sexual discrimination. While it is important to be aware of this possibility, it may not always be possible to know why one parent chooses to donate over another. While transplant teams must attend to the possibility of compromised autonomy on the part of women donors, they also must weigh the risks and benefits that the women face.

Economically disadvantaged persons

Finally, at least one more vulnerable group deserves attention: economically disadvantaged persons. Persons unable to obtain adequate food, clothing or shelter are not likely to be able to "freely" consent to the sale of one of their kidneys (64). Because of this, the sale of solid organs by living persons is illegal in most developed countries. However, in other countries, this practice is quite common, especially in third world countries such as India (62) and Egypt (65), although even in these countries this practice is beginning to come under intense scrutiny. For example, in Egypt unrelated persons are no longer allowed to "donate" kidneys to others, because the government felt the practice had become exploitative (65).

By banning the sale of kidneys, governments act paternalistically. As we discussed earlier, such paternalism is justified to protect people from harm. Yet it seems unfair to prevent poverty stricken people from doing something to improve their lot. If we can justify donation for no money on the grounds that the risks to the donor are acceptable, how can we preclude those from donating who probably stand to gain even more by donating (66)?

We justify such paternalism by arguing that once sale of organs is permitted, it is likely to be used to discriminate against the weakest members of society. Although it is unfair to suffer from abject poverty, and seems hypocritical to forbid people from selling kidneys (thereby helping themselves and those with kidney disease), we should not permit a practice which ultimately will be used primarily to take advantage of these same people. The only alternative would be to allow reimbursement for the pain, suffering and inconvenience of donation within a system regulated to prevent the practice from becoming exploitative (67).

RELATED VERSUS UNRELATED DONATION

The debate over whether to allow the sale of kidneys is not over. Thus, it is helpful to clarify the relevance of whether donors are related or not related to those receiving the donation.

We have said nothing so far that would preclude a practice of accepting kidneys from unrelated donors. However, in weighing the factors we outline above, related donors will be more likely to be acceptable. This is because, as Singer et al (68) point out, the risk/benefit ratio improves with related donation, for donors are likely to receive greater happiness by the improved health of a loved one than of a perfect stranger. The more intimately involved one is with the recipient, the more one benefits by donating.

Related donation is even more compelling if it is assumed that we have a special obligation toward relatives. Sommers (69) puts forth such an ethic under the category of "filial duty". We are not expected to treat all people the same, but are morally required to give special attention to the needs of our parents, siblings or other close relatives. This contrasts with the position of many prominent philosophers. For example, Kant (70) places moral duty on an impartial ethical imperative, without making any distinction between strangers and relatives. Mill (71) bases all moral decisions on measurements of pleasure and pain that do not give special weight to relatives. Sommers (69) argues that systems like these fail to account for real duties that we must acknowledge. And to the extent that she is correct, the case for related donation strengthens.

Friedman (72) takes this logic a step further, arguing that friendships also carry moral significance. This fits well with our earlier statements, because close friends of recipients also gain from the recipients' improved health. Both Sommers and Friedman's accounts are consistent with the phenomenon that, without financial incentive, people who feel compelled to donate to relatives and loved ones do not usually volunteer to donate organs to strangers.

Neither of these positions, however, precludes strangers from donating kidneys. In fact, for Sommers and Friedman such a donation would be beyond what duty would require. Thus, Fellner (21) argues that we should stop being suspicious of unrelated donors, and recognize that they also gain psychological benefits by donating. He thinks organ donation should be looked upon as an act of the highest morality. Whether related or unrelated, friend or stranger, donors stand both to help other people and to improve their image of themselves by donating.

CONCLUSION

The factors we discussed above can be used to decide when to override an autonomous person's desire to donate a kidney. Transplant teams, primary care physicians, family members and other interested parties must assess the types of risks and benefits we outline above. Potential donors may have good intentions by offering to donate, but transplant teams must balance the potential donors' altruism and autonomy against the factors described above. Thus, transplant teams must try to determine whether a person is competent to decide to donate. If the potential donor is sick, the transplant team must decide whether the risks of nephrectomy are too high to justify donation (73). In cases where the risks are uncertain, the team can explain the uncertainty to the potential donor so that he or she can decide (74).

Autonomy requires physicians to respect their patients' desires, but it does not force them to perform operations on patients that are not warranted by a fair assessment of the risks and benefits. Ultimately, the decision rests with the transplant team, for only they can perform the required operations. However, these teams may want help on difficult cases, and should freely consult with ethicists, ethics committees, or institutional review boards when needed. In this process, a few key considerations must not be forgotten. Every attempt must be made to preserve donors' autonomy and privacy. Donors must.be given adequate opportunity to reflect on the risks and benefits of donating. Finally, the medical evaluation of donors should be undertaken by physicians unassociated with the transplant team, who can act solely as advocates of the potential donors' best interests (75).

Starzl's words remain relevant (5). The relative benefits of living donor kidney transplantation over other forms of therapy for ESRD are increasingly hard to identify.

We think this should encourage transplant teams to become aware of the special categories of vulnerable donors and to decline to accept potential donors when doubts arise about the balance of risks and benefits or about the existence of free, informed consent.

REFERENCES

1. Beauchamp TL, Walters L: Contemporary issues in bioethics, 2nd Edition. Wadsworth Publishing Company, Belmont, 1982.
2. Speake J: A dictionary of philosophy. Pan Books Ltd, London, 1979.
3. MacIntyre A: Egoism and altruism. In: "The encyclopedia of philosophy",(Ed P Edwards), Macmillan Publishing Co, Inc & The Free Press, New York, 2: 462-466, 1967.
4. Kreis H: Why living related donors should not be used whenever possible. Transpl Proc, 17 (1): 1510-1514, 1985.
5. Starzl TE: Will live organ donations no longer be justified? Hastings Center Report, 15 (2): 5, 1985.
6. Siegler M, Lantos JD: Ethical justification for living liver donation. Cambridge Quarterly Journal of Health Care Ethics, 1992 (in press).
7. Woodruff MFA: Ethical problems in organ transplantation. Br Med J, 1: 1457-1460, 1964.
8. Merril JO, Murray JE, Harrison JH, et al: Successful homotransplantation of the human kidney between identical twins. JAMA, 160: 277-282, 1956.
9. Murray JE, Merrill JP, Dammin GJ, et al: Kidney transplants in modified recipients. Ann Surg, 156: 337-355, 1962.
10. Murray JE, Merrill JP, Harrison JH, et al: Prolonged survival of human kidney homografts by immunosuppressive drug therapy. N Eng J Med, 268: 1315-1323, 1963.
11. McGeown MG: Ethics for the use of live donors in kidney transplantation. Am Heart J, 75 (5): 711-714, 1968.
12. Bergan JJ: Current risks to the kidney transplant donor. Transpl Proc, 5 (2): 1131-1134, 1973.
13. Ringden O, Friman L, Lundgren G, Magnusson G: Living related kidney donors: complications and long-term renal function. Transplantation, 25 (4): 221-223, 1978.
14. Weiland D, Sutherland DER, Chavers B, Simmons RL, Ascher NL, Najarian JS: Information on 628 living-related kidney donors at a single institution, with long-term follow-up in 472 cases. Transpl Proc, 16 (1): 5-7, 1984.
15. Vincenti F, Amend WJC, Kaysen G, et al: Long-term renal function in kidney donors: sustained compensatory hyperfiltration with no adverse effects. Transplantation, 36 (12): 626-629, 1983.
16. Miller IJ, Suthanthiran M, Riggio RR, et al: Impact of renal donation: long-term clinical and biochemical follow-up of living donors in a single center. Am J Med, 79: 201-208, 1985.
17. Anderson CF, Velosa JA, Frohnert PP, et al: The risks of unilateral nephrectomy: status of kidney donors 10 to 20 years postoperatively. Mayo Clinic Proc, 60: 367-374, 1985.
18. Levey AS, Hou S, Bush H: Kidney transplantation from unrelated living donors: time to reclaim a discarded opportunity. N Engl J Med, 314 (14): 914-916, 1986.
19. Fellner CH, Marshall JR: Twelve kidney donors. JAMA, 206 (12): 2703-2707, 1968.
20. Fellner CH, Marshall JR: Kidney donors - The myth of informed consent. Am J Psych, 126 (9): 1245-1251, 1970.
21. Fellner CH: Organ donation: for whose sake? Ann Int Med, 79 (4): 589-592, 1973.
22. Marshall JR, Fellner CH: Kidney donors revisited. Am J Psych, 134 (5): 575-576, 1977.
23. Evans RW, Rader B, Manninen DL: The quality of life of hemodialysis recipients treated with recombinant human erythropoietin. JAMA, 263 (6): 825-830, 1990.
24. Bay WH, Herbert LA: The living donor in kidney transplantation. Ann Int Med, 106: 719-727, 1987.
25. Kamstra-Hennen L, Beebe J, Stumm S, Simmons RG: Ethical evaluation of related donation: the donor after five years. Transpl Proc, 13 (1): 60-61, 1981.
26. Fassbinder W, Brunner FP, Brynger H, et al: Combined report on regular dialysis and transplantation in Europe. Nephrol Dial Transpl, 6 (Suppl 1): 5-35, 1991.

27. Khauli RB, Novick AC, Steinmuller DR, et al: Comparison of renal transplantation and dialysis in rehabilitation of diabetic end-stage renal disease patients. Urology, 27 (6): 521-525, 1986.
28. Bradley JR, Evans DB, Calne RY: Long-term survival in haemodialysis patients. Lancet, I: 295-296, 1987.
29. Silins J, Fortier L, Mao Y, et al: Mortality rates among patients with end-stage renal disease in Canada, 1981-86. Canad Med Ass J, 141: 677-682, 1989.
30. Burton PR, Walls J: Selection-adjusted comparison of life-expectancy of patients on continuous ambulatory peritoneal dialysis, haemodialysis, and renal transplantation. Lancet, I: 1115-1119, 1987.
31. Johnson JP, McCauley CR, Copley JB: The quality of life of hemodialysis and transplant patients. Kidney Int, 22: 286-291, 1982.
32. Evans RW, Manninen DL, Garrison LP, et al: The quality of life of patients with end-stage renal disease. N Engl J Med, 312 (9): 553-559, 1985.
33. Kutner NG, Brogan D, Kutner MH: End-stage renal disease treatment modality and patients' quality of life: longitudinal assessment. Am J Nephrol, 6: 396-402, 1986.
34. Parfrey PS, Vavasour H, Bullock M, Henry S, Harnett JD, Gault MH: Symptoms in end-stage renal disease: dialysis vs transplantation. Transpl Proc, 19 (4): 3407-3409, 1987.
35. Parfrey PS, Vavasour H, Gault MH: A prospective study of health status in dialysis and transplant patients. Transpl Proc, 20 (6): 1231-1232, 1988.
36. Morris PLP, Jones B: Life satisfaction across treatment methods for patients with end-stage renal failure. Med J Australia, 150: 428-432, 1989.
37. Bremer BA, McCauley CR, Wrona RM, Johnson JP: Quality of life in end-stage renal disease: a reexamination. Am J Kidney Dis, 13 (3): 200-209, 1989.
38. Koch U, Muthny FA: Quality of life in patients with end-stage renal disease in relation to the method of treatment. Psychotherapy and Psychosomatics, 54:161-171, 1990.
39. Deniston OL, Carpenter-Alting P, Kneisley J, Hawthorne VM, Port FK: Assessment of quality of life in end-stage renal disease. Health Services Research, 24 (4): 555-578, 1989.
40. Evans RW: Recombinant human Erythropoietin and the quality of life of end-stage renal disease patients: a comparative analysis. Am J Kidney Dis, 18 (4): 62-70, 1991.
41. Sayag R, De-Nour AK, Shapira Z, Kahan E, Boner G: Comparison of psychosocial adjustment of male nondiabetic kidney transplant and hospital hemodialysis patients. Nephron, 54: 214-218, 1990.
42. Smith AY, VanBuren CT, Lewis RM, Kerman RH, Kahan BD: Factors determining renal transplant outcome at the University of Texas at Houston. In: "Clinical transplants" (Ed P Terasaki), Los Angeles, UCLA Tissue Typing Lab, 1987, pp 155-166.
43. Imagawa DK, Cecka JM: Renal regrafts. In: "Clinical transplants" (Ed P Terasaki), Los Angeles, UCLA Tissue Typing Lab, 1988, pp 387-398.
44. Lidz CW, Meisel A, Zerubavel E, Carter M, Sestak RM, Roth LH: Informed consent: a study of decisionmaking in psychiatry. New York, The Guilford Press, 1984.
45. Fost N: Children as renal donors. N Engl J Med, 296 (7): 363-367, 1977.
46. Strunk vs Strunk.(Ky. 1969), 445 S.W.2d 145
47. Hart vs Brown.(Super. 1972), 29 Con. Supp. 368
48. In re Richardson.(La App 1073), 284 So2d 185
49. Lausier vs Pescinski.67 Wis2d 4, 226 NW2d 180
50. Bernstein DM, Simmons RG: The adolescent kidney donor: the right to give. Am J Psych, 131 (12): 1338-1343, 1974.
51. Simmons RG, Hickey K, Kjellstrand CM, Simmons RL: Family tension in the search for a kidney donor. JAMA, 215 (6): 909-912, 1971.
52. Evans RW, Orians CE, Ascher NL: The potential supply of organ donors: an assessment of the efficiency of organ procurement efforts in the United States. JAMA, 267 (2): 239-246, 1992.
53. Manninen DL, Evans RW, Dugan MK, Rader B: The costs and outcome of kidney transplant graft failure. Transpl Proc, 23 (1): 1312-1314, 1991.
54. Fost N: Organs from anencephalic infants: an idea whose time has not yet come. Hastings Center Report, Oct, 5-10, 1988.
55. Cranford RE: The persistent vegetative state: the medical reality (Getting the facts straight). Hastings Center Report, Feb, 27-32, 1988.
56. Shewman DA: Anencephaly: selected medical aspects. Hastings Center Report, Oct, 11-19, 1988.

57. Peabody JL, Emery JR, Ashwal S: Experience with anencephalic infants as prospective organ donors. N Engl J Med, 321: 344-350, 1989.
58. Holzgreve W, Beller F, Buchholz B, Hansmann M, Kohler K: Kidney transplantation from anencephalic donors. N Engl J Med, 316: 1069-1070, 1987.
59. Truog RD, Fletcher JC: Can organs be transplanted before brain death? N Engl J Med, 321 (6): 388-390, 1989.
60. Associated Press: Organ donations barred by judge: vital organs of doomed girl can't be given to others. A Florida Court rules. New York Times, Mar, 28: 6, 1992.
61. Starzl TE: The changing mores of biomedical research. Ann Intern Med, 67 (Suppl. 7): 56, 1967.
62. Moore FD: Three ethical revolutions: ancient assumptions remodeled under pressure of transplantation. Transpl Proc, 20 (Suppl 1): 1061-1067, 1988.
63. Koka P, Cecka JM: Sex and age effects in renal transplantation. In: "Clinical transplants" (Ed P Terasaki), Los Angeles, UCLA Tissue Typing Lab, 1990, pp 437-445.
64. Annas GJ: Life, liberty and the pursuit of organ sales. Hastings Center Report, Feb, 22-23, 1984.
65. Hedges C: Egypt's doctors impose kidney transplant curbs. New York Times, 1992, Thurs, Jan 23.
66. Andrews LB: My body, my property. Hastings Center Report, 16 (5): 28-38, 1986.
67. Lantos JD, Siegler M: Re-evaluating donor criteria: live donors. In: "The surgeon general's workshop on increasing organ donation: background papers", Washington DC, US Department of Health and Human Services, 1991, pp 271-290.
68. Singer PA, Siegler M, Whitington PF, et al: Ethics of liver transplantation with living donors. N Engl J Med, 321 (9): 620-622, 1989.
69. Sommers CH: Filial morality. The Journal of Philosophy, 83 (8): 439-456, 1986.
70. Kant I: Foundations of the metaphysics of morals. Indianapolis, The Bobbs-Merrill Company Inc, 1959.
71. Mill JS: Utilitarianism.1863.
72. Friedman M: Feminism and modern friendship: dislocating the community. Ethics, 99 (2): 275-290, 1989.
73. Singer PA, Lowance D, Siegler M: Whose kidney is it anyway? Ethical considerations in living kidney donation. Am Kidney Found, 5 (1): 16-20, 1988.
74. Spital A, Spital M: Donor's choice or Hobson's choice? Arch Intern Med, 145: 1297-1301, 1985.
75. Caplan AL, Siegler M: Risks, paternalism, and the gift of life. Arch Intern Med, 145: 1188-1190, 1985.

DIAGNOSTIC METHODS IN NEPHROLOGY

Chapter 18

NON-INVASIVE MEASUREMENT OF BODY FLUID DYNAMICS

PETER M. KOUW, PETER M.J.M. DE VRIES AND AB J.M. DONKER

Department of Internal Medicine, Free University Hospital, Amsterdam, The Netherlands.

INTRODUCTION

The fluid balance is an important aspect in nephrology. A variety of nephrological diseases presents itself with symptoms of overhydration such as oedema and hypertension. A complete loss of fluid balance regulation is a feature of most forms of chronic renal failure. Fluid can be withdrawn during dialysis, but the physician is confronted with the difficulty to assess post-dialysis dry weight. Moreover, dialysis leads to a fall in extracellular (EC) osmolality. It has been speculated that this fall is significant enough to induce an osmotic dysequilibrium between the EC- and intracellular (IC) compartment. The resulting cellular swelling might be related to some of the adverse effects of dialysis therapy. Thus, it will be advantageous to chart fluid balance both in renal disease and renal replacement therapy.

In recent years the conductivity technique has evolved to a method suitable to monitor dynamic changes in fluid balance non-invasively.

In this review a description will be given of the most important aspects of this technique. Before that, the impossibility to use isotopic dilution methods for this purpose will be discussed.

ISOTOPIC DILUTION TECHNIQUES TO MEASURE FLUID VOLUMES

Since no direct techniques to explore body fluid spaces are available, study of body fluid spaces was always performed with indirect methods.

Of these, methods based on the tracer dilution principle have been the most widely applied. The theory of this principle is simple. A marker whose volume of distribution is equal to the volume of the fluid space under investigation can be used. When a known quantity of such a marker substance is injected into the body, it will be distributed according to its volume of distribution. After an appropriate period of equilibration, the serum concentration has to be measured. Distribution volume is calculated as the quantity injected, divided by the measured serum concentration. For most volume studies based on this principle, radioactive tracers are used.

It must be remembered that the human body is an inhomogeneous system, composed of various compartments that interchange substances at varying rates. In tracer studies it is generally assumed that the tracer is confined to the respective compartment measured.

Two isotopes of water, deuterium oxide and tritiated water, widely used to detect total body water (TBW), demonstrate well-defined borders (1). Other tracers, however, exhibit poorly defined borders, for example those used for the determination of extracellular fluid volume (EFV). EC water is divided over several compartments: plasma, lymph, connective tissue, cartilage and bone, and the transcellular fluids. There is no marker that equally equilibrates among these many compartments.

Most investigators have chosen to measure the physiologically important EFV. One of the most useful and widely accepted tracers to determine this EFV is ^{82}Br (2). The major disadvantage of bromide is its cellular penetration (3). Other indicators and radioactive tracers that have been employed to measure EFV are inulin (4), thiocyanate (5), thiosulphate (6), ^{24}sodium (7), and ^{35}S-sulphate (8). However, they all cross cell membranes to a significant but variable extent and thereby introduce errors in the measurement of EFV. Intracellular fluid volume (IFV) is calculated as the difference between measured TBW and measured EFV. Errors occurring during the two determinations therefore accumulate in the calculation of IFV.

Besides radioactivity, isotopic dilution techniques have some other disadvantages that handicap their clinical application. The mentioned EC methods all contain errors as a consequence of natural dissociation of the used isotope and leakage of tracer to other compartments of the body (e.g. IFV). For the water isotopes there is also an exchange between the labeled hydrogen atoms and labile hydrogen atoms of organic molecules. Last but not least, these methods need a period of equilibration before a measurement can be performed. Therefore, the application is restricted to steady state situations and can't be applied repeatedly in short time periods. Thus, in order to study dynamic changes in body fluid state, other techniques are warranted.

CONDUCTIVITY MEASUREMENTS

History

The electrical phenomena of biological systems have intrigued scientific investigators for many years. One of these phenomena is the electrical conductivity of human tissues and its relation to body water. Its history started in 1940, when Barnett demonstrated that changes in resistance and capacitive reactance of the body closely followed clinically induced changes in a subject's hydration state (9). Shortly afterwards, Nijboer et al illustrated the relationship of impedance changes to cardiac and respiratory activity (10).

Over the years many applications of conductivity measurements have been established. Whole body impedance is used to determine body composition. Cardiac stroke volume can be detected by impedance cardiography and monitoring of the electrical impedance response of a leg to venous occlusion is used to diagnose venous thrombosis. As this review will focus on fluid balance, only the application of conductivity measurements in the field of fluids will be discussed further.

Terminology

In the field of bio-electrical research, terminology is rather confusing. Expressions like impedance, conductivity, admittance, bio-electrical frequency analysis, and bioimpedance can be read. In this review the following terms will be employed.

- Resistance [in Ohm(Ω)];
- Conductivity [in Siemens(S)]; the reciprocal value of resistance.
- Impedance [in Ohm(Ω)]; the resistance for alternating currents.
- Admittance [in Siemens(S)]; the reciprocal value of impedance.
- Specific conductivity [in 1/(Ω.cm)]; the conductivity value standardized for length and diameter of the measured medium.

Multiple frequency measurements

It has been shown that measurement of the conductivity at a fixed frequency (50 or 100 kHz) of parts of the human body makes it possible to measure accumulation of fluid, for example inside the thorax (11-13). The method has also been used to register changes in fluid content inside the body during and after haemodialysis (14, 15). Afterwards, it was shown that measurement of the electrical admittance at various frequencies offered the possibility of evaluating both IC and EC conductivities (16-18).

A simplified model is suitable to explain how these variables are obtained. The model consists of an EC and an IC path for an electrical current (Figure 1). The EC path is characterized by the frequency-independent resistance Re, representing the total resistance of the EC fluid. The IC path consists of a capacitor Cm, representing the total cell membrane capacity, and a frequency-independent resistance Ri, representing the total resistance of the cell contents.

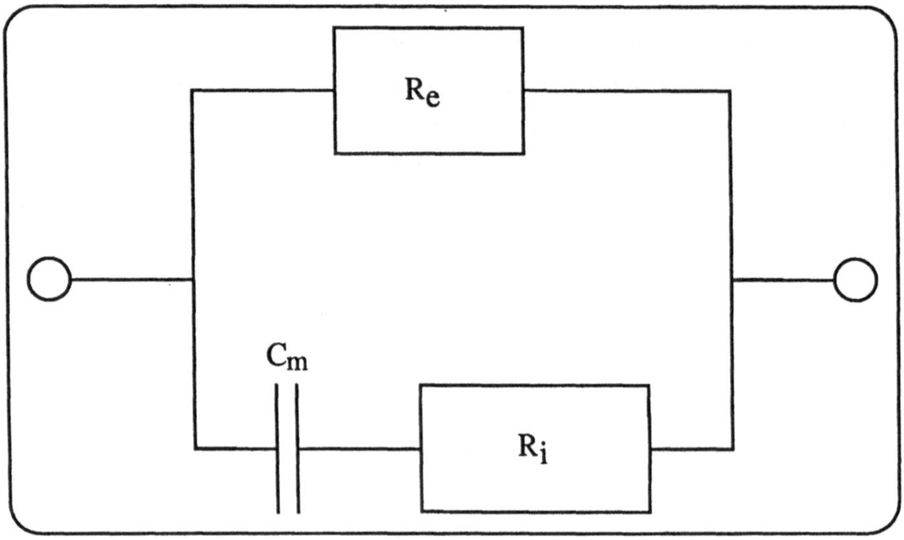

Figure 1. A simplified model for the conduction of electrical currents in biological tissues. Re is the EC resistance, Ri is the IC resistance, and Cm is the cell-membrane capacity.

Translation of the model to the physiological situation implies that at low frequencies, at which the resistance of the membrane capacity is high compared to the resistance of the EC fluid (< 5kHz), the electrical current only flows through the EC fluid. At intermediate frequencies (5-250 kHz) the current flows through the EC and a part of the IC fluid. At sufficiently high frequencies (>250 kHz), the resistance of the cell membrane becomes negligibly small relative to the EC and the IC resistances. The current then flows through the EC and the IC fluid.

According to the model, a plot of the frequency-response of the measured admittance values reveals an S-shaped curve (Figure 2). The low frequency limit expresses the EC conductivity. Subtraction of the low frequency limit from the high frequency limit yields the IC conductivity. It is assumed that IC and EC conductivities are related to IFV and EFV, respectively.

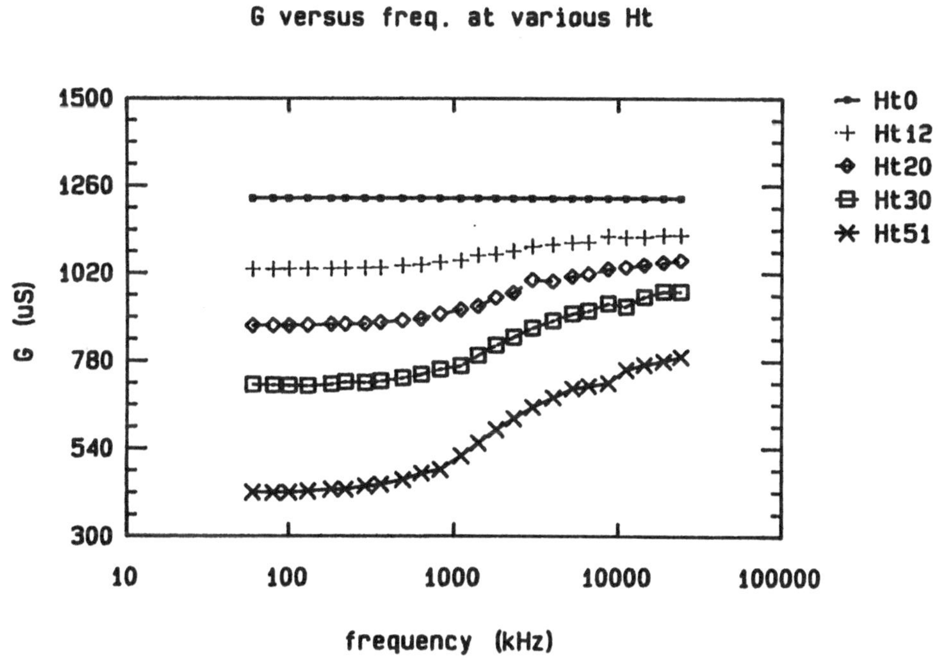

Figure 2. Characteristic S-shaped, frequency dependent admittance (Y) curves measured at various haematocrits. The intracellular conductivity (high frequencies values minus low frequencies values) is clearly related to the haematocrit.

Segmental conductivity measurements

A major point of concern in segmental conductivity measurements is the arrangement of the electrodes. It is necessary to use four electrodes (Figure 3). Two electrodes are used to generate an electrical field. A second pair is placed between the current-passing electrodes for voltage measurement. Conductivity is calculated as the ratio of current strength to voltage.

When only two electrodes are used, current conduction and voltage measurement are performed with the same electrode. The impedance measured in this way partly consists of the impedance of the skin-electrode junction. A tetrapolar (or four electrode) system is slightly more complicated but almost insensitive to the electrode-skin impedance.

It is essential that the current also penetrates the deeper tissue layers of the investigated segment. To ensure this, the distance between the current conducting- and the measuring electrodes has to be sufficient (19). Secondly, the configuration of the electrodes is important to insure an optimum distribution of current through the tissue. Circumferential electrodes have to be used in order to prevent the current from flowing only superficially (20).

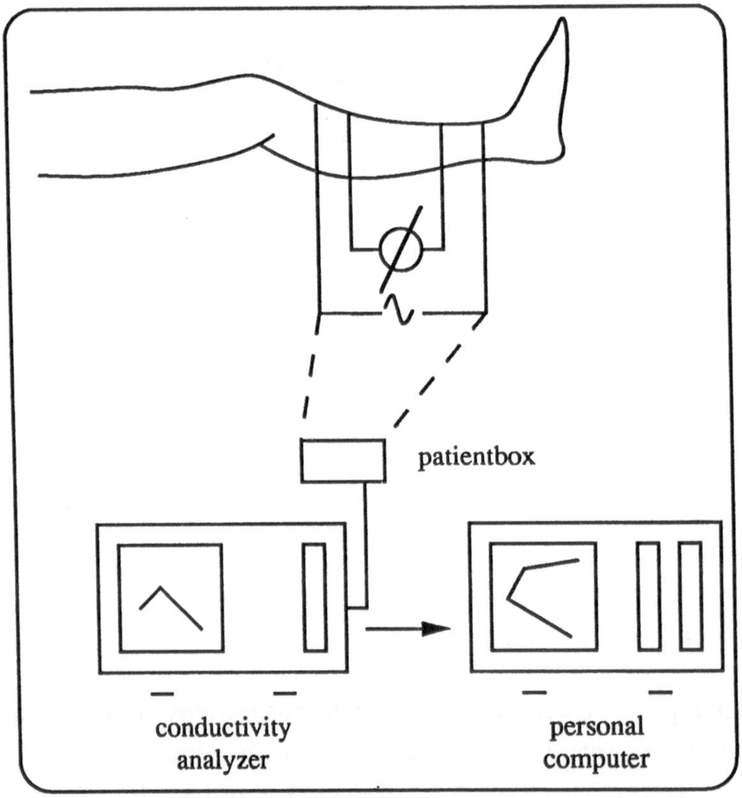

Figure 3. A schematical representation of the experimental set-up of segmental conductivity measurements.

An additional advantage of a homogeneous electrical field distribution by circumferential electrodes is that it simplifies standardization. For example, the lower leg resembles a cone. The volume can be inferred from circumferences and length of this geometrical body. Therefore, the measured IC and EC conductivities can be expressed as conductivities per cubic centimeter tissue. These figures reflect the fluid content of tissue. Comparison of values in patients with values obtained in normal individuals provides a gauge for the IC and EC hydration state (21).

Validation

The validity of the postulated model has been shown in different ways.

In vitro experiments were performed at blood samples with varying haematocrit values in a conductivity cell (Figure 2). Not only the expected S-shaped curves could be demonstrated, but also a good correlation between IC conductivity and the corresponding haematocrit value, and thus, IFV (22). Furthermore, EC conductivity depended on the amount of plasma, and thus EFV, in the conductivity cell. A formula has been composed describing the close relation of percentage EC fluid in the conductivity cell to measured EC conductivity (23). All in all, there is circumstantial evidence that the model is valid *in vitro*.

In order to validate the method *in vivo*, multiple frequency conductivity measurements have been performed at the lower limb. Again, the predicted characteristic frequency response was revealed (24, 25). In another study, regional conductivity measurements at the upper leg were performed in 16 growth hormone deficient patients. At the same site, the upper leg was scanned by means of computer tomography, yielding a transsectional view of the upper leg. A subcutaneous non-conducting fat layer, a region of conducting muscle tissue, and the centralized non-conducting femoral bone were recognized. A good relation ($r = 0.80$; $p<0.001$) could be shown between measured high-frequency conductivity and the area of body water containing muscle tissue that was visualized by these CAT-scans (submitted for publication).

Furthermore, conductivity figures are reproducible. Assessment of segmental intra- and extracellular conductivities in a group of individuals twice a week yielded coefficiencies of variance of 8 and 4%, respectively.

EFV and IFV computed from whole body impedances at various frequencies appeared to be closely related to EFV and IFV assessed by means of isotopic dilution techniques (26). These latter data document the validity of the conductivity technique in steady state. However, it has been stated that the conductivity method is also a sound method to detect changes in fluid balance, that cannot accurately be assessed by means of isotopic dilution techniques. In order to prove this postulate, a study was designed to validate the technique under dynamic circumstances. In healthy subjects isotonic diuresis was induced by the intravenous injection of 40 mg furosemide. The resulting depletion of EFV was calculated from concurrently performed, segmental conductivity measurements. The decrease in EFV appeared to be closely related to the urine production in each individual (submitted for publication). Thus, conductivity measurements can be used to chart EC fluid dynamics.

Unfortunately, comparable procedures to induce reproducable changes in IFV in order to validate the conductivity method as a tool to record IC fluid dynamics are not available.

In vitro, however, it is easy to manipulate cell volume by stressing the cell osmotically. Again, these experiments have been carried out in a conductivity cell containing blood samples. Osmotically induced changes in haematocrit, and thus in IFV, were accurately detected by IC conductivity measurements (27). Thus, experimental data advocating the validity of conductivity measurements to monitor IC fluid dynamics have not been derived *in vivo*, but *in vitro*.

Translation of extra- and intracellular conductivities to fluid volumes

Although biological fluids are the principle conductors of electrical currents in tissue, water itself is an extremely poor conductor. The conducting properties of biological fluids result from the conducting properties of their solutes. Of these solutes, electrolytes are by far the best conductors (22). Therefore, the EC and IC conductivities not only depend on the amount of fluid, but also on the electrolyte concentrations of their respective compartments.

During dynamic fluid monitoring, changes in conductivity directly reflect changes in fluid volume if electrolyte concentrations are not changed. Otherwise, conductivity figures have to be corrected. Unfortunately, it is hardly possible to derive IC or interstitial fluid to study changes in electrolyte concentration.

Although the IC and EC fluids are dominated by different electrolytes, their total electrolyte concentrations are comparable to that of plasma or serum (27). Since IC and EC electrolyte concentrations are mirrored by the electrolyte concentration in serum, serum specific conductivity equals that of EFV and IFV (28).

Serum conductivity can be determined in two ways. The most accurate one is to assess the conducting property of serum in a conductivity cell (22). Another option is to calculate serum conductivity from the serum electrolyte concentrations (28). Since each ion represents a certain amount of conductivity which has been established accurately, the conductive properties of serum can be simply calculated from the nature and concentration of its electrolytes (22).

Thus, if intra-individual serum conductivity changes are known, changes in volume can be accurately calculated during dynamic fluid monitoring. The same holds true for comparison of interindividual fluid volumes. If conductivity measurements are performed to establish EFV and IFV, as in measurement of whole body impedance, the deviation of electrolyte concentration from normal values has to be considered and integrated in the calculations.

Whole body impedance

Thomasset (25) was the first to study the use of whole body impedance as a measure for TBW. For this purpose two electrodes were placed at the ankle and two at the contralateral wrist. It was demonstrated that the measured impedance was inversely proportional to TBW (25, 26, 29). By means of regression analysis the best correlation between TBW and impedance values was determined. Later on, the changes in TBW during haemodialysis were also studied (30). These impedances were measured at one single frequency.

As has been mentioned above, measurements at various frequencies are necessary to differentiate between IC and EC conductivity, and consequently between IFV and EFV.

Jenin and coworkers were the first to use two frequencies for this purpose (31). Tedner and Lins reported the same technique and applied it to haemodialysis patients (32, 33). However, their motive to perform a low and a high frequency measurement was to calculate TBW more accurately.

Thoracic fluid monitoring

A large number of investigators has studied the monitoring of chest fluid using impedance measurements (11-13). Nijboer and Sedensky were the first to use the tetrapolar electrode method to monitor thoracic impedance changes (34). The outer two were the current electrodes and the inner two the measuring electrodes. This technique was refined by Kubicek et al. (35).

The development of differential impedance plethysmography greatly improved the technique (15). For thoracic measurements the electrodes are applied around the thorax and the neck. All these studies have been performed with a fixed excitation signal frequency: in most cases 50 or 100 kHz. Since thoracic fluid is EC, measurements at a single frequency do not seriously disturb the outcome of these studies.

Whole body impedance versus segmental impedance

Although assessment of whole body impedance suggests that information concerning total body fluid is obtained, this is not entirely true. Whole body impedance consists of three serially connected impedances, namely the impedances of arm, trunk and leg, and is equal to the sum of these impedances (Ohm's law). The magnitude of each of these impedances can be calculated according to the formula:

[1] $$R = \rho * \frac{l}{A}$$

in which A is the cross-sectional area and l the length of arm, trunk and leg, respectively, ρ being the tissue-specific impedance.

Since A of the trunk is relatively large compared to A of the limbs, whole body impedance mainly embodies the sum of the local impedances of arm and leg. Indeed, it has been shown that this concept is correct (36). Therefore, there is little reason to prefer assessment of whole body impedance to segmental impedance.

Although whole body impedance mainly includes impedance of the limbs, it has been shown that it accurately predicts whole body EFV or TBW (26). This indicates that normally fluid is fairly equally dispersed between trunk and limbs, or that fluid is mainly distributed in the limbs. Since trunk impedance has relatively little impact on whole body impedance, pathological accumulation of fluid in the trunk is less easy to detect by assessing whole body impedance. In case of pathological accumulation of fluid in the thoracic cavity it is, therefore, more appropriate to perform thoracic fluid monitoring. Although no current information is available, we propose that in order to detect ascites it is more convenient to place electrodes proximal at the limbs, guaranteeing a measurement of trunk impedance.

DYNAMIC FLUID MONITORING IN THE FIELD OF NEPHROLOGY

Transcellular fluid shift

A clinical application of the conductivity measurements is found in the survey of IFV and EFV during haemodialysis. Some authors assessed whole body impedance during dialysis (33). Other authors performed segmental conductivity measurements in order to monitor IFV and EFV during dialysis (37).

Haemodialysis is associated with a pronounced fall in serum osmolality, due to removal of metabolic waste products, e.g, urea. It is believed that a serum osmolality change almost instantaneously equilibrates with the interstitial space. So, the fall in osmolality that appears during conventional haemodialysis not only accounts for the intravascular, but also for the extravascular compartment. Little is known about the interaction between EFV and IFV during dialysis. Sodium can not freely penetrate the cell membrane but urea can. Since the permeability of the cell membrane for urea is less than for water, an osmotic gradient over the cell membrane may nevertheless result (38). Water movement by osmosis will neutralize this gradient at the expense of IC oedema. This situation can cause side effects in two ways. First, the cellular swelling can give rise to the so-called disequilibrium syndrome causing complaints like headache, nausea, vomiting, or muscle cramps. Secondly, the fluid shift from the EC to the IC compartment restricts the ability of the tissues to mobilize fluid into the intravascular space by decreasing the hydrostatic pressure of the interstitium. Evidence for this concept was found in a study in which dialysis patients were treated with three different dialysate sodium concentrations successively (39). As a consequence, hypovolaemia due to fluid withdrawal will be more severe or will appear sooner during treatment.

It is well known that hypovolaemia favours the emergence of intradialytic hypotension. Several investigators developed two-pool models describing the course of the concentration gradient between EFV and IFV as a function of IC generation rate, cell wall permeability and dialyzer clearance (40, 41). Although these models simplify the real situation in the body, some conclusions can be drawn and application of the models to haemodialysis shows that a transcellular concentration gradient will develop during treatment.

This postulate can be substantiated by the survey of the fluid balance by conductivity measurements. Furthermore, the magnitude of the transcellular fluid shift can be assessed and its physiological importance can be studied. EFV comprises both interstitial and blood volume (BV). A handicap of the conductivity method is, that it is incapable to differentiate between BV and interstitial fluid. Therefore, some method has to be applied concurrently in order to chart BV. Changes in BV are inversely related to the grade of haemoconcentration. Although no on-line method to monitor BV is commercially available yet, changes in BV can be assessed by studying haemoglobin concentration in serial blood samples during treatment (42). Erythrocyte counts, serum albumin concentrations and haematocrits can also be used to serve this purpose, but one has to keep in mind that ensuing changes in mean cellular volume of erythrocytes during dialysis introduce errors in the estimation of BV based on haematocrit changes.

In conclusion EFV, IFV and BV can be studied simultaneously by combining the conductivity technique and the assessment of the degree of haemoconcentration. In the next paragraphs a summary of the current results of studies on the fluid balance will be provided.

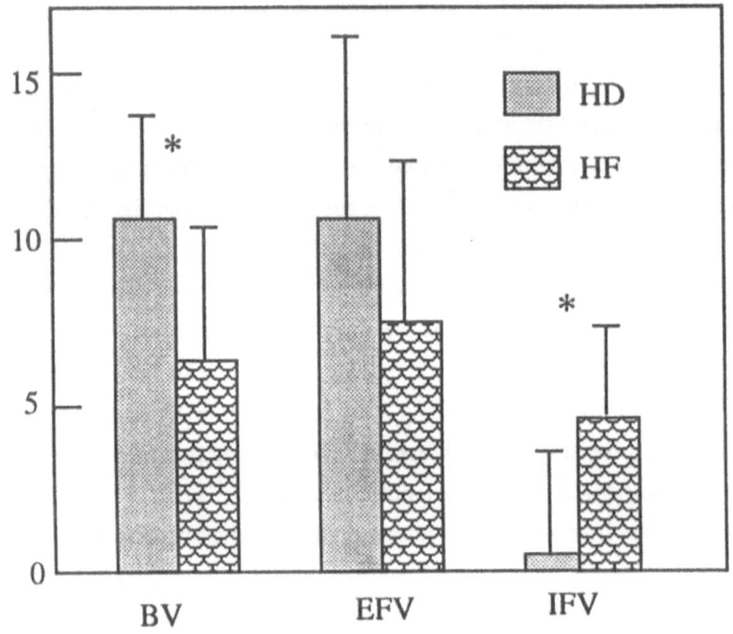

Figure 4. Percentage decrease in IFV, EFV and BV during haemofiltration (HF) and haemodialysis (HD) (* significantly different between HF and HD; $p<0.05$).

Haemofiltration versus conventional haemodialysis

It is well-known that haemofiltration (HF) leads to a less effective removal of low molecular weight substances than conventional haemodialysis (HD)(43). However, the rate of subjective symptoms of dysequilibrium during HF is far less than during HD. The question arises whether the response of the fluid balance to HF explains the increased tolerance to therapy.

In order to study this concept, fluid balance has been monitored during HF and HD (44).

As a result of the greater fall in EC osmolality during HD, IFV during HF and HD contrasted. HD led to a slight increase in IFV, whereas IFV declined during HF. As a result, fluid withdrawal tended to deplete EFV less during HF (Figure 4). The transcellular fluid shift to the interstitial space promoted refilling of the intravascular space and led to a better BV preservation during HF.

It is questionable whether the pronounced fall in IFV during HF has to be interpreted as 'more physiological' than the stable IFV during HD. An argument that supports this view is that the fall in osmolality during HF was far less than during HD. Furthermore, the observed recruitment of IC fluid towards the intravascular space improved cardiovascular tolerance to fluid withdrawal during HF, while less complaints were registered.

In another study the recovery of IFV and EFV after HF and HD was investigated too (45). Again HF was characterized by a marked decline in IFV and a better BV preservation. The observed decrease in IFV appeared to be transitory and disappeared after a recovery period that was significantly shorter than after HD. In conclusion, transient cellular shrinkage is a hallmark of HF that coincides with better BV preservation and less complaints during and after treatment.

Influence of dialysate sodium concentration on fluid balance

During renal replacement therapy the decrease in urea concentration is the main contributor to the fall in EC osmolality. It has been clearly established that the maintenance of a constant serum osmolality is a major protective factor for blood pressure stability during dialysis (46-49). Therefore, replacement of urea by a non-toxic osmolar substance during dialysis might raise EC osmolality and consequently reduce dialysis-induced morbidity. Since sodium is a natural constituent of EC fluid and cell membranes are relatively impermeable to sodium, high sodium dialysate is the best alternative to meet this requirement. Furthermore, it is easy to vary serum sodium concentration by calibrating dialysate sodium concentration.

In order to study this concept, fluid balance has been monitored during dialysis with high or low dialysate sodium concentrations (50). A clear relation between IFV and serum sodium could be demonstrated ($r = 0.51$, $p<0.005$). In contrast to dialysis treatment with low sodium, high sodium dialysate led to a decrease in IFV and, consequently, appeared to be an effective instrument to manipulate IFV. As might be expected, the ensuing interstitial fluid expansion enhanced refilling of the intravascular compartment and resulted in a reduced susceptibility to hypotensive episodes.

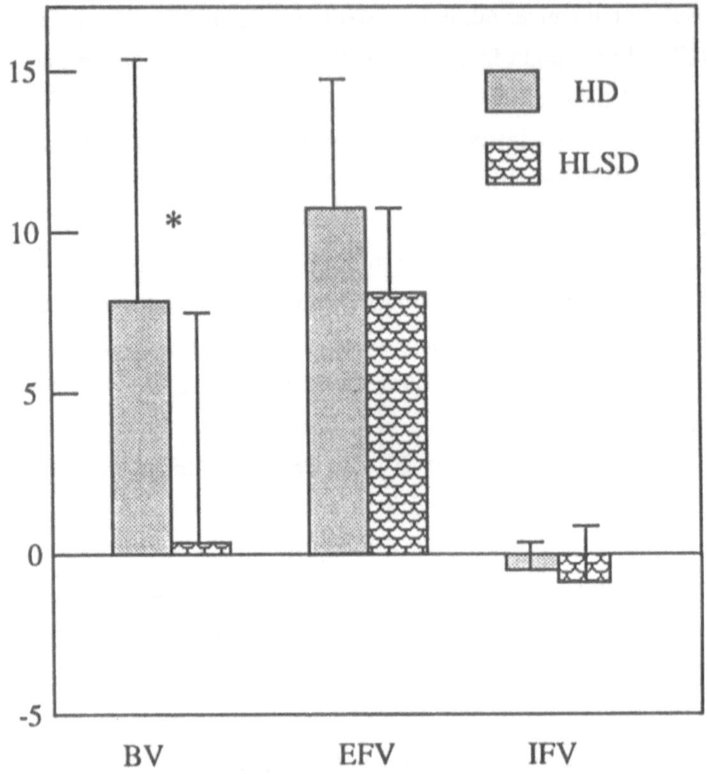

Figure 5. Percentage decrease in IFV, EFV and BV during dialysis with sequential high and low sodium dialysate (HLSD) and haemodialysis (HD) (* significantly different between HLSD and HD, $p<0.05$).

Although the application of a dialysate high in sodium seems worthwhile, post-dialysis hypernatriaemia, associated with thirst and increased interdialytic weight gain, might complicate the next dialysis session (51). This latter problem might be overcome by alternating dialysate sodium concentration during dialysis (52, 53). In theory, it leads to fluctuations in serum sodium concentration and consequently, in interstitial osmolality. The created transcellular osmotic gradient will induce a transcellular fluid shift. By repeating this procedure, alternating swelling and shrinking of cells might result. Consequently, in addition to diffusive mass transfer of urea, a convective mass transfer across the cell membrane will be induced, facilitating osmotic equilibration across the cell membrane and reducing symptoms of dialysis disequilibrium.

In order to test this hypothesis, fluid balance has been monitored by conductivity measurements during conventional dialysis and dialysis with sequential high and low sodium dialysate (HLSD)(54). Although fluctuations in plasma sodium concentration were induced, no oscillation in IFV or EFV could be shown compared to HD. Furthermore, after treatment IFV and EFV did not differ between the two strategies (Figure 5). These data indicate that no variations in interstitial sodium concentration occurred, making the concept of a shrinking and swelling cell highly debatable. Interestingly, BV was much better preserved than during conventional HD, which could be explained by an osmotic gradient, not across the cell membrane, but across the capillary membrane instead. Additional evidence to support this explanation was found in the fact that calculated distribution volume of sodium during the high and low dialysate sodium periods appeared to approximate plasma volume much closer than interstitial fluid volume. Thus, it appears that sodium accumulates in the plasma volume during a high sodium episode, instead of dispersing over the total EFV. So, it is an osmotic substance that is suitable to enhance refilling of the BV.

Assessment of post-dialysis dry weight

As mentioned above, conductivity measurements are advocated to survey changes in EFV and IFV during renal replacement therapy. Since low and high frequency conductivities are related to total EFV and TBW, respectively (26), these variables can also inform about tissue hydration and might be used to assess dry weight. During HD fluid is withdrawn directly from the BV, ultimately leading to hypovolaemia and hypotension. Refilling of the intravascular compartment from the overhydrated tissues neutralizes hypovolaemia. If the tissues are underhydrated, the fluid deficit restricts the process of refilling and patients will be liable to suffer from hypotension during treatment. During dialysis, fluid is withdrawn mainly from the EFV (21, 50). In order to test the hypothesis that regional EC conductivity predicts tissue hydration, EC conductivity after dialysis was studied (21). EC conductivity appeared to be comparable and within narrow limits in different groups of healthy volunteers. Interestingly, in a group of haemodialysis patients who were dialysed until their clinically determined dry weight was reached, the same average EC conductivity was found. It was concluded that this average EC conductivity value was characteristic for normally hydrated tissue.

An expression of the regional, individual EFV after dialysis as percentage of EFV in healthy volunteers was derived by dividing EC conductivity of each patient by the average EC conductivity in healthy volunteers. The relation between post-dialysis EFV and the impact of fluid withdrawal on BV during 46 standard haemodialysis sessions with a duration ranging from 3 to 5 hours, is expressed in Figure 6.

BV decrease was associated with a small EFV. No BV decrease was manifest if a large EFV was still present after dialysis. Thus, refilling of the BV was in proportion to the remaining EFV after dialysis and corresponded with the physiology of refilling.

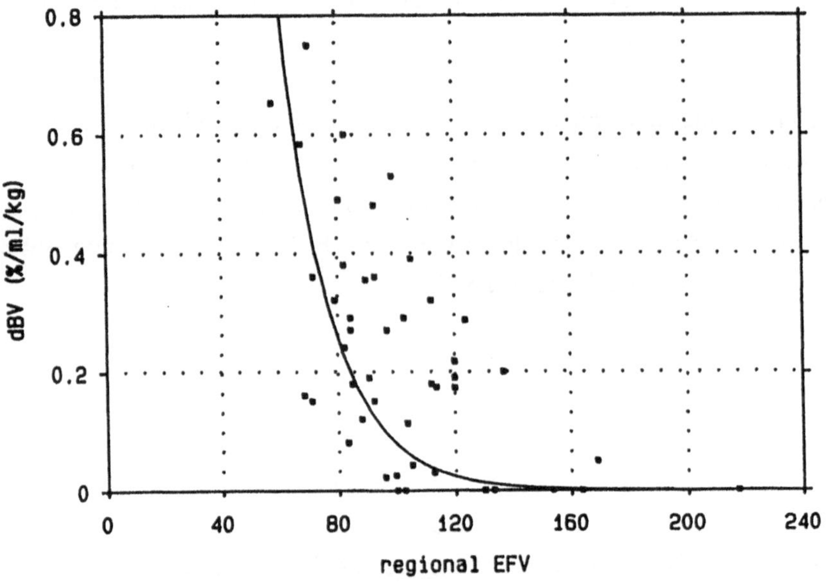

Figure 6. The relation between BV decrease (dBV) per unit fluid withdrawal (%/ml/kg) and remaining regional EFV (in percentage of the mean values obtained in volunteers) after dialysis ($r = 0.62$, $p<0.0001$).

Subsequently, haemodynamic variables such as pulse rate, stroke volume (SV), and left ventricular end-diastolic diameter (LVED) have been studied during dialysis (submitted for publication). A sharp decrease in SV and LVED, matching underhydration, was seen in the patients, diagnosed as underhydrated by means of conductivity measurements. These results yielded additional evidence that the conductivity method is a valid instrument to interpret tissue hydration.

CONCLUSIONS

Non-invasive conductivity measurements can be used to chart IFV and EFV. The technique has been validated both *in vitro* and *in vivo*. Since no equilibration time is required and measurements can be repeated unlimited, the method is superior to isotopic dilution techniques in assessing fluid dynamics. Furthermore, conductivity measurements can be used to determine tissue hydration state and deserve a place in the assessment of post-dialysis dry weight.

REFERENCES

1. Woodbury DM: Physiology of body fluids. In: "Physiology and Biophysics", vol. II (Eds TC Ruch and HD Patton), Saunders, Philadelphia, 1974, pp 130-156.
2. De Planque BA, Geyskes GG, Van Dongen R, Dorhout Mees EJ: Simultaneous determination of extracellular volume and blood volume with the Volémetron. Clin Chim Acta, 11: 270-277, 1965.
3. Boer P: Estimated lean body mass as an index for normalization of body fluid volumes in humans. Am J Physiol, 247: F632-F636, 1984.
4. Gaudino M, Levitt MR: Inulin space as a measure of extracellular fluid. Am J Physiol, 157: 387-393, 1949.
5. Herbst CA: Simultaneous distribution rate and dilution volume of bromide-82 and thiocyanate in body fluid overload. Ann Surg, 179: 200-208, 1974.
6. Cardozo RH, Edelman IS: The volume of distribution of sodium thiosulfate as a measure of the extracellular fluid space. J Clin Invest, 31: 280-290, 1952.
7. Miller H, Wilson GM: The measurement of exchangeable sodium in man using the isotope Na-24. Clin Sci, 12: 97-111, 1953.
8. McGrath BP, Tiller DJ, Horvath JS, Johnson JR: Measurement of extracellular fluid volume in patients on maintenance hemodialysis. Kidney Int, 9: 57-59, 1976.
9. Barnett A: Electrical method for studying water metabolism and translocation in body segments. Proc Soc Exp Biol Med, 44: 142-148,1940.
10. Nijboer J, Bagno S, Barnett A, Halsey RH: Radiocardiograms - the electrical impedance changes of the heart in relation to electrocardiograms and heart sounds. J Clin Invest, 19: 963-983, 1940.
11. Korsten HHM, Meijer JH, Hengeveld SJ, Delamarre JBVM, Leusink JA, Schurink GA, Schneider H: Continuous monitoring of intrathoracic fluid. In: "Computing in anesthesia and intensive care", (Ed O Prakash), Martinus Nijhof, The Hague, 1983, pp 141-152.
12. Pomerantz M, Delgado F, Eiseman B: Clinical evaluation of transthoracic electrical impedance as a guide to intrathoracic fluid volumes. Ann Surg, 171: 686-694, 1970.
13. Van de Water JM, Mount BE, Barela JR, Schuster R, Leacock FS: Monitoring the chest with impedance. Chest, 64: 597-603, 1973.
14. Meijer JH, Oe PL: Osmotic aspects in artificial kidney dialysis. In: "Exogenous and endogenous influences on metabolic and neural control", Vol 1, (Eds ADF Addink and N Spronk), Pergamon Press, Oxford, 1982, pp 351-362.
15. Meijer JH, Reulen JPH, Oe PL, Allon W, Thijs LG, Schneider H: Differential impedance plethysmography for measuring thoracic impedances. Med Biol Eng Comput, 20: 187-194, 1982.
16. Gebhard MM, Gersing E, Brockhoff CJ, Schnabel PhA, Bretschneider HJ: Impedance spectroscopy: a method for surveillance of ischemia tolerance of the heart. Thorac Cardiovasc Surgeon, 35: 26-32, 1987.
17. Kanai H, Haeno M, Sakamoto K: Electrical measurement of fluid distribution in legs and arms: estimation of extra-cellular and intra-cellular fluid. IEEE Frontiers of Eng in Health Care, 7: 273-276, 1982.
18. Haeno M, Tagawa H, Sakamoto K, Kanai H: Estimation of intra- and extracellular fluid volume in living tissues during dialysis. In: "Progress of bio-impedance study in Japan", Research Group of Bio-Impedance, Tokyo, Japan, 1987, pp 81-83.
19. Corten PMJ: Continuous registration of segmental stroke volume and wall movement of the left ventricle by means of electrical impedance measurements with an intraventricular multi-electrode catheter. Thesis (Krips Repro), Meppel, The Netherlands, 1980.
20. Jossinet J, Kardous G: Physical study of the sensitivity distribution in multi-electrode systems. Clin Phys Physiol Meas, 8: 33-37, 1987.
21. Kouw PM, Olthof CG, Ter Wee PM, Oe PL, Donker AJM, Schneider H, de Vries PMJM: Assessment of post-dialysis dry weight: an application of the conductivity measurement method. Kidney Int, 41: 440-444, 1992.

22. De Vries PMJM, Meijer JH, Vlaanderen K, Visser V, Oe PL, Donker AJM, Schneider H: Measurement of transcellular fluid shift during haemodialysis. Part II. *In vitro* and clinical evaluation. Med Biol Eng Comp, 27: 152-158, 1989.
23. Hanai T: Electrical properties of emulsions. In: "Emulsion science" (Ed Ph Sherman), Acad Press, London, 1968, pp 354-477.
24. Meijer JH, De Vries PMJM, Goovaerts HG, Oe PL, Donker AJM, Schneider H: Measurement of transcellular fluid shift during haemodialysis. Part I. Method. Med Biol Eng Comput, 27: 147-151, 1989.
25. Thomasset A: Bio-electrical properties of tissue impedance measurements. Lyon Med, 207: 107-118, 1962.
26. Segal KR, Burastero S, Chun A, Coronel P, Pierson RN, Wang J: Estimation of extracellular and total body water by multiple-frequency bioelectrical-impedance measurement. Am J Clin Nutr, 54: 26-29, 1991.
27. Guyton AC: Textbook of Medical Physiology, 8th edition, Saunders, London, 277, 1991.
28. De Vries PMJM: Determination of intracellular and extracellular fluid volume by means of non-invasive conductivity measurements. Thesis, Free University Press, Amsterdam, The Netherlands, 1989.
29. Lukaski HC, Bolonchuk WW: Estimation of body fluid volumes using tetrapolar bioelectrical impedance measurements. Aviat Space Environ Med, 1988, pp 1163-1169.
30. Spence JA, Baliga R, Nijboer J, Seftick J, Fleischmann L: Changes during hemodialysis in total body water, cardiac output and chest fluid as detected by bioelectrical impedance analysis. Trans Am Soc Artif Intern Organs, 25: 51-55, 1979.
31. Jenin P, Lenoir J, Roullet C, Thomasset AL, Ducrot H: Determination of body fluid compartments by electrical impedance measurements. Aviat Space Environ Med, 46: 152-155, 1975.
32. Tedner B: Equipment using an impedance technique for automatic recording of fluid-volume changes during haemodialysis. Med Biol Eng Comput, 21: 285-290, 1983.
33. Tedner B, Lins LE: Fluid volume changes during hemodialysis monitored with the impedance technique. Artif Organs, 9: 416-427, 1985.
34. Nijboer J, Sedensky JA: Bioelectrical impedance during renal disease. Proc Dialysis Transplant Forum, 1: 214-219, 1974.
35. Kubicek WG, Karnegis JN, Patterson RP, Witsoe DA, Mattson RH: Development and evaluation of an impedance cardiac output system. Aerosp Med, 37: 208-212, 1966.
36. Baumgartner RN, Cameron Chumlea W, Roche AF: Estimation of body composition from bioelectric impedance of body segments. Am J Clin Nutr, 50: 221-226, 1989.
37. Kanai H, Sakamoto K, Haeno M: Electrical measurement of fluid distribution in human legs: estimation of extra- and intra-cellular fluid volume. J Microwave Power, 18: 233-243, 1983.
38. Guyton AC: Textbook of Medical Physiology, 8th edition, Saunders, London, 40, 1991.
39. Van Stone JC, Bauer J, Carey J: The effect of dialysate sodium concentration on body fluid distribution during hemodialysis. Trans Am Soc Artif Intern Organs, 26: 383-386, 1980.
40. Frost TH, Kerr DNS: Kinetics of hemodialysis: a theoretical study of the removal of solutes in chronic renal failure compared to normal health. Kidney Int, 12: 41-50, 1977.
41. Popovich RP, Hlavinka DJ, Bomar JB, Moncrief JW, Decherd JF: The consequences of physiological resistances on metabolite removal from the patient-artificial kidney system. Trans Am Soc Artif Intern Organs, 21: 108-116, 1975.
42. Schallenberg U, Stiller S, Mann H: A new method of continuous haemoglobinemetric measurement of blood volume during haemodialysis. Life Support Systems, 5: 293-305, 1987.
43. Baldamus CA, Pollok M: Ultrafiltration and haemofiltration, practical applications. In: "Replacement of renal function by dialysis" (Ed JF Maher), Kluwer Acad Publ, Dordrecht, 1989, pp 327-346.
44. De Vries PMJM, Olthof CG, Solf A, Schuenemann B, Oe PL, Quellhorst E, Schneider H, Donker AJM: Fluid balance during haemodialysis and haemofiltration: the effect of dialysate sodium and a variable ultrafiltration rate. Nephrol Dial Transplant, 6: 257-263, 1991.
45. Olthof CG, de Vries PMJM, Kouw PM, Oe PL, Gerlag PGG, Schneider H, Donker AJM: The recovery of the fluid balance after haemodialysis and haemofiltration. Clin Nephrol, 37: 135-139, 1992.
46. Henrich WL, Woodard TD, McPhaul JJ: The chronic efficacy and safety of high sodium dialysate: double-blind cross-over study. Am J Kidney Dis, 2: 349-353, 1982.

47. Kjellstrand C, Rosa A, Shideman J: Hypotension during hemodialysis. Osmolality fall is an important pathogenetic factor. J ASAIO, 3: 11-19, 1980.
48. Raja R, Henriquez M, Kramer M, Rosenbaum JL: Intradialytic hypotension - role of osmolar changes and acetate influx. Trans Am Soc Artif Intern Organs, 25: 419-421, 1979.
49. Swartz RC, Somermeyer MH, Hsu CH: Preservation of plasma volume during hemodialysis depends on dialysate osmolality. Am J Nephrol, 2: 189-194, 1982.
50. De Vries PMJM, Kouw PM, Olthof CG, Solf A, Schuenemann B, Oe PL, Quellhorst E, Donker AJM: The influence of dialysate sodium and variable ultrafiltration on fluid balance during hemodialysis. Trans Am Soc Artif Intern Organs, 36: 821-824, 1990.
51. Barre PE, Brunelle G, Gascon-Barre M: A randomized double blind trial of dialysate sodiums of 145 mEq/L, 150 mEq/L and 155 mEq/L. Trans Am Soc Artif Intern Organs, 34: 338-341, 1988.
52. Dumler F, Grondin G, Levin NW: Sequential high/low sodium hemodialy-sis: an alternative to ultrafiltration. Trans Am Soc Intern Organs, 25: 351-353, 1979.
53. Martin-Malo A, Perez R, Gomez J, Burdiel LG, Andres E, Castillo D, Moreno E, Aljama P: Sequential hypertonic dialysis. Nephron, 40: 458-462, 1985.
54. Kouw PM, Olthof CG, Gruteke P, de Vries PMJM, Meijer JH, Oe PL, Schneider H, Donker AJM: The influence of high and low sodium dialysis on blood volume preservation. Nephrol Dial Transplant, 6: 876-880, 1991.

INDEX

[Page numbers following (T) refer to Tables; page numbers following (F) refer to Figures]